Sleep
Disorders

An Alternative Medicine Definitive Guide

by HERBERT ROSS, D.C., *and* KERI BRENNER, L.Ac.,

with BURTON GOLDBERG

ALTERNATIVEMEDICINE.COM BOOKS
TIBURON, CALIFORNIA

AlternativeMedicine.com, Inc.
1640 Tiburon Blvd., Suite 2
Tiburon, CA 94920
www.alternativemedicine.com

Editor: John W. Anderson
Associate Editor: Ellen Cavalli
Art Director: Janine White
Production Manager: Gail Gongoll
Production Assistance: Victoria Swart

Manufactured in Canada.

10 9 8 7 6 5 4 3

Library of Congress Cataloging-in-Publication Data

Ross, Herb
    Sleep disorders: an alternative medicine definitive guide / by Herb Ross and
Keri Brenner; with Burton Goldberg.
        p. cm.
    Includes bibliographical references and index.
    ISBN 1-887299-20-3 (pbk.)
    1. Sleep disorders—Alternative treatment. 2. Insomnia— Alternative treat-
ment.
I. Brenner, Keri. II. Goldberg, Burton, 1926- III. Title.

RC547.R66 2000
616.8'498—dc21
                                                                    00-038581

                                                                        CIP

Contents

About the Authors

Herbert Ross, D.C., is an internationally known authority on alternative solutions to sleep disorders and founder of the Aspen Sleep Institute, in Colorado. Dr. Ross is a certified acupuncturist and a neuro-emotional (NET) therapist. He lectures extensively on sleep disorders on television and in person throughout the U.S. and abroad. Dr. Ross is personal chiropractor to motivational speaker Anthony Robbins.

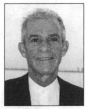

Keri Brenner, L.Ac., is a licensed acupuncturist and writer based in Fairfax, California. Keri holds a master's degree in acupuncture and Oriental medicine from the Oregon College of Oriental Medicine. She began her journalism career as a reporter for newspapers on both the East and West coasts, and currently provides editorial content for a self-help-oriented website in San Francisco.

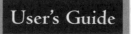

User's Guide

One of the features of this book is that it is interactive, thanks to the following icons:

This means you can turn to the listed pages elsewhere in this book for more information.

Many times the text mentions a medical term that requires explanation. We don't want to interrupt the text, so instead we put the explanation in the margins under this icon.

This tells you where to contact a physician, group, or publication mentioned in the text. This is an editorial service to our readers. All items are based on recommendations from the clinical practice of physicians in this book. The publisher has no financial interest in any clinic, physician, or product discussed in this book.

This sign tells you there may be some risks, uncertainties, side effects, or special contraindications regarding a procedure or substance.

Here we refer you to our best-selling book, *Alternative Medicine: The Definitive Guide*, for more information on a particular topic.

This icon will alert you to an article published in our bimonthly magazine, *Alternative Medicine*, that is relevant to the topic under discussion.

Here we refer you to our book *Alternative Medicine Definitive Guide to Cancer* for more information on a particular topic.

Here we refer you to our book *The Enzyme Cure* for more information on enzymes and how they can be used to relieve health problems.

Here we refer you to our book *The Supplement Shopper* for more information on nutritional supplements for various health conditions.

Important Information

Burton Goldberg and the editors of *Alternative Medicine* are proud of the public and professional praise accorded AlternativeMedicine.com's (formerly Future Medicine Publishing) series of books. This latest book in the series continues the groundbreaking tradition of its predecessors.

Your health and that of your loved ones is important. Treat this book as an educational tool which will enable you to better understand, assess, and choose the best course of treatment when a health problem arises, and how to prevent health problems such as sleep disorders from developing in the first place.

Remember that this book on sleep disorders is different. This book is about alternative approaches to health—approaches generally not understood and, at this time, not endorsed by the medical establishment. We urge you to discuss the treatments described in this book with your doctor. If your doctor is open-minded, you may actually educate him or her. We have been gratified to learn that many of our readers have found their physicians open to the new ideas presented to them.

Use this book wisely. As many of the treatments described in this book are, by definition, alternative, they have not been investigated, approved, or endorsed by any government or regulatory agency. National, state, and local laws may vary regarding the use and application of many of the treatments discussed. Accordingly, this book should not be substituted for the advice and care of a physician or other licensed health-care professional. Pregnant women, in particular, are urged to consult a physician before commencing any therapy. Ultimately, you must take responsibility for your health and how you use the information in this book.

AlternativeMedicine.com and the authors have no financial interest in any of the products or services discussed in this book, with two exceptions. Pure Energies is a company that sells EMF-protective devices—Dr. Herb Ross is the CEO of Pure Energies. The book also makes references in the text to AlternativeMedicine.com's other publications. All of the factual information in this book has been drawn from the scientific literature. To protect privacy, all patient names have been changed. Branded products and services discussed in the book are evaluated solely on the independent and direct experience of the health-care practitioners quoted. Reference to them does not imply an endorsement nor a superiority over other branded products and services which may provide similar or superior results.

Don't Suffer Through More Sleepless Nights

SLEEPLESS NIGHTS are not something you have to live with—alternative medicine has practical solutions for identifying and treating the underlying causes and can bring lasting relief to those with insomnia and other sleep disorders. Many people have learned this the hard way, tossing and turning at night for years before discovering that there is another option. Alternative medicine recognizes that sleep disorders do not have one cause, but multiple factors that together overload your body systems. Looking at illness and health in this way makes for more effective treatment than the single cause focus of conventional medicine. In this book, you will learn that once you identify the hidden factors that are combining to produce your sleep problem, you can treat each one and permanently eliminate it. Patient success stories throughout the book provide practical details on how others were able to reverse their sleep disorders.

Today, an estimated 60 million Americans have a sleep disorder, making it one of the most prevalent chronic health problems. For many of those with problems sleeping, the consequences are falling asleep on the job, inability to concentrate, and increased susceptibility to other illnesses because of an immune system compromised by lack of rest. And it is estimated that Americans spend $16 billion each year on sleep-related medical care. Much of this money is poorly spent, because conventional sleeping aids— potentially addictive sedatives—ultimately create more sleep disturbances than they eliminate.

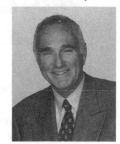

Alternative medicine physicians, on the other hand, focus on finding the root causes, rather than merely trying to alleviate symptoms. Our practitioners can make sure that finding the right treatment protocol doesn't turn into a nightmare. They realize that sleep disorders, including insomnia, sleep apnea, restless legs syndrome, and narcolepsy, often arise from poor diet, toxic overload, disrupted circadian rhythms, geopathic and emotional stress, and hormonal and structural imbalances. The majority of sleep problems are symptoms of an unhealthy body, not diseases in and of themselves. Most people with disturbed sleep will find relief by taking steps to promote their overall health: improving diet,

This book is here to tell you that you don't have to live with sleep problems, or with a continuing cycle of drugs and their side effects. By treating what is actually causing the condition, not only can sleep disorders be reversed but your overall health will be improved.

reducing stress, balancing hormones, and detoxifying the body, among others.

In this book, we show you how to prevent and reverse sleep disorders using safe, noninvasive, and proven alternative therapies. Alternative medicine looks at the whole person, considering the individual's symptoms, health history, diet, and underlying imbalances. You can then use a combination of alternative treatments to heal these underlying causes leading to sleep problems, bringing lasting relief, not a simple masking of symptoms. This is the basic principle of alternative medicine and the reason why it succeeds where conventional medicine often fails in treatment of chronic disease.

You'll learn more about these self-help options:

■ How to avoid foods that aggravate sleep disorders and how to improve your diet to support restful sleep.

■ Detoxification strategies to cleanse your body of sleep-disrupting poisons.

■ Herbs, vitamins and minerals, and homeopathic remedies to help you sleep.

■ Exercises and physical therapies to correct structural imbalances and muscle tension that may be contributing to your sleepless nights.

■ The role of stress in sleep disorders and effective mind/body therapies to cope with emotional imbalances.

This book is here to tell you that you don't have to live with sleep problems, or with a continuing cycle of drugs and their side effects. By treating what is actually causing the condition, not only can sleep disorders be reversed but your overall health will be improved. The alternative therapies in this book will start you on your way to restful nights and better health. God bless.

—Burton Goldberg

Visit our website at
www.alternativemedicine.com

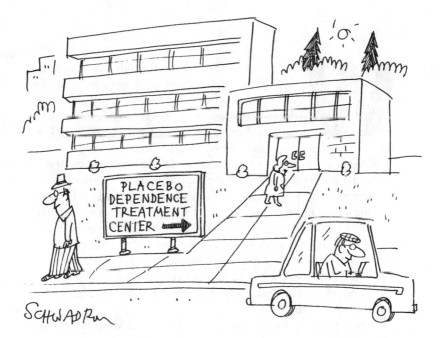

CHAPTER

1

The Basics of Sleep

WE SPEND UP TO one-third of our lives asleep. Although some hard-driven people may view sleep as an inconvenience that curtails productivity and leisure activities, slumber is certainly no waste of time. In fact, sleep may play a more crucial role than diet or exercise in fostering optimal health.

Sleep is a natural restorative, an antidote to the damage done to our bodies during the course of the day. It allows the body to replenish its immune system, eliminate free radicals, and ward off heart disease and mood imbalances. The mechanisms of sleep are as remarkable as its physiological function. You may think that merely closing your eyes signals the slumbering instinct, but the process of falling—and staying—asleep requires an elaborate cerebral orchestration of hormones, biological rhythms, and environmental cues. And as with any other bodily function, sleep requires a balance of all factors to ensure proper health.

When sleep is disrupted—due to insomnia, sleep apnea, narcolepsy, restless legs syndrome, jet lag, sleepwalking, night terrors, or other disorders—emotional and physiological health suffers. If you're among the 60 million Americans suffering from chronic or intermittent sleep disorders each year,[1] tossing and turning all night has likely beset you with a host of potentially debilitating conditions, including an inability to concentrate, fatigue, and poor immune function. But you don't have to accept sleep deprivation and the ills that accompany it. And you don't have to resort to pharmaceutical sleeping aids that come with their own set of disabling side effects.

This book provides practical alternative therapies proven to induce and maintain a deep, regenerative sleep. Before you take a tranquilizer that invariably masks your symptoms, consider trying natural remedies that treat the underlying causes of your disorder. Diet modification, detoxification, stress management, and environmental controls can gently and effectively help you snooze your way back to health.

Success Story: Lifestyle Changes Restore Sleep

Jerry, a 47-year-old print shop owner, had not slept more than three hours a night for years. Lately, he started having spasms in his legs at night, which further interfered with his sleep. During the waking hours, he was tired all the time and looked ten years older. He was also irritable and snapped at his employees and his family. He had chronic bloating and gas in his digestive tract, and he frequently alternated between constipation and diarrhea. His energy level was erratic, sometimes feverish and other times dropping lower than normal. He was very concerned about falling asleep while driving.

Jerry had tried numerous types of sleeping pills, but nothing had worked. He was desperate to get some sleep. Before even scheduling any tests with Jerry, we looked at his lifestyle. Jerry started every day by drinking the first of many cups of coffee. He worked straight through lunch, grabbing a sandwich at his desk. Then, he worked through dinnertime, finally quitting around 10 p.m. After that, he had dinner, washing it down with two or three glasses of wine. After dinner, Jerry immediately fell sound asleep, only to awaken at 2 a.m., unable to fall back to sleep for the rest of the night. Jerry never exercised and was under constant stress from the deadlines and schedules that were the nature of his business. He had become totally driven by the business and left no time for himself.

We told Jerry that the only way we could work with him is if he were willing to change his lifestyle. We made it clear that his sleeping problems were only a sign that all his vital body functions—circulatory, digestive, nervous, and hormonal systems—were beginning to fail. It had been so long since they were supported with proper nutrition and rest that they could no longer maintain the internal balance nec-

For more information about **exercise and acupuncture for sleep disorders**, see Chapter 9: Correcting Structural Imbalances, pp. 224-247.

essary to good health. Jerry initially resisted the suggestions but finally agreed, realizing that another sleeping pill was not the answer. He agreed to begin an exercise program. We referred him to a personal trainer who had him begin with aerobic and resistance weight training. We also referred him to an acupuncturist for a series of treatments to help balance his system.

We analyzed Jerry's nutrition and found that he had what is called a "leaky gut," a condition in which bacterial toxins from his intestinal tract were "leaking" into the rest of his body through his intestinal wall and depositing toxins into the bloodstream, tissues, cells, and lymph. Also, Jerry's digestive system was deficient in hydrochloric acid and enzymes, both of which are needed to break down nutrients in food so they can be absorbed. He did not have enough of the beneficial bacteria in his intestines to digest his food properly. To counter this digestive dysfunction and ease the toxic load on his body, we started Jerry on a liver detoxification program. A saliva test showed that Jerry was low on the hormone DHEA (dehydroepiandrosterone), which is important for metabolism, so we prescribed DHEA supplements.

We also examined Jerry's diet, looking for stimulants that impair sleep. We suggested that Jerry reduce caffeine. He did that by substituting decaffeinated coffee for regular coffee in gradually increasing proportions until it was all decaffeinated. He stopped consuming wine and salt and agreed to eat three balanced meals a day and not eat snacks on the run. Jerry also began eating dinner between 6 p.m. and 7 p.m., and went to bed by 10 p.m.

For more on **poor diet and sleep disorders**, see Chapter 3: Improve Your Diet, pp. 56-85. For more on **liver detoxification**, see Chapter 4: Detoxify Your Body, pp. 86-119. For more on **meditation and counseling**, see Chapter 6: Resolve Emotional Issues, pp. 146-173. For more on **chiropractic**, see Chapter 9: Correcting Structural Imbalances, pp. 224-247.

For many insomniacs, stress management is very important to encourage the body to heal and allow it to respond to its natural internal cues. Stress management for Jerry meant hiring a consultant to organize his business and to teach him how to communicate better with his employees and family. To further reduce his daily stress levels, Jerry learned how to meditate and committed himself to meditating twice a day for 15 minutes at a time. Jerry also received weekly chiropractic treatments to correct structural imbalances that were impinging on his nervous system. He was also counseled, supported, and encouraged on all of his lifestyle changes.

By the end of three weeks, Jerry was sleeping through the night. In addition, he enjoyed renewed energy and vitality. In a short time, he had lost 20 pounds, was no longer irritable, and found he was able to leave the office at 5 p.m. and the work would still get done. At the end of three months, Jerry's digestive system was normal and he was feeling relaxed and happy. He had regained his spark and was more youthful. Jerry's sleep continued to be deep, uninterrupted, restful, and restorative.

The Physiological Function of Sleep

For years, scientists have debated the purpose of sleep. According to some evolutionary scientists, sleep evolved primarily as a survival mechanism. Before the discovery of fire, our early human ancestors were unable to see and avoid approaching dangers at night, such as stalking animals or precarious cliffs. Thus, humans—as well as all other animals—slept to keep themselves safe.

While this evolutionary approach partly explains the reasons for when we sleep (see "Circadian Rhythms and the Body's Clock, p. 27), it doesn't answer why we sleep. The obvious clue is to ameliorate their feelings of exhaustion. But researchers have struggled with the missing link between the desire for and the purpose of sleep: Why can't the body replenish its vitality without delving into a netherworld of dreams and diminished consciousness? What is it about sleep that enables the body to fix itself? At present, it appears that sleep—particularly the sleep-inducing hormone melatonin—plays a crucial role in keeping the brain free of free radicals and in stimulating the immune system. Studies prove that without sleep, the body would break down and die.

Zzz's Against Free Radicals

During the waking and sleeping hours, our bodies are exposed to numerous free radicals (SEE QUICK DEFINITION). Free radicals are normal products of metabolism and are also derived from pesticides, industrial pollutants, smoking, alcohol, viruses, most infections, allergies, stress, even certain foods and excessive exercise. Free radicals create oxidation, the same process that turns iron to rust and the exposed surfaces of sliced apples brown. They are "free" in the sense of being unattached: molecular loose cannons that combine with oxygen in the air to initiate the process of spoilage. Internally, the same sort of deterioration occurs. Free radicals attack cell membranes, often in a matter of minutes. To counter the effects of free radicals, our bodies manufacture or rely on outside sources of antioxidants (SEE QUICK DEFINITION), whose purpose is to scavenge for free radicals, bind with them, and eliminate them before they contaminate healthy cells. Toxins, however, impede this process by

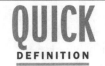

creating too many free radicals, which quickly deplete the body's reserve of antioxidant nutrients.

If free radicals are left to roam unimpeded throughout the body, the brain suffers many of the consequences. The brain, which consumes approximately 20% of the oxygen we breathe, is composed mostly of unsaturated fatty acids, complex molecules that are highly susceptible to free-radical damage because they have a "loose" hold on their electrons. Also, brain tissue is rich in iron, which can transform hydrogen peroxide, a byproduct of oxygen metabolism, into hydroxyl radicals, which are particularly dangerous forms of free radicals.[2] Hydroxyl radicals can cause irreversible damage in the brain, because neurons (brain cells) cannot be regenerated. Neuronal damage can lead to memory impairment, loss of motor control, Alzheimer's disease, Lou Gehrig's disease, multiple sclerosis, and Parkinson's disease.[3]

Fortunately, the brain is protected by the blood-brain barrier, a layer of modified capillaries that makes access to the brain less permeable. This barrier keeps many toxins out of the brain, reducing (but not eliminating) the load of free radicals. However, it also prevents many antioxidants from entering the brain, allowing free radicals to accumulate.

Sleep can stem the influx of free radicals. When we sleep, the pineal gland in our brain produces a hormone called melatonin. Melatonin is best known for its hypnotic or sleep-inducing powers (see "The Role of Melatonin," p. 28), but numerous scientific studies have shown that melatonin is a powerful antioxidant as well. And because melatonin is produced within the brain, it does not have to contend with the blood-brain barrier.

Studies prove that melatonin is a highly effective scavenger of hydroxyl radicals and peroxyl radicals, another type of toxic free radical. In fact, melatonin has been shown to be more effective in scavenging hydroxyl radicals than other well-known antioxidants such as glutathione.[4] Melatonin appears to inactivate free radicals on a subcellular level, reaching the free radicals in DNA, proteins, and lipids.[5] It also seems to stimulate important antioxidant enzymes, including superoxide dismutase, glutathione peroxidase, and glutathione reductase.[6]

In experiments, melatonin has reduced the neuronal damage associated with Alzheimer's disease and Parkinson's disease.[7] It has also been shown to prevent cataracts (caused by free-radical damage in the eye lens), as well as counteract the free-radical effects of toxins such as paraquat, carbon tetrachloride, and safole.[8] Further studies have shown that prolonged periods of sleep deprivation—that is, prolonged periods without elevated production of melatonin—cause neuronal damage in animal subjects.[9]

For information on **treating sleep disorders with melatonin**, see Chapter 5: Resetting the Body Clock, pp. 120-145.

The Immune System: Don't Snooze, You Lose

Antioxidants are not the body's only defense against harmful substances roaming the body. The body is equipped with a potent immune system (SEE QUICK DEFINITION) that identifies, attacks, and ultimately eliminates invading pathogens (antigens). During an immune response, white blood cells called T cells neutralize pathogens; other cells called B cells produce antibodies (SEE QUICK DEFINITION); and still other immune cells release chemicals (such as histamine) into the bloodstream to aid in the removal of antigens from the body.

In the context of sleep, it is important to understand the immune function of T cells. Though they are produced in the bone marrow, T cells mature in the thymus gland. The thymus programs each of the billions of T cells for a special immune duty. Some T cells are trained to become "killer" cells, which engulf or attack invading antigens. Types of killer cells include natural killer (NK) cells, which destroy hard-to-detect virus-infected and cancer cells; phagocytes, which immobilize and kill antigens through ingestion; and cytotoxic cells, which inject a poison into antigenic cell membranes to kill them. Other T cells are called "helper" cells, which act as mission control for the immune system. When antigens invade the body, T-helper cells coordinate the activation and deactivation of killer and other immune cells by producing intercellular signaling chemicals called cytokines. The major cytokines are interleukins, interferons, colony-stimulating factors, and tumor necrosis factors.

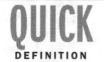

DEFINITION

The **immune system** guards the body against foreign, disease-producing substances. Its "workers" are various white blood cells including one trillion lymphocytes and 100 million trillion antibodies produced and secreted by the lymphocytes. Lymphocytes are found in high numbers in the lymph nodes, bone marrow, spleen, and thymus gland.

An **antibody** is a protein molecule made from amino acids by white blood cells in the lymph tissue and set in motion by the immune system against a specific foreign protein, or antigen. An antibody is also referred to as an immunoglobulin and may be found in the blood, lymph, saliva, and the gastrointestinal and urinary tracts, usually within three days after the first encounter with an antigen. The antibody binds tightly with the antigen as a preliminary for removing it from the system or destroying it.

19

Research has found that T-helper cells contain receptors specifically designed to fit melatonin molecules. During sleep, melatonin attaches to these receptors and stimulates the production of a factor (substance) similar to interleukin-4 (IL-4). This factor then stimulates the activation of NK cells, phagocytes, and cytotoxic cells, as well as immune cells found in the bone marrow.[10] One study found that increasing nighttime melatonin levels with 2 mg of melatonin led to a 240% increase in production of NK cells.[11] Another study found that the amount of melatonin normally found in the bloodstream during sleep increased the ability of a certain phagocyte (called a monocyte) to destroy skin cancer cells by 73%.[12]

The immune-stimulating properties of sleep may explain why we sleep more when suffering from an infectious disease, such as a cold or flu.[13] Experiments have shown that animals deprived of sleep for prolonged periods become severely ill and generally die from common viral infections that ordinarily have no affect on animals allowed to sleep.[14]

Other Health Benefits of Sleep

Researchers have also found melatonin to significantly reduce levels of LDL ("bad") cholesterol. In fact, one study showed that melatonin could decrease LDL cholesterol by up to 42%.[15] Melatonin also has been proven to lower high blood pressure.[16] Low blood levels of melatonin have been implicated in patients with manic depression and schizophrenia; in these cases, restoring patients to normal nighttime levels of melatonin reversed their disorders.[17] Stress and the associated adrenal hormone cortisol may have been contributing factors in reducing the patients' amounts of melatonin.

For more on **stress and sleep problems**, see Chapter 6: Resolve Emotional Issues, pp. 146-173.

The pineal gland isn't the only gland functioning during sleep. The endocrine glands (SEE QUICK DEFINITION) secrete human growth hormone (HGH) and a variety of other hormones during sleep. Also, physiological processes that occur during the dream stage of sleep have been shown to improve cognitive health (see "In Dreams: Memory and Forgetting," p. 24).

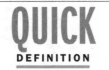

DEFINITION

Endocrine glands, including the testicles, ovaries, pancreas, adrenals, thyroid, parathyroid, and pituitary, are central to the regulation and normalization of all the body's complex, interconnected systems, from metabolism and heat production to spermatogenesis and uterine preparations for pregnancy.

The Stages of Sleep

In the early days of sleep research, scientists believed that all but the most essential bodily and cerebral functions would shut down during

Awake–low voltage–random, fast

50 µV

1 sec

Stage 1 – 8 to 12 cps – alpha waves

Stage 2 – 3 to 7 cps – theta waves

Theta waves

Stage 3 – 12 to 14 cps – sleep spindles and K complexes

Sleep spindle

K Complex —

Stage 4 – ½ to 2 cps – delta waves > 75 µV

REM Sleep – low voltage – random, fast with sawtooth waves

Sawtooth waves   Sawtooth waves

Types of Brain Waves:
Beta: 14 to 30 cycles per second; brain is awake and concentrating.
Alpha: 8 to 13 cycles per second; brain is awake but relaxed.
Theta: 4 to 7 cycles per second; brain is sleeping lightly.
Delta: 1 to 3 cycles per second; brain is sleeping deeply with no dreams.

The Five Stages of Sleep

Stage	Degree of Sleep	Duration
1	"Dozing," very light	30 seconds to 7 minutes
2	Light	45 to 50 minutes in first cycle, decreasing to 25 minutes in last
3	Moderately deep	7 to 15 minutes in first 2 or 3 cycles, then disappears
4	Very deep	12 minutes in first 2 or 3 cycles, then disappears
REM	Dreaming	10 minutes at first, increasing to 15 to 30 minutes as cycles continue

sleep. It wasn't until the advent of the electroencephalograph (EEG) in the late 1920s that researchers began to realize that sleep involves a startling amount of brain activity. By monitoring brain waves (see "Types of Brain Waves," p. 21), scientists discovered five cyclic stages of alternately low and high brain-wave function. It generally takes 90 to 110 minutes for the brain to complete one cycle.

The first four stages are called NREM (non–rapid eye movement) sleep; the fifth stage is REM (rapid eye movement). The NREM phases comprise approximately 75% of the sleep cycle (50% in infants) and are characterized by very restful sleep, in which body movements,

Level of Consciousness	Brain Wave Activity	Physiological Processes
Drifting in and out of sleep; awakened easily by all stimuli	Irregular, rapid alpha waves	Muscles relax; smooth, even breathing; body temperature and heart rate begin to drop
Awakened easily by sounds and movement	Irregular theta waves, with intermittent rapid alpha activity and bursts of delta waves	Breathing, temperature, heart rate continue to decrease; muscles further relax; eyes may roll slowly
Difficult to awaken with stimuli	Brain waves slow drastically, mostly large delta waves	Breathing and heart rate continue to drop but stabilize; very relaxed; may sweat
Very difficult to awaken with stimuli	Large, slow delta waves	Breathing and heart rate stable but slow; very relaxed; may sweat
May be awakened easier but difficult to adjust to reality	Smaller, more regular alpha waves resembling those of Stage 1	Eyes roll back and forth; muscles freeze except for some twitching in face, toes, fingers; breathing, heart rate irregular; penile erections in men

blood pressure, breathing, and basal metabolic rates are reduced by as much as 30% from normal wakeful levels.[18] There may be some dreaming during NREM sleep though you're unlikely to recall them.[19] The majority of remembered dreaming occurs during the REM phase.

In everyone except for infants, narcoleptics, and people deprived of sleep for more than 200 hours, NREM stages precede REM. However, you may skip around from various light and deep stages or completely omit the deep sleep stages after the second or third cycle of the night. Additionally, people commonly experience a period of up to two hours of "quiet wakefulness" between four-hour periods of regular sleep cycles.

In Dreams: Memory and Forgetting

Most scientists believe that dreams are the result of neurons (brain nerve cells) transmitting electrical impulses into the brain's long-term memory bank, at which time electrons are released that trigger hallucinations in the cortex. But the purpose of dreams—like the purpose of sleep—has been hotly debated by both sleep researchers and psychiatrists.

A century ago, Sigmund Freud postulated that dreams allow the repressed mind a chance to act out its darkest urges. Others believe dreams impart meaningful lessons we can apply to our waking lives. While there may be some credence to both theories, some sleep researchers believe dreaming improves our memory and capacity to learn. According to this theory, REM sleep allows the brain to transfer new material into the memory, specifically by increasing the efficiency of the left brain hemisphere, which during waking hours is active in collecting new language skills and other information.[20] The precise mechanisms of this memory consolidation process are still under investigation. One study links REM-induced blood flow through a part of the brain called amygdaloid complexes (containing the left thalamus and pontine tegmentum) to the processing of some types of memory.[21] Brain catecholamines (chemicals such as dopamine and epinephrine)—which may be diminished by sleep deprivation—help transfer new information from the intermediate-term, high-capacity buffer in the hippocampus (a part of the brain) into the long-term memory storage in the neocortex.[22] Regardless of the mechanism, several studies confirm the correlation between dream sleep and long-term learning retention.

In one study, scientists introduced test subjects to basic visual discrimination tasks and then allowed some of the subjects to sleep normally overnight, while the rest were permitted to sleep during all stages of sleep except for REM dream sleep. The subjects who had dreamed performed significantly better on the new tasks than those subjects who were dream-deprived.[23] Another study found that subjects taking a French language course reported better learning retention if their dreams contained references to the French class.[24] Sleeping and dreaming immediately after learning a new task has proven more effective on long-term recognition memory than sleeping hours after learning the task.[25] Other studies suggest that not only do dreams help us learn better, they help us develop new solutions or adaptations to problems.[26] Studies have shown that people deprived of REM sleep are more irritable and anxious in the waking hours—and thus, less able to cope with daily problems—than those who are allowed to dream.[27]

Ironically, we often forget the content of most of our dreams. This may be due to vasotocin, a chemical released by melatonin during sleep that acts as an amnesic agent, erasing recent memory from the hippocampus during dreams.[28] Or, as sleep expert William Dement, M.D., Ph.D., hypothesizes, we may forget dreams so as to avoid confusing ourselves. "If we remembered every dream clearly," he says, "it might become difficult to sort out what really occurred and what was a dream."[29]

During this interval, sleepers are neither fully awake nor fully asleep, but resting, reviewing their dreams, their thoughts turned off.

Stage 1—This is the shortest phase, in which slowing alpha waves prepare you for the sleep state. As you drift in and out of wakefulness, your breathing, heart rate, metabolic rate, and body temperature begin to drop. Muscles start to relax; you may experience a sensation of falling, followed by sudden muscle contractions called hypnic myoclonia. You may experience hypnagogic (the act of falling asleep) dreams. You are easily awakened by external stimuli, at which point you may only remember a few fragments of hypnagogic images and thoughts.

Stage 2—This is the longest sleep phase, marked by a light level of sleep. The brain slows down into theta waves, with intermittent surges of rapid brain waves (spindles) followed by large, slow bursts of delta waves. Breathing, heart rate, metabolic rate, and body temperature continue to decline. You may be awakened easily by sound and movement.

Stage 3—As the brain progressively slows down to large, slow delta waves, you enter a deeper stage of sleep. Muscles go limp and breathing is slow and even. The sleeper may begin to sweat. During this stage and Stage 4, the body begins to restore itself. In people under 30, the endocrine glands release human growth hormone (HGH), which promotes cell division and organ growth. Awakening a person in Stage 3 sleep is fairly difficult to do, and the sleeper may experience grogginess for a few seconds or minutes after awakening. After two or three sleep cycles, this stage may disappear and you may go directly from Stage 2 to REM sleep.

Stage 4—This is the deepest stage of sleep. Delta waves become larger and much slower than in Stage 3, and breathing, heart rate, metabolism, and temperature reach their lowest levels. Muscles continue to be inactive and the sleeper may sweat, but the body continues its restorative activities. Some sleepers may experience night terrors or sleepwalking. Toward the end of this stage, sleepers may readjust their position and may experience a muscular contraction as they enter the next stage. Rousing sleepers from this phase takes a great deal of effort. Once awakened, people feel groggy and may require several minutes to orient themselves. After two or three cycles, this stage may disappear for the duration of the night.

Stage 5 (REM)—This is the dreaming phase, marked by small, rapid alpha waves that resemble those indicating wakefulness and sensory awareness of external stimuli. However, in this stage our brains are reacting to internally generated stimuli from our dreams. All other muscles seize up to prevent us from reacting to the action in the dreams, but the sleeper may experience some slight twitching in the face, fingers, and toes. Men experience penile erections. Breathing and heart rate speed up and slow down in reaction to dream content. A sleeper in the REM stage is difficult to rouse and, if awakened, they will have a hard time adjusting to reality. This stage becomes progressively longer with each cycle, possibly lasting 60 minutes in the fifth cycle.

How Much Sleep Do You Need?

The average person sleeps 7.5 hours per night and completes four to five sleep cycles.[30] A person's sleep requirements for good health vary according to age and gender, as well as level of activity during the day. Contrary to conventional wisdom, it is not necessary for all adults to get eight hours of sleep every night to maintain good health. Some people function well with only five hours of sleep, while others may need ten to feel revived in the morning. On the whole, though, most experts recommend approximately eight hours of sleep per day. Infants require the most sleep at 16 to 18 hours a day and young adults generally need about 7.0 to 8.5 hours of shut-eye. As people age, they tend to sleep more lightly and for a shorter duration. The amount of sleep older people need has been debated over the years, but since people over age 55 spend fewer and fewer minutes in Stages 3 and 4, they may need more than eight hours of sleep to experience the restorative powers of deep sleep.

The modern American lifestyle can deter people from getting the sleep they need to function properly. Late nights at the office, shift work, and multiple social and familial obligations eat away from the time dedicated to slumber. Many high school students are sleep-deprived—due to the early start times of some schools or trying to do too many activities along with homework—and this may affect their academic abilities. Such factors can run up a high sleep debt, the cumulative amount of time needed to make up for loss of sleep. If you need eight hours of sleep but get only six hours two nights in a row, your total sleep debt will be four hours (2 nights x 2 hours). If you neglect to pay off your sleep debt, you will likely experience mood problems as well as poor cognitive function, which can be detrimental to your health and the health of those around you. According to the National Highway Traffic Safety Administration, driver fatigue (due to sleep deprivation) is responsible for an estimated 100,000 motor vehicle accidents and 1,500 deaths each year.[31]

For information on **self-administered and diagnostic sleep tests**, see Chapter 2: Sleep Disorders and Their Causes, pp. 34-55.

Though there are tests that doctors use to assess whether you're meeting your sleep requirements, if you feel alert and emotionally stable with good memory recall and reaction times, you're probably getting enough sleep. Another clue is sleep latency, the normal length of time it takes you from the time you lie down to the moment you fall asleep. While most people can't pinpoint the actual moment they fall asleep, you can still estimate. The average sleep latency is between 15 and 20 minutes; falling asleep within five minutes of hitting the sack indicates sleep deprivation. "Microsleeps," very brief periods of sleep (as little as a fraction of a second), are another sign of sleep deprivation. Most people who experience microsleeps aren't aware of it, but a minor lapse in attention may tip you off to their occurrence. Additionally, feeling drowsy during the day, even during tedious activities, likely means that you haven't had enough sleep.

Circadian Rhythms and the Body's Clock

As mentioned earlier, sleeping during the night likely evolved to keep animals, including the human species, out of harm's way. Supporting this theory is the fact that most of us still follow the sun's cycles, sleeping when the sun is down and waking when it's up. In fact, we possess innate cycles similar to those of the sun, called circadian rhythms. Scientists believe that these rhythms are guided partly by genes that have evolved in many species, from fruit flies to humans.[32]

Circadian rhythms are regularly recurring, biological changes in our mental and physical behaviors over the course of the day. As indicated by the term *circadian* (Latin for "around a day"), these rhythms repeat approximately every 24 hours and are primarily controlled by the body's biological "clock." Circadian rhythms are most commonly linked to sleep/wake patterns and account for the fluctuations of alertness and drowsiness throughout the day. People with normal circadian rhythms are most alert during the morning and afternoon, but tend to get drowsy toward evening and feel the need for sleep at nighttime. Research shows that circadian rhythms occur in other physiological processes as well, including blood pressure, body temperature, hormone levels, and the immune system.[33]

The body clock is actually part of the hypothalamus, an area of the brain just above the point where the optic nerves cross. Specifically, the

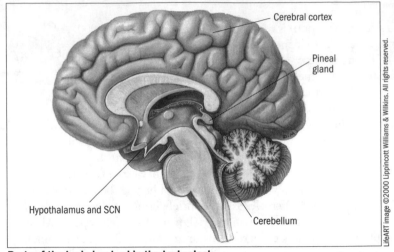

Parts of the brain involved in the body clock.

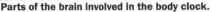

clock is a cluster of hypothalamic nerve cells called the suprachiasmatic nuclei (SCN). As with other precise timepieces, researchers believe the body clock operates on the principle of oscillation. In much the same way that a grandfather clock keeps time with the evenly spaced swings of a pendulum, the body clock tells time with the slow ebb and flow of protein molecules in the SCN. In controlled conditions where test subjects are deprived of light and other time cues, a "day" by body clock standards is close to 25 hours. However, we do not exist in a dark vacuum. Light, from both the sun and artificial devices, as well as environmental cues (called *zeitgeber*—"time-giver" in German) such as alarm clocks, influence our circadian rhythms and set our body clocks to follow the 24-hour cycle of the sun.

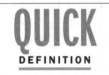

DEFINITION

Hormones are the chemical messengers of the endocrine system that impose order through an intricate communication system among the body's estimated 50 trillion cells. Examples include the "male" sex hormone (testosterone), the "female" sex hormones (estrogen and progesterone), melatonin (pineal), growth hormone (pituitary), and DHEA (adrenal).

How light manages to sway our internal timepieces also depends on the SCN nerves in the hypothalamus. The optic nerves relay information about external light levels to the SCN, which in turn sends the light signals to several regions of the brain, including the pea-sized pineal (pronounced pie-NEEL) gland. The pineal gland is instrumental in sleep, because it secretes melatonin, the sleep-inducing hormone (SEE QUICK DEFINITION).

The Role of Melatonin

As discussed above, melatonin has been shown to have numerous health benefits, as an immune stimulant, antioxidant, and cardiovascular ally. But it is crucial in the induction of sleep and the regulation of the circadian rhythm.

When it's dark, the pineal gland secretes melatonin in extremely minute amounts—blood levels of melatonin are measured in picograms, that is, trillionths of a gram. The actual amounts depend on age and other factors, but between five and ten times more melatonin is released at night than during the day.[34] Melatonin is the antithesis of another hormone, adrenaline, produced by the adrenal glands. As melatonin enters the bloodstream, it begins to slow down the waking (alpha) brain waves. Subsequently, the heart rate decreases, muscles relax, blood pressure drops, and the body begins to enter the stages of sleep.

The average blood levels of melatonin throughout the day mirrors typical circadian rhythms. Low amounts of melatonin correspond to the periods of heightened alertness; high amounts of melatonin relate to periods of drowsiness and sleep. Between 7 a.m. and 2 p.m., melatonin is at its lowest level, below ten picograms per milliliter (pg/ml) of blood. From 2 p.m. to about 8 p.m., melatonin levels rise slightly, as the pineal gland begins production of the sleep hormone. Melatonin reaches its peak (70 pg/ml) in most people at approximately 2 a.m., flattens for a couple of hours, then around 4 a.m. begins a dramatic drop to its lowest levels.

Production of melatonin not only varies during the 24-hour cycle, it also fluctuates during our life span. Newborns produce very low amounts of melatonin, usually sleeping 16 to 18 hours a day, spread out over six to

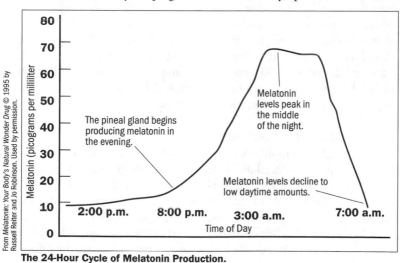

The pineal gland begins producing melatonin in the evening.

Melatonin levels peak in the middle of the night.

Melatonin levels decline to low daytime amounts.

The 24-Hour Cycle of Melatonin Production.

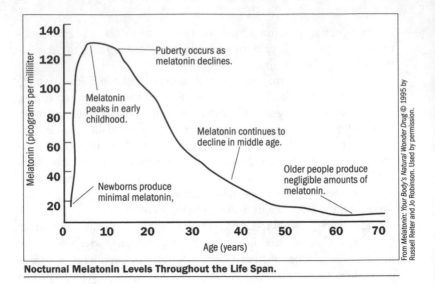

Nocturnal Melatonin Levels Throughout the Life Span.

From *Melatonin: Your Body's Natural Wonder Drug* © 1995 by Russell Reiter and Jo Robinson. Used by permission.

seven naps. By the age of three months, they begin producing greater levels of the hormone; it is also during this time that babies begin to sleep through the night and become more alert during the day. Melatonin levels surge from then on, peaking before the age of ten at about 125 pg/ml. Children during this time sleep ten or more hours a night and undergo a dramatic growth spurt, which is aided by sleep.

When adolescents reach puberty, a time when high levels of sex hormones are being released, melatonin levels begin to decline and continue thus for the rest of the person's life. Simultaneously, for reasons scientists are still researching, other hormones begin to dip, including testosterone, estrogen, growth hormone, and DHEA. Between the ages of 20 and 30, melatonin levels are about 40-60 pg/ml; by age 50, levels are below 20 pg/ml. People over 60 produce neglible amounts of melatonin, below 10 pg/ml.

The Precursors to Melatonin

The pineal gland simply doesn't make melatonin out of thin air. For melatonin to be produced, the brain needs an adequate supply of tryptophan, an amino acid that cannot be created by the body. We can only obtain this essential amino acid through our diet, in protein foods such as meat, fish, dairy products, and some legumes. The brain is surrounded by the blood-brain barrier, so tryptophan requires the aid of a special type of protein called a carrier, which transports the amino acid across the protective layer.

A Brief Glossary of Brain Chemical Terms

Amino acids are the building-blocks of the 40,000 different proteins in the body, including enzymes, hormones, and the brain chemical messengers called neurotransmitters. Eight amino acids cannot be made by the body and must be obtained through the diet; others are produced in the body but not always in sufficient amounts. The body's main "amino acid pool" consists of: alanine, arginine, aspargine, aspartic acid, carnitine, citrulline, cysteine, cystine, GABA, glutamic acid, glutamine, glycine, histidine, isoleucine, leucine, lysine, methionine, ornithine, phenylalanine, proline, serine, taurine, threonine, tryptophan, tyrosine, and valine.

Enzymes are specialized living proteins fundamental to all living processes in the body, necessary for every chemical reaction and the normal activity of our organs, tissues, fluids, and cells. Enzymes are essential for the production of energy required to run cellular functions. There are hundreds of thousands of these "Nature's workers." Enzymes enable the body to digest and assimilate food. There are special enzymes for digesting proteins, carbohydrates, fats, and plant fibers. Enzymes also assist in clearing the body of toxins and cellular debris.

A **neurotransmitter** is a brain chemical with the specific function of enabling communications between brain cells, called neurons. Electrical thought impulses are changed into neurotransmitters at the dendrites, the branching tips of a nerve cell; then they are passed on to the next nerve cell. Chief among the 100 neurotransmitters identified to date, there are six involved in most mental activities. Acetylcholine is required for short-term memory, concentration, and all muscle contractions. GABA is a calming agent that works to stop excess nerve signals (stimulation) and thus keeps brain firings from getting out of control. Serotonin does the same and helps produce sleep, regulate pain, and influence mood—it's called the "feel good" neurotransmitter—although too much serotonin can produce depression. Dopamine regulates physical movements and muscular control, and it influences mood, sex drive, and memory retrieval. L-glutamate is essential for laying down new memories and the recall of existing ones; it also inhibits the chronic stress response and the excess secretion of cortisol. Norepinephrine causes the brain to be more alert; it helps carry memories from short-term "storage" to long-term and it enables one to maintain a positive mood.

Once tryptophan has entered the brain, a specialized enzyme helps brain cells convert the amino acid into another substance called 5-hydroxy-tryptophan, or 5-HTP. Another enzyme then helps convert 5-HTP into a neurotransmitter called serotonin. Once again, an enzyme called N-acetyl-transferases, or NAT, reacts with some of the serotonin to make a chemical called N-acetyl-serotonin (NAS). With the help of another specialized enzyme, the pineal gland is able to convert NAS into melatonin.[35]

Melatonin and the Light Paradox

Light plays a crucial—and seemingly paradoxical—role in sleep, as it both inhibits and promotes melatonin production. The NAT enzyme necessary in melatonin synthesis is mostly or completely inactivated by exposure to any light.[36] Studies have shown that being exposed to even a fairly dim light at night can significantly reduce the synthesis of melatonin;[37] a 100-lux light (a 100-watt bulb from a distance of five feet) has been shown to inhibit melatonin secretion.[38] At the same time, studies have shown that bright light also significantly boosts melatonin production.[39]

Why are these findings so contradictory? The truth is, they're not. What matters with light is when you and your nervous system—and thus your body clock—are exposed to it. During the daytime hours—when the circadian rhythm is at its more alert stages—the brain requires bright light. This promotes the increased synthesis of serotonin, which in turn means more melatonin will be produced at night. During the nighttime hours, when the circadian rhythm is nearing its lowest level, the brain needs to produce melatonin, to prepare the body for sleep. Thus, the brain requires darkness—even a nightlight a few feet from the bed can be detrimental to melatonin production.

Factors That Can Disrupt Your Body Clock

Many people with sleep disorders have disrupted circadian rhythms, often due to melatonin imbalances, in which the natural sleep/wake patterns are interrupted or reversed. Many Americans spend up to 90% of their days indoors, in buildings with fluorescent lights. This lack of exposure to bright sunlight or its artificial cousin, full-spectrum light, is a major contributor to disrupted circadian rhythms and concurrent reduced melatonin levels. Lack of regular exercise, structural imbalances, and chronic stress are also common factors. So, too, is a poor diet, often marked by overconsumption of stimulants such as alcohol, coffee, spicy foods, sugar, and over-the-counter medications. Electromagnetic fields, both natural and artificial, also play a role in diminishing the function of the pineal gland, resulting in decreased melatonin production and an imbalanced body clock.

For more about the **factors that disrupt circadian rhythms** and **seasonal affective disorder (SAD)**, see Chapter 5: Resetting the Body Clock, pp. 120-145.

Seasonal Affective Disorder (SAD)

One of the most prevalent consequences of a disrupted circadian rhythm is an illness called seasonal affective disorder (SAD). Individuals who receive little natural light during the day often experience an imbalance in their serotonin and melatonin levels—specifically, a rise in melatonin and a

Organizations for Sleep Information

American Sleep Apnea Association
2025 Pennsylvania Avenue NW
Washington, DC 20006
tel: 202-293-3650

American Sleep Disorder Association
1610 14th Street NW, Suite 300
Rochester, MN 55901
tel: 507-287-6006

Association of Professional Sleep
Societies
1610 14th St. NW, Suite 300
Rochester, MN 55901
tel: 507-287-6006

Better Sleep Council
333 Commerce Street
Alexandria, VA 22314
tel: 703-683-4503

The National Commission on
Sleep Disorders Research
701 Welch Road, Suite 2226
Palo Alto, CA 94304
tel: 415-725-6484

National Center on Sleep
Disorders Research
Two Rockledge Centre, Suite 10038
6701 Rockledge Drive, MSC 7920
Bethesda, MD 20892-7920
tel: 301-435-0199

National Sleep Foundation
1522 K Street, NW, Suite 500
Washington, D.C. 20005
fax: 202-347-3472
website: www.sleepfoundation.org

corresponding decline in serotonin. When low-light exposure is chronic, it can lead to SAD. Often called "winter depression," SAD frequently occurs during the fall and winter months, when days grow shorter and natural light is limited.

The symptoms of SAD's winter doldrums are no doubt familiar to many. In fact, it's estimated that over ten million Americans experience SAD every year, according to the National Institute of Mental Health (NIMH), and another 25 million get some milder depressive symptoms on a seasonal basis. What does SAD feel like? Typically, there is chronic depression and fatigue that may leave you bedridden; hypersomnia (increased sleep by as much as four hours or more per night) and reduced quality of the sleep, leaving you feeling less refreshed; and cravings for carbohydrates and candy, which can lead to sometimes significant weight gain. Women with SAD may report that their premenstrual symptoms are aggravated. Similar seasonal behavioral changes, particularly increased sleep and variations in appetite, are seen in other mammals.

Sleep Disorders & Their Causes

If you're tired as you read this, you're not alone. In a 2000 survey, 30% of adults admitted to being so drowsy during the day that it interfered with their daily activities.[1] Sleep deprivation is usually to blame. The average adult sleeps just under seven hours per night during the work week;[2] most people function best on at least eight hours of shut-eye. Sometimes sleep deprivation is self-imposed—you choose to stay up late working or socializing or watching TV, and get up early to exercise or make the morning commute. But others can't get enough sleep, no matter how hard they try. According to the National Institute of Neurological Disorders and Stroke, approximately 40 million Americans suffer from long-term chronic sleep disorders, while another 20 million experience occasional sleep problems. But those statistics may underestimate the prevalence of slumber woes; according to the survey referred to above, 62% of American adults reported that they had experienced a sleep problem at least a few times a week during the previous year. In fact, it is estimated that 95% of sleep disorders are not diagnosed.[3]

Altogether, Americans spend about $16 billion each year on sleep-related medical care. Unfortunately, much of this money is poorly spent, because conventional sleeping aids—potentially addictive sedatives—ultimately create more sleep disturbances than they eliminate. Conventional physicians are beginning to realize this fact, however, and are increasingly likely to suggest that their patients make lifestyle changes to remedy sleep disorders. But knowing exactly which changes to make for your particular condition can be difficult, and conventional doctors are poorly trained in recognizing the underlying causes of sleep problems.

Alternative medicine practitioners can make sure that finding the right treatment protocol doesn't turn into a nightmare. They realize that sleep disorders, including insomnia, sleep apnea, restless legs syndrome, and narcolepsy, often arise from poor diet, toxic overload, disrupted circadian rhythms, geopathic and emotional stress, and hormonal and structural

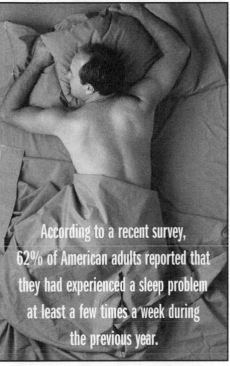

According to a recent survey, 62% of American adults reported that they had experienced a sleep problem at least a few times a week during the previous year.

imbalances. In short, the majority of sleep problems are symptoms of an unhealthy body, not diseases in and of themselves. Most people with sleep disorders will find relief by taking steps to promote overall health: improving their diet, reducing stress, balancing hormones, and detoxifying the body, among others. This chapter will introduce you to the primary underlying causes of sleep problems and provide you with an overview of alternative therapies proven to help restore normalcy to your sleep—and your life.

Types of Sleep Disorders

Sleep disorders fall under two categories, dyssomnias and parasomnias. Dyssomnias are conditions characterized by the difficulty in falling or maintaining sleep or by excessive sleepiness during the day. Insomnia, sleep apnea, narcolepsy, restless legs syndrome, periodic limb movements in sleep, hypersomnia, and delayed and advanced sleep phase syndromes are dyssomniac conditions. Parasomnias are behavioral abnormalities that occur during sleep, including sleepwalking, night terrors, and REM behavior disorder.

Sleep researchers sometimes further classify sleep disorders as primary or secondary. Primary disorders are unrelated to any existing medical conditions, and secondary disorders arise as the result of some other illness or hormonal change, such as menopause, pregnancy, depression, or fibromyalgia. Alternative medicine practitioners may not make such distinctions, because the underlying causes are often the same.

Insomnia

Insomnia is a broad term, casually used to describe the inability either to fall asleep or to remain asleep during the course of the night. Insomniacs usually do not feel rested the next morning and may experience excessive drowsiness, irritability, and poor cognitive function during the day. Fifty-eight percent of U.S. adults report bouts of insomnia recurring at least a few times each week, with shift workers experiencing insomnia more frequently than regular day workers do (66% compared to 55%).[5] Sleep researchers classify insomnia in terms of the time of night that it effects: sleep-onset insomnia, sleep-maintenance insomnia, and early-morning-awakening insomnia.

Most researchers also characterize insomnia based on frequency. Transient insomnia lasts one or several nights and is usually triggered by stress, excitement, and traveling across time zones (jet lag). Intermittent insomnia occurs sporadically over a long course of time; it, too, is generally set off by stress. Chronic insomnia occurs on most nights and lasts a month or more, and may arise from various medical conditions, including depression, arthritis, asthma, heart disease, hyperthyroidism, kidney disease, and Parkinson's disease.[6] Postmenopausal women and older people tend to suffer from some type of insomnia.

Conventional treatment for transient and intermittent insomnia is usually with over-the-counter sleeping pills, or benzodiazepine prescription sedatives. Chronic insomnia rarely responds positively to sleeping pills.

The Sleepiness Scale

Sleep researchers at Stanford University in Palo Alto, California, have developed a way to document your sleep habits. Called the Stanford Sleepiness Scale, this simple questionnaire allows you and your doctor to determine if you are getting enough sleep and whether any of your sleep or daytime habits indicate a sleep disorder.[4] It is particularly useful if you also keep a "sleep diary," a record of your sleep patterns, including what time you go to bed each night (and nap during the day), how long it takes you to fall asleep, and when you get up.

To complete the Stanford scale, simply make a notation of the number that best corresponds to how you feel at different times of the day. Make notations an hour or two after you wake up in the morning (when you're usually at your peak of alertness), at around 2 p.m. (when circadian rhythms are at their sleepiest daytime levels), and again at 7 p.m. or 8 p.m. (typically the most alert time in the evening). By comparing your responses over a course of days or even weeks, you'll be able to tell if your sleepiness/wakefulness patterns coincide with the norm, or if your circadian rhythms are off track.

1) Almost in a reverie, hard to stay awake
2) Sleepiness, prefer to be lying down
3) Fogginess, losing interest, slowed down
4) A little foggy, not at peak, let down
5) Relaxed, not full alertness, responsive
6) Functioning at a high level, not at peak
7) Feeling active, vital, alert, wide awake

■ Sleep-Onset Insomnia—People suffering from sleep-onset insomnia take 30 or more minutes to fall asleep, after which they enjoy a relatively normal night of sleep. Of the adults who complain of having insomnia, 22% report experiencing this type.[7] People suffering from sleep-onset insomnia often exacerbate their situation by focusing on the fact that they are not sleeping; this is called psychophysiological insomnia. In this case, a person's normal pre-sleep rituals, behavior, or sleeping environment trigger insomnia. The more the sleeper worries about falling asleep, the worse the insomnia becomes.

■ Sleep-Maintenance Insomnia—This type of insomnia is characterized by waking up one or more times during the course of the night. It takes more than 30 minutes to fall back asleep after each awakening. This is the most common type of insomnia, accounting for 34% of insomnia cases.[8]

■ Early-Morning-Awakening Insomnia—If you awaken before dawn and can't get back to sleep, you have early-morning-awakening insomnia. Twenty-two percent of insomniacs reportedly suffer from this type.[9]

Jet Lag and Shift Work: Insomniac's Nightmares

If you've ever flown across country or across the ocean, you are probably very familiar with jet lag. Jet lag is a type of insomnia caused by traveling between time zones. If you fly from California to New York, you have to move your watch three hours ahead to match the Eastern time zone—but your body clock is still running on Pacific time. So at 10 p.m., while New Yorkers (most of them anyway) are starting to get ready for sleep, your body feels as though it's only 7 p.m. You're still wide awake and unable to get to sleep. Another factor in jet lag is exposure to electromagnetic fields during the flight, which can affect the pineal gland's ability to produce melatonin.

Shift work can cause the same kinds of problems as jet lag. People who are constantly disrupting their body's internal rhythm by changing shifts, or working night shifts for five nights and then trying to have a normal schedule on the weekends, can develop insomnia.

For information about **sleep apnea**, contact: The American Sleep Apnea Association, 2025 Pennsylvania Avenue NW, Washington, DC 20006; tel: 202-293-3650; website: www.sleepapnea.org.

Sleep Apnea

An estimated 18 million Americans suffer from sleep apnea, a potentially life-threatening disorder in which the sleeper experiences intermittent cessation of breathing.[10] The more common form of this condition is obstructive sleep apnea, in which the air passages become blocked, causing respiratory distress. Obstruction may be caused when the throat muscles and tongue relax during sleep, allowing the tongue and uvula (the small, fleshy tissue hanging from the back of the throat) to sag and block the airway. Excessive tissue in the airways (prevalent among overweight people) and excess swelling and mucus production in the nose (often caused by childhood allergies) can also narrow and substantially obstruct breathing during sleep.[11] Central sleep apnea is less common and is triggered when the brain fails to signal the respiratory muscles to breathe.

In an episode of sleep apnea, the sleeper involuntary stops breathing for ten to sixty seconds, resulting in decreased blood levels of oxygen and increased amounts of carbon dioxide. This change in blood gases alerts the brain to begin breathing. To do so, the brain must awaken the body from deep sleep. The sleeper then resumes breathing, usually with a loud snort or gasp, and then quickly falls back to light sleep. People with obstructive sleep apnea usually snore heavily before and after the breathing pauses.

These apneic events can occur up to 30 times each hour, although the sleeper rarely realizes this because the awakenings are so brief. However, these constant arousals prevent patients from getting enough deep sleep, and lead

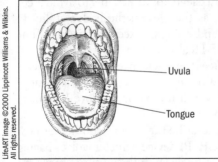

Uvula

Tongue

In obstructive sleep apnea, the air passages become blocked when the throat muscles and tongue relax during sleep, allowing the tongue and uvula (the small, fleshy tissue hanging from the back of the throat) to sag and block the airway.

Snoring and Sleep Apnea

Snoring is a common sign of sleep apnea, but it does not necessarily indicate that you're suffering from this disorder. Although 30% to 40% of adults snore, only 1% of snorers have sleep apnea.[12] So if you snore, how do you know whether it is sleep apnea or not?

Snoring, unlike most cases of sleep apnea, does not involve obstruction of the airways. Instead, the sawing-wood sound is caused by vibrations of the soft palate and uvula during the source of breathing during sleep. If snoring is not accompanied by pauses in breathing, you can be assured that your snoring is not indicative of sleep apnea. To be sure, you may want to consult your doctor about testing for sleep apnea.

Snoring unrelated to sleep apnea has not been found to pose any health risk and doesn't cause daytime drowsiness for the sleeper (though the bed partner may be awakened by loud snoring).[13] To prevent snoring, sleep experts recommend that people sleep on their sides. If you tend to roll on your back at night, sew a pocket into the back of your pajamas and put a tennis ball or golf balls inside—that'll keep you on your side. Dental appliances are also sometimes used.

to excessive daytime sleepiness, morning headaches (from lack of oxygen), depression, irritability, sexual dysfunction, learning and memory difficulties, and falling asleep during daily activities. Sleep apnea has also been linked to irregular heartbeat, heart attack,[14] high blood pressure, and stroke, as well as sudden infant death syndrome (SIDS),[15] so it is prudent that people who suspect that they or their children suffer from this disorder get medical care. However, the American Sleep Apnea Association contends that up to 83% of those people don't realize they suffer from this serious sleep disorder, due to the sleepers' inability to detect their own problem.[16] Sleeping partners often observe the apneic episodes and can provide valuable information as to whether you suffer from the symptoms of sleep apnea. Doctors usually use the polysomnography test and/or the Multiple Sleep Latency Test (see "Diagnosing Sleep Disorders," p. 46) to diagnose this problem.

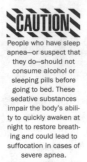
Doctors often advise sleep apnea patients to avoid alcohol and sleeping pills, as they lessen the body's ability to awaken from sleep, and to lose excessive weight. The National Institutes of Health reports that even a 10% weight loss can reduce the incidence of sleep apnea.[17] Sleeping in a side position and wearing a dental appliance that repositions the jaw and tongue may prove helpful in relieving mild sleep apnea.

Doctors may also prescribe the use of a continuous positive airway pressure (CPAP) device, which involves having the sleeper wear a mask that forces air through the nose and keeps the throat from collapsing. In some cases, doctors recommend surgery to remove adenoids and tonsils (most effective in young children), nasal polyps, and other tissue blocking the airway. In another surgical procedure, excess tissue in the back of the throat is removed using surgical instruments (uvulopalotopharygnoplasy) or lasers (uvulopalatoplasty). This procedure may eliminate sleeping problems but not sleep apnea itself; additionally, the long-term effects are unknown. The most drastic conventional measure is tracheostomy, in which a small hole is made in the windpipe, allowing the sleeper to breathe uninterrupted during the night. This procedure works, but it is rarely used.

Restless Legs Syndrome (RLS)

Restless legs syndrome is an unpleasant sleep disorder, in which sufferers often feel creeping, crawling, prickling, burning, itching, or tugging sensations in the legs while resting or sitting for extended periods of time. Sometimes the arms may be affected as well. At night, the sensations can be so bothersome that RLS patients feel the need to move the legs and often cannot get to sleep until the discomfort subsides. The RLS Foundation, in Rochester, Minnesota, estimates that 80% of the 12 million Americans with RLS also experience periodic limb movements in sleep (PLMS—see below). RLS patients often suffer from sleep-onset or sleep-maintenance insomnia and extreme daytime drowsiness.

For information on **restless legs syndrome**, contact: Restless Legs Syndrome Foundation, Inc., P.O. Box 7050, Dept. WWW, Rochester, MN 55903-7050; tel: 507-287-6465; website: www.rls.org; e-mail: RLSFoundation@rls.org.

RLS sufferers generally find temporary relief by stretching, rubbing, or massaging their legs. Conventional doctors may prescribe dopaminergic agents (which modulate or increase levels of the brain chemical dopamine), benzodiazepines (nervous system sedatives), opioids (narcotic pain-killers), and anticonvulsant drugs.

Most cases of RLS are diagnosed in people between the ages of 50 and 60, but symptoms of this sleep disorder usually manifest earlier. Some children who experience "growing pains" or are labeled hyperactive because they cannot sit still may actually be suffering from RLS. According to the RLS Foundation, up to 15% of pregnant women, usually in the third trimester, experience RLS, which often disappears after delivery. Some cases of RLS appear to be hereditary. Anemia, diabetes, kidney failure, and rheumatoid arthritis are associated with the onset or provocation of RLS. Doctors usually diagnose RLS by taking a detailed family history and sometimes polysomnograph tests, in which increased number of brain-wave spikes called K-complexes, followed by bursts of alpha brain waves, indicate RLS.[18]

Periodic Limb Movements in Sleep (PLMS)

Periodic limb movements in sleep is a disorder that often but not necessarily co-exists with restless legs syndrome. PLMS is characterized by sudden, involuntary, and repetitive leg jerking that occurs at the onset of sleep as well as during the course of sleep. These movements can happen every ten to 60 seconds, perhaps hundreds of times, usually in the first half of the night during NREM sleep. PLMS, like RLS, is responsible for cases of sleep-onset and sleep-maintenance insomnia, and often disturbs the sleep of bed partners as well. As with RLS sufferers, PLMS patients often feel excessively sleepy during the day.

Conventional doctors may prescribe dopaminergic agents or opioids to PLMS patients. Some physicians may recommend 15- to 30-minute sessions of transcutaneous electric nerve stimulation (TENS; applying electrical charges to leg nerves) before bed to alleviate nighttime leg jerking.

Narcolepsy

Narcolepsy is a chronic sleep disorder in which patients experience daytime sleepiness so excessive that they fall asleep at inappropriate times for a few seconds up to 30 minutes. These sleep "attacks" can occur repeatedly in the course of normal daily activities—talking, eating, working, walking—even after a full night's sleep. Other classic symptoms of narcolepsy are cataplexy (SEE QUICK DEFINITION); sleep paralysis, in which the person is temporarily unable to talk or move when falling asleep or waking up; and hypnagogic hallucinations, often-frightening dreamlike experiences that sometimes

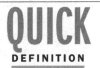

QUICK DEFINITION

Cataplexy is an episodic disorder marked by the sudden loss of muscle function. The severity varies: patients may experience slight weakness, such as limpness of the neck or knees, sagging facial muscles, or an inability to speak distinctly; or they may suffer complete body collapse. Cataplexy, which is a common symptom in narcolepsy, may be triggered by sudden emotional reactions, such as anger, fear, and laughter, and can last anywhere from a few seconds to several minutes. During these events, patients remain conscious.

occur in Stage 1 sleep. Of the estimated 200,000 Americans with narcolepsy, only 20% to 25% suffer from all four symptoms; the rest experience only sleep attacks or a combination of attacks and other symptoms.[19]

Sleep researchers have discovered that people with narcolepsy experience a reversal of sleep stages. As discussed in Chapter 1, the majority of people begin the sleep cycle with NREM stages and then end with REM, the dream state. Narcoleptics, however, begin with REM sleep—an abnormality that extends into the waking hours. In narcolepsy, common aspects of normal REM sleep—lack of muscle tone, sleep paralysis, and vivid dreams—inappropriately occur during periods of wakefulness.

Narcolepsy may be genetic; the National Institutes of Health estimates that 8% to 12% of narcoleptics have a close relative with the disorder.[20] Symptoms usually manifest in the early teen or adult years. Doctors use polysomnogram tests as well as the Multiple Sleep Latency Test to diagnose narcolepsy (see "Diagnosing Sleep Disorders," p. 46). However, since some cases of narcolepsy are infrequent and mild, and others are mistaken for symptoms of depression or epilepsy or as side effects of medications, this sleep disorder is underdiagnosed. As a result, fewer than 50,000 people are aware that they suffer from narcolepsy.[21] Conventional treatment involves stimulant drugs, such as Ritalin, as well as low-dose antidepressants. Doctors also advise patients to supplement their nighttime sleep with two to three short naps (lasting 10 to 15 minutes each) during the day.

Delayed Sleep Phase Syndrome (DSPS)

Delayed sleep phase syndrome is a condition in which the patient chronically stays up quite late, usually until 3-4 a.m., and then sleeps all morning, getting up at 10-11 a.m. If DSPS sufferers must arise earlier in the morning, they do so with great difficulty, experience daytime drowsiness and impaired performance, but still cannot go to sleep until the early morning hours. Usually teenagers or young adults are affected and as many as 15% to 20% of college students may suffer from DSPS.[22] Eastbound travelers may experience transient DSPS as part of jet lag.

Advanced Sleep Phase Syndrome (ASPS)

Advanced sleep phase syndrome is the direct opposite of DSPS, in which a person tends to always fall asleep very early in the evening, usually between 6 p.m. and 9 p.m., and wakes up before dawn, sometimes as early as 1 a.m. People suffering from ASPS may fall asleep at dinner parties and other evening social functions, but may force themselves with

Owls and Larks:
Do You Have a Sleep Phase Disorder?

We're all familiar with "night owls" and "morning larks"—people who tend to prefer waking and sleeping at different hours than most other people. Owls are at their most alert during the late evening and nighttime hours and don't fall asleep until past midnight. Larks, in contrast, function best in the morning hours and fall asleep fairly early in the night. Individual variations in circadian rhythms generally determine whether you're an owl, lark, or regular robin—someone who experiences peak performance in the normal nine to five schedule.

So how do you know whether your sleep personality is actually indicative of advanced or delayed sleep phase syndrome? These disorders may appear to closely resemble owl (delayed) and lark (advanced) characteristics; however, sleep phase syndromes are extremes. Owls typically have rhythms that are approximately two hours later than their regular robin peers—not six or eight hours, as is the case in DSPS. And larks are about two hours ahead of everyone else, again not six or eight hours. Moreover, owls and larks, if they get adequate sleep, generally function normally during the day. People suffering from a sleep phase disorder find it difficult to synchronize their wakeful hours with the activities of the rest of the population.

great difficulty to stay awake later in the evening. However, they may experience sleep deprivation as they continue to arise very early in the morning. About one-third of adults over 65 tend to fall into this pattern, reports James Perl, Ph.D., author of *Sleep Right in Five Nights*.[23]

Hypersomnia

Hypersomnia describes sleep disorders in which people sleep too much—either for prolonged periods at night or during the day. Some people normally sleep longer than others—ten or more hours a day—but this does not necessarily indicate a disorder.[24] Seasonal affective disorder (SAD), described in the previous chapter, is a type of hypersomnia, in which people sleep in late, among other symptoms. Other variations of hypersomnia are as follows:

■ Recurrent Hypersomnia—This disorder, which includes Kleine-Levin Syndrome, lasts several weeks and can recur periodically. Some cases are marked by binge eating and hypersexuality; it usually occurs in adolescent males.

■ Idiopathic Hypersomnia—This type of hypersomnia has symptoms that may be mistaken for narcolepsy, including excessive daytime sleepiness and sleep attacks—except it does not include cataplexy.

- Posttraumatic Hypersomnia—People who have had head injuries may develop this type of disorder, usually immediately after the traumatic incident. Other symptoms include headaches and concentration and memory problems.

Parasomnias

Parasomnias are abnormal physical behaviors that occur during sleep. Usually these conditions involve arousal during the slow-wave stages of NREM sleep, Stages 3 and 4. Parasomniacs aren't actively conscious of their actions and, upon awakening, often cannot recall what happened during the nocturnal episodes. Parasomnias tend to be more common in children and often run in families. Research indicates that parasomniac conditions may be triggered by malfunctions in the brain mechanism that regulates the stages of sleep.[25] Conventional physicians usually treat all disorders with medications, including benzodiazepines. Evaluation at a sleep disorder clinic is recommended if the problem is chronic or if the sleeper becomes violent during an episode.

Sleepwalking (Somnambulism)—Sleepwalking, or somnambulism, usually occurs in Stage 4, the deepest sleep stage, during the first third of the night. This parasomnia, as its name suggests, typically involves walking, sitting, or other repetitive, routine motions. Sleepers, however, are not acting out their dreams; each episode generally lasts between five and 15 minutes.[26] Sleepwalkers appear to be conscious during the episodes: their eyes are usually open and pupils dilated, and they're often able to safely navigate around obstacles, such as furniture. But they are not actively conscious of their actions and don't recall the episode upon waking. In fact, EEGs reveal that the brain waves of sleepwalkers alternate between waking (alpha) waves and sleeping (delta) waves; sleepwalkers are literally half awake and half asleep.[27]

An estimated 4% of American adults have consulted doctors about their sleepwalking[28] and approximately 10% to 15% of children between the ages of five and 12 have experienced sleepwalking.[29] Stress, fever, sleep deprivation, and even epilepsy have been shown to trigger sleepwalking. Conventional physicians sometimes prescribe sedatives or even stimulants to counter this disorder. Doctors generally advise against waking sleepwalkers, as they are very difficult to arouse and, if awakened, may become alarmed. Instead, guide them gently back to bed and let them wake up on their own. Also, make sure sharp or fragile objects are removed from the sleepwalker's bedroom to prevent property damage or physical injury.

Night Terrors—Night terrors (also called sleep terrors) are frightening episodes for both sleepers and their housemates. People experiencing this parasomnia suddenly let out a piercing scream or cry, and may even jump out of bed, run out of the house, and do bodily harm to themselves or others. These actions are accompanied by heavy sweating and heart palpitations. Though the sleepers may appear conscious of their acts—their pupils are dilated—they may not awaken until after the episode. Night terrors are not nightmares, because patients have no dream recall; in fact, episodes occur during the deep, NREM (nondream) stages of sleep.

As with sleepwalking and other parasomnias, young children tend to suffer from night terrors; only 3% of adults experience this disorder.[30] Night terrors are believed to be associated with a disruption in the nervous system. Stress, sleep deprivation, or sleeping in a different bed may spark night terrors. This disorder generally disappears as children mature. Some adults may be prescribed medication; doctors may also recommend exercise and getting more sleep.

REM Behavior Disorder (RBD)—REM behavior disorder is a potentially dangerous parasomnia. As indicated by its name, this disorder occurs during the REM (dream) stage of sleep. Normally, most of our muscles become paralyzed during the REM phase to prevent us from acting out our dreams. In RBD, however, it appears the brain does not properly signal the paralysis function and sleepers physically engage in their dreams without being actively conscious of their behavior. RBD patients have been known to become violent during dreams, injuring themselves and others, even killing people. Three-quarters of RBD patients repeatedly hurt themselves during RBD episodes.[31]

This disorder usually affects middle-aged and older men and is often associated with some type of nerve problem or brain damage. The primary conventional drug used to treat REM-sleep disorders is a benzodiazepine called clonazepam.

Rhythmic Movement Disorder (RMD)—This disorder involves head-banging, head-rolling, body-rocking, body-rolling, or other repetitive movements of the head and neck during sleep. It typically occurs immediately prior to sleep onset and is sustained into light sleep (Stages 1 and 2).[32] RMD may also last into the deep sleep stages.[33] RMD usually develops in infants at nine months of age and disappears by the age of ten years; if it persists, it is often associated with autism and mental impairment.[34] Some adults also suffer from this disorder.

Benzodiazepines, tranquilizers, and tricyclic antidepressants are usually prescribed by conventional physicians for persistent, severe forms of this sleep disorder.

Teeth-Grinding (Bruxism)—This sleep disorder, clinically called bruxism, is characterized by the grinding of teeth during sleep. Approximately 5% of adults and 15% of children experience chronic bruxism.[35] Usually this condition doesn't cause sleep deprivation or associated health and psychological problems unless it is very severe. However, any teeth-grinding can damage the teeth, bones, gums, and jaw joint.

Many people believe teeth-grinding serves as an outlet for releasing stress experienced during the day. However, doctors contend that bruxism is the body's way of trying to correct structural problems in the mouth. Nocturnal chewing action may be an attempt to grind upper and lower teeth for a better fit. Teeth-grinding may also be the result of temporomandibular joint (TMJ) syndrome. Dentists often prescribe a mouth guard, which, although it does not eliminate the grinding instinct, protects the teeth from damage.

Bed-Wetting (Sleep Enuresis)—Bed-wetting is a common occurrence in toddlers and is only recognized as a disorder after the age of five. It is estimated that 3% of youths between the ages of 12 and 18 suffer from chronic sleep enuresis.[36] This uncontrollable loss of bladder control during the night happens in all sleep stages and is believed to be hereditary; less than 1% of sleep enuresis is attributed to emotional problems.[37] Physiological abnormalities and disorders, including a small bladder, metabolic or hormonal imbalances, allergies, bladder infections, and obstructive sleep apnea are associated with the development of this disorder.

Diagnosing Sleep Disorders

Diagnosing sleep disorders is, at best, an imprecise process—first, because scientists are still learning about the physiology of sleep and, second, because patients are unable to provide clues about problems that occur while they're sleeping. However, there are two standard tests that help doctors identify sleep disorders: polysomnography and the Multiple Sleep Latency Test. Your doctor may also want you to undergo tests that analyze your biochemical characteristics, such as a blood test called a radioimmunoassay (RIA), which measures levels of melatonin. If your physician suspects you have obstructive sleep apnea, you may take a breathing test, during which technicians use an oximeter to measure your breathing patterns, blood oxygen levels, and respiration rates as you sleep.

■ Polysomnography—This test monitors bodily functions, including electrical activity of the brain, eye movement, muscle activity, heart rate, air flow, and blood oxygen levels, during sleep. This test is often used to diagnose sleep apnea, narcolepsy, restless legs syndrome (RLS), and periodic limb movements in sleep (PLMS), but may be employed to test for other sleep disorders.

■ Multiple Sleep Latency Test (MSLT)—The test measures how long it takes a person to fall asleep at any point during the day as drowsiness occurs. Generally, people without sleep disorders fall asleep in ten to 20 minutes; those who fall asleep in less than five minutes are categorized as experiencing sleep deprivation and a sleep disorder of some type. This test is typically used to diagnose sleep-onset insomnia, sleep apnea, and narcolepsy.

Why Sleeping Pills Don't Work

More than 13 million Americans take prescription sleeping medications, primarily benzodiazepine tranquilizers (such as Valium®, Klonopin®, and Xanax®) and antidepressants (Elavil® and Sinequan®).[39] The number of people taking readily available over-the-counter (OTC) sleeping pills (antihistamines such as Unisom®, Nytol, and

How Big is Your Sleep Debt?

One clue as to whether you have a sleep disorder is a large sleep debt, the cumulative amount of sleep you've missed due to choice or to sleep problems. The Multiple Sleep Latency Test (MSLT) is the gold standard by which doctors measure sleep debt, but the Epworth Sleepiness Scale below will give you a good idea of how much sleep you're missing.[38] Ask yourself how likely you are to doze off or fall asleep in the scenarios below. Rate your response according to the following scale and add the total score for an evaluation of your sleep debt.

(Scale: 0 = Would never doze; 1 = Slight chance of dozing; 2 = Moderate chance of dozing; 3 = High chance of dozing)

____ Sitting and reading
____ Watching TV
____ Sitting inactive in one place (theater, meeting, etc.)
____ As a passenger in a car for an hour without a break
____ Lying down to rest in the afternoon when circumstances permit
____ Sitting and talking to someone
____ Sitting quietly after a lunch without alcohol
____ In a car, while stopped for a few minutes in traffic

Total Score:
0-5 = Slight or no sleep debt
6-10 = Moderate sleep debt
11-20 = Heavy sleep debt
21-25 = Extreme sleep debt

Tylenol® PM) may be even greater. While these drugs may provide a moderate amount of relief for a short period of time, they ultimately do more harm than good.

All types of sleeping "aids" function by sedating or depressing the brain. Benzodiazepines slow the brain waves; antidepressants manipulate the levels of brain chemicals; and OTC drugs block histamine and other chemical reactions in the brain and body. These processes temporarily alleviate insomnia and other sleep disorders. However, most sleeping pills have a deleterious effect on your sleep cycle, increasing the time spent in light, Stage 2 sleep and diminishing the time spent in deep sleep and REM sleep. As discussed in Chapter 1, deep and REM sleep are required for optimal cerebral, immune, cardiovascular, and mental health. Chronic use of sedative medications impairs these functions and can open the door to illness. All of these drugs may also adversely interact with alcohol and other medications, slowing heart rate and breathing to potentially dangerous levels.

Additionally, sleeping pills, especially tranquilizers and antidepressants, can become addictive. Since the efficacy of all drugs diminishes with use, you'll require higher and higher dosages in order to feel the sedating effects, fueling the dependency on these drugs. If you stop taking them, you may experience "rebound insomnia," in which insomnia recurs, often more severely. Rebound insomnia may also disrupt REM sleep, triggering nightmares.

OTC drugs, even if used for a short time, have many adverse side effects, including drug-induced "hangovers" or stupor. "Research that has investigated performance on mental tasks (such as learning and decision-making) and on motor tasks (such as driving a car) on days after the use of sleeping pills finds that people usually do worse after taking a pill than they do after a night of insomnia," states sleep expert Russel J. Reiter.[40] The reason this happens is that your body still retains some of the medication the next day and its sedating effects linger. Peter Hauri, Ph.D., director of the Mayo Clinic Insomnia Research and Treatment Program, says this is particularly problematic for older adults—who tend to have more sleep disorders anyway—because they metabolize medications more slowly. OTC drugs can also provoke anxiety, dizziness, restlessness, confusion, amnesia, blurred vision, nausea, digestive upset, and frequent urination.[41]

Patients suffering from sleep apnea are warned not to take any sleeping medications, as they impair the body's ability to arouse itself and restore normal breathing.

What Alternative Medicine Can Do for Sleep Disorders

Alternative medicine offers patients lasting relief from sleep disorders. While certain extreme disorders have genetic underpinnings and may require continued medical care, even cases of narcolepsy have been reversed by eliminating food allergies and following other alternative therapies. According to the alternative medicine approach, sleep disorders result from multiple causes, many of them with a less-than-obvious connection to the disorder or not easily detectable. As you will discover in this book, a number of underlying imbalances, with accompanying physical, mental, and environmental factors, contribute to all forms of sleep problems.

It is essential to understand the factors that went into creating the sleep disorder in each person, because sleep disorders are rarely caused by one thing alone and no two people have exactly the same causal factors. Alternative medicine employs a battery of diagnostic tools—sleep tests, physical examination, dietary assessment, tests for digestive, detoxification, and hormonal function, and emotional evaluation—to build an individualized picture of the patient's condition. Skilled alternative practitioners take the time needed to find the root causes of sleep disorders and the patient also becomes actively involved in their treatment. Alternative medicine not only respects differences among individuals, but concentrates its diagnosis and treatment plan on this "customized" approach. With alternative medicine, health is restored to the whole patient, rather than simply providing superficial symptom relief. The goal is to help each person achieve a balance among physical healing and the emotional, mental, and even spiritual aspects of their life.

Alternative medicine draws upon a wide range of therapies to help treat—and even prevent—sleep disorders. The primary keys are proper diet and nutrition, detoxification, stress reduction, and environmental controls. Diet and nutrition can have a significant impact on sleep and special care should be taken to avoid substances that might overly stimulate the brain. Vitamins, minerals, herbs, and other natural supplements such as melatonin can provide effective relief without the side effects of conventional drugs.

Removing toxins from the body has shown to be therapeutic for patients—alternative medicine offers a number of safe and effective detoxification strategies. Meditation, biofeedback, hypnotherapy, and other mind/body techniques can help reduce stress. Skeletal problems

Sleep Problems Don't Have to Be Part of Aging

It is commonly believed that as we get older, we should expect to sleep poorly. On the contrary, how well you will sleep as you age depends on your lifestyle. If you spend most of your life drinking alcohol, eating poorly, and not exercising, it is likely you will experience sleep difficulties. Many people in their 60s, 70s, and 80s sleep soundly because they maintain healthy lifestyles.

Sleep problems are not an automatic accompaniment to aging, emphasizes H. Vafi, M.D.[42] "Although uninterrupted sleep may be more difficult to achieve [with aging], insomnia may not be as much a factor in growing older as it is a by-product of a negative attitude about aging," says Dr. Vafi. While it's true that older people tend to spend less time in deep sleep, possibly due to reduced levels of melatonin, exercise, proper diet, melatonin supplementation, and light therapy can help seniors—and everyone else—sleep like a baby again.

can also be addressed through a variety of other modalities, including bodywork, exercise, and yoga. Environmental imbalances can be regulated with magnet therapy and feng shui. Light therapy is especially helpful for people with disrupted circadian rhythms.

Seven Reasons Why You Can't Sleep

Sleep disorders develop as a result of a combination of poor diet and food allergies; an accumulation of toxins in the body (from the environment, food, drugs, and other sources); biomechanical stress and imbalances; poor stress-coping abilities and other emotional factors; hormonal imbalances; and geopathic irregularities. All of these factors may also disrupt the circadian rhythms, leading to such problems as sleep phase syndromes and insomnia.

Poor Diet and Food Allergies

Ingested stimulants such as caffeine, sugar, and spicy foods, are major contributors to sleep disorders. Caffeine—found in coffee, non-herbal teas, soft drinks, and many over-the-counter drugs—can remain in the body from 12 to 20 hours, thwarting sleep.[43] Sugar creates uneven blood sugar levels (hypoglycemia) that can disrupt your sleep in the middle of the night. Another side effect is called insulin rebound, in which the body is overwhelmed with an influx of simple sugars and is no longer able to digest food properly. This condition causes an emergency stress reaction in the body that prevents sleep. It can also result in food addictions, a vicious cycle of bingeing on sugary or caffeinated foods, keeping blood sugar levels and sleep patterns out of balance. Food allergies are also implicated in promoting food addictions and often are found in children with obstructive sleep apnea.

Seemingly relaxing substances such as alcohol and nicotine also impair the ability to sleep deeply and continuously through the night. Nicotine is actually a stimulant, similar to caffeine. Although drinking alcohol may appear to help induce sleep, it often will create shortened, lighter sleep.[44] Liquor is a very strong diuretic and may prompt you to awaken throughout the night to urinate. Sleep problems may also be caused by vitamin or mineral deficiencies, including B vitamins, copper, iron, and zinc.

Toxic Colon and Liver

While it may not seem readily apparent, the role of the liver and colon are important for establishing and maintaining regular, restful sleep. Both the colon and the liver remove toxins (in air, water, and food) and waste from the body. If either system is not working properly, the body can become dangerously toxic, resulting in conditions such as food allergies and bacterial overgrowth that have been shown to disturb sleep. Heavy metals such as mercury are particularly toxic to the body and can directly cause insomnia. Toxic load can also deplete vitamins and minerals essential to inducing a good night's sleep.

Disrupted Circadian Rhythms

Seasonal affective disorder (SAD), advanced and delayed sleep phase syndromes, and some cases of insomnia are caused by disruptions in circadian rhythms. Inadequate exposure to bright light and sunlight is a major contributor to upsetting our body clocks, but so is traveling across time zones and shift work. Poor diet, heavy use of stimulants, lack of exercise, and unmanaged stress can also upset our natural sleep patterns. An often-overlooked cause of circadian rhythm disruptions is extremely low frequency electromagnetic fields (EMFs), which have been found to diminish the pineal gland's ability to produce melatonin. Electrical power lines, home appliances, commercial airplanes, and computers generate EMFs.

Stress and Psychological Factors

Stress and pent-up emotional issues can wreak havoc on the brain, deregulating brain chemicals and organs that are instrumental in procuring a good night's rest. Unmanaged daily stress can deplete your hormonal and nutrient reserves and create a vicious cycle of less sleep and more stress. Additionally, unresolved psychological issues, such as deep-seated internal fears or relationship conflicts, can disturb brain chemistry and hinder deep sleep.

Geopathic Stress and Environmental Toxins

Geopathic stress is defined as an abnormal energy field, often of an electromagnetic nature, created deep underground by large mineral deposits, water streams, or geological faults. Accumulated exposure to these discordant energies (usually due to the location of our homes) can create illnesses, including cancer, migraines, depression, and disrupted sleep. We are exposed to other environmental problems inside our homes that ruin our chances for normal sleep. Toxic household chemicals, disruptive noise levels, and electromagnetic fields from power lines and appliances can impair melatonin production, nullify attempts at relaxation, and interfere with our sleep.

Hormonal Imbalances

Hormonal imbalances in both men and women can disrupt sleep. While women undergo hormonal shifts throughout their lifetime, it is now known that men undergo a similar shift, referred to as andropause or "male menopause." In both cases, primary sex hormones, such as estrogen and progesterone in women and testosterone in men, shift and decline, resulting in a host of emotional, psychological, and physical changes. Sleep is often disrupted during these transitions. As these hormonal shifts are taking place, it is common for melatonin levels to also drop.

Structural Imbalances

Sleep can be disrupted if you have structural imbalances, particularly in the spine. Such conditions block the flow of nerve impulses, either causing pain that keeps us awake at night or impinging on the nervous system's ability to send sleep signals. The lack of regular exercise can lead to sleep disorders as well, because it causes muscular tension and allows stress to build up in the body.

How This Book Can Help You Sleep Again

Alternative medicine is about getting back to a natural balance. Only when you have addressed and resolved the imbalances in your life can you enjoy deep, restorative sleep. This book will help you understand the causes underlying your sleep problems and guide you to therapies that can get your sleep patterns and your life back on track.

Improve Diet and Eliminate Food Allergies—In Chapter 3: Improve Your

Diet, you will learn how food-related problems—including hypo-glycemia, insulin rebound, and food addictions—cause sleep disorders. We detail strategies on avoiding stimulants in your diet and eliminating food allergies. This chapter also provides recommendations for nutrient supplementation and integrating a whole-foods diet into your life.

Detoxify Your Colon and Liver—In Chapter 4: Detoxify Your Body, we detail valuable detoxification therapies for your colon and liver. You will learn the importance of detoxification diets and be introduced to organ-cleansing methods, such as enemas and colonics. We also pro-vide dietary, herbal, and supplement remedies for bacteria overgrowth (such as candidiasis, overgrowth of the *Candida albicans* fungus) and parasites, two factors that further impair the intestine's ability to elim-inate toxins, which ultimately disrupts sleep.

Reset Your Body Clock—The importance of balanced circadian rhythms will be emphasized in Chapter 5: Resetting the Body Clock. People suffering insomnia due to travel and shift work as well those experi-encing sleep phase syn-dromes will learn how to reprogram their body clocks to adjust to new sleep/wake schedules. Those suffering from seasonal affective dis-order will learn valuable

> Alternative medicine is about getting back to a natural balance. Only when you have addressed and resolved the imbalances in your life can you enjoy deep, restorative sleep.

ways to improve their mood during the winter months. Light therapy and melatonin supplementation will be described in detail. Additionally, we highlight some behavioral adjustments that can reset your body clock, including napping, relaxation techniques, and auto-genic suggestion.

Resolve Emotional Issues—In Chapter 6: Resolve Emotional Issues, we discuss how lingering psychological problems can adversely affect sleep. We explore different ways emotional issues can be resolved, including diet modification, cognitive therapy, hypnotherapy, and stress management techniques such as meditation. We also discuss how you can establish "sleep rituals" that will allow you to unwind at day's end and fall asleep easily.

Restore Harmony to Your Home—Chapter 7: Protection from a Toxic Environment describes how environmental pollution and geopathic

Assessing Your Sleep History

As part of an examination for your sleep problem, a physician will generally ask about your sleep habits. These questions are also helpful for self-assessment of your own sleep problems.

- Do you have a history of sleep problems?
- How much sleep do you get, on average, in a 24-hour period?
- When do you normally sleep? When do you consider the best time for sleeping?
- What time do you go to bed? And what time do you wake up?
- How long does it normally take for you to fall asleep?
- Is your bedroom noisy? Is it dark enough?
- Do you frequently awaken during the night and why?
- Do you feel refreshed after a night's sleep?

- Are you often sleepy or fatigued during the day?
- Do you take naps during the day, and how often?
- When did you last have a good night's sleep?
- Has anyone ever told you that you snore or stop breathing during the night?
- Have you ever been told that you walk in your sleep?
- Have you ever been told that you exhibit jerking leg or arm movements during the night?
- Have you ever fallen asleep suddenly while driving or at work?
- Do you exercise regularly?
- What types of foods do you eat and when?
- Do you smoke or drink alcohol frequently?
- Are you taking sleeping aids or other medications?

stress contribute to poor sleep, and provides suggestions on minimizing these factors. You will learn how to reduce your exposure to harmful toxins and chemicals at home, and you'll also find out how magnet therapy protects you from harmful electromagnetic fields. This chapter also introduces the principles of feng shui, an ancient Japanese tradition that aims to improve health through the appropriate placement of household items. By simply rearranging some of your furniture, you can create a peaceful and sleep-promoting sanctuary in your bedroom.

Balance Your Hormones—Melatonin isn't the only hormone that plays a role in our sleep patterns. In Chapter 8: Balancing Your Hormones, you will learn how changes in sex hormones contribute to sleep disruptions. The primary focus will be on menopause and andropause, and what women and men going through these transitional times can do to improve their sleep. You will learn how to correct hormonal imbalances through traditional Chinese medicine, diet, and lifestyle modifications, and stress reduction.

Correct Structural Imbalances—In Chapter 9: Correcting Structural Imbalances, you will learn how physical disharmonies in your body can rob you of sleep. This chapter also describes how spinal and other structural misalignments can be reversed through chiropractic, acupuncture, and reflexology. Additionally, we describe special relaxation techniques that help induce sleep. Regular exercise such as *qigong* and yoga will also be examined as a means to reduce stress and restore deep sleep.

3 Improve Your Diet

WHAT YOU EAT will definitely influence the quality of your sleep. Unhealthy eating patterns, including excess levels of stimulants such as caffeine, sugar, and alcohol, along with eating too many nutrient-depleted, processed foods, can disturb sleep. Food allergies can also cause sugar and chemical imbalances in the body that may be interrupting your sound sleep. Alternative medicine recognizes the importance of diet for healthy function and has a variety of recommendations for improving your sleep and your health. In this chapter, we look at the factors in your diet that may be contributing to irregular or disrupted sleep. We also recommend dietary and nutritional strategies that will help you get a good night's rest.

The Connection Between Diet and Sleep

Diet is a primary consideration in sleep disorders. Consumption of stimulants like caffeine and sugar, food allergies, the intake of drugs and alcohol, and poor dietary choices are all factors that can disrupt sleep.

Caffeine

Konrad Kail, N.D., notes that caffeine can have a pronounced effect on sleeping habits. "Even a few cups of coffee in the morning can interfere with the quality and quantity of sleep at night," says Dr. Kail. "Caffeine consumption has been associated with insomnia, periodic leg movements syndrome, and restless legs syndrome." If you drink coffee daily, even one or two cups, the caffeine can easily disrupt your sleep.

After you drink a cup of coffee, the caffeine enters your bloodstream quickly, resulting in an immediate burst of energy. Many coffee drinkers are familiar with some of the temporary stimulant effects of caffeine, including nervous "jitters" and irritability. This is because caffeine stimulates your central nervous system, leading to an increase in brain activity and overall energy. It also increases blood pressure, heart rate, respiration, and metabolism. More specifically, caffeine causes the adrenal glands to produce hormones, such as adrenaline, norepinephrine, and cortisol, that activate and energize the body.[1] Normally, these hormones are secreted in daily cycles, peaking in the morning and having the lowest values at night. High amounts of cortisol are linked with muscle dysfunction, thyroid dysfunction, immune system depression, and sleep disorders.

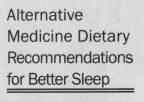

Alternative Medicine Dietary Recommendations for Better Sleep

- Eliminate Stimulants from Your Diet
- Eliminate Allergenic Foods
- Eat a Whole Foods Diet
- Supplementation for Better Sleep

Caffeine is also a diuretic, meaning that it promotes fluid loss from the body. This can lead to deficiencies in nutrients important for sound sleep, particularly the B vitamins, calcium and magnesium, zinc, and iron.[2] Some people are more sensitive to the effects of caffeine, because their bodies require more time to metabolize the caffeine (clear it from the body), a function handled primarily by the liver. Caffeine can remain in the body up to 20 hours, so even caffeine ingested early in the day can inhibit your ability to get to sleep.

Coffee is not the only source of caffeine in the diet—chocolate contains caffeine as well as other stimulants. The hot chocolate that many people drink before bedtime may actually keep them awake. Tea and soft drinks are other common sources of caffeine. In addition, many over-the-counter medications (cold and cough preparations, weight-loss drugs, pain relievers) contain caffeine or caffeine-related substances and can also increase sleep disorders.

Sugar

Much like caffeine, sugar is often consumed because it gives the body an immediate source of energy. As effective as caffeine for providing a short burst of energy, sugar's high is also short-lived. Once consumed,

Although we generally feel satisfaction or relief after eating a sugary snack, the sensation does not come directly from the glucose that enters our bloodstream, but rather from the corresponding surge in insulin. This is because, in addition to managing glucose, insulin is used by the body to transport the amino acid tryptophan, a building block of the neurotransmitter (SEE QUICK DEFINITION) serotonin, to the brain. Serotonin is sometimes referred to as the "happiness" chemical due to its influence on mood. High levels of serotonin in the brain produce feelings of self-confidence, calm, satisfaction, and composure. However, when levels start to decline, we start to feel anxious, cannot concentrate, and become depressed.

When tryptophan is scarce, serotonin is in similarly short supply. This creates an intolerable condition for the brain, which demands immediate action, hence our cravings for sugar. Sugar causes quick satisfaction by initiating the release of insulin, which delivers tryptophan to the brain and restores serotonin levels.[4] In effect, sugar works like an antidepressant. "If serotonin levels are depressed, you're depressed," says Michael Phillips, D.C., who compares sugar's action to that of the drug Prozac. "Prozac, so commonly prescribed for depression, works by elevating levels of serotonin. The emotional aspects of blood sugar imbalances are rooted in a [similar] physiological response."

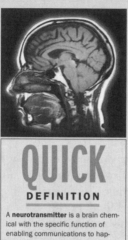

QUICK
DEFINITION

A **neurotransmitter** is a brain chemical with the specific function of enabling communications to happen between brain cells. Chief among the 100 identified to date are acetylcholine, gamma-aminobutyric acid (GABA), serotonin, dopamine, and norepinephrine. Acetylcholine is required for short-term memory and muscle contractions. GABA works to stop excess nerve signals; serotonin helps produce sleep, regulate pain, and influence mood. Norepinephrine is an excitatory neurotransmitter.

sugar creates uneven blood sugar levels that can disrupt your sleep in the middle of the night as your body metabolizes the sugar and demands more.

Sugar induces hypoglycemia during the night, according to Kenneth Rifkin, N.D., of Lake Oswego, Oregon.[3] Hypoglycemia, or low blood sugar (glucose), is a condition often associated with diabetes. Symptoms of hypoglycemia include anxiety, weakness, sweating, rapid heart rate, dizziness, headache, irritability, and poor or double vision, among others. Glucose is the primary source of fuel for the brain (although too much glucose in the blood can create health problems). Following a meal, glucose levels rise sharply, and the pancreas responds by releasing insulin, a substance that helps the cells absorb glucose from the blood. In healthy people, the release of insulin acts to keep blood sugar levels fairly constant; when the pancreas produces too much insulin, however, blood glucose levels drop suddenly, depriving the brain of needed fuel.

A diet high in simple sugars and refined carbohydrates can lead to nighttime hypoglycemia. Blood levels of glucose drop and the body releases adrenaline, cortisol, and other hormones to stimulate the brain and indicate that it is time to eat. This can awaken you or prevent you from entering a deep sleep state.

Food Allergies

We tend to think of allergies in terms of pollens, dust, and animal hair—the things that make us sneeze or give us a rash. However, the truth is that we can be allergic to many different types of substances, including foods, and suffer a wide variety of symptoms. "The majority of Americans suffer from allergies," says James Braly, M.D., of Fort Lauderdale, Florida. "This is particularly true of food allergy, which, along with undernutrition, is the most commonly undiagnosed condition in the United States today." Allergies to foods can cause a number of reactions in the body that disturb sleep.

An allergy is the immune system's abnormal reaction to a substance that is harmless to most people. The immune system usually responds to only dangerous invaders, such as bacteria or viruses, and ignores "normal" substances such as foods. People develop allergies when the immune system has become weakened or compromised and can no longer distinguish between harmful and harmless substances. In response to these otherwise normal substances, the immune system releases chemicals, such as histamines, resulting in many of the symptoms associated with allergies. Dr. Braly has identified 88 possible food allergy symptoms, including stomach pains, joint pain, insomnia, weight gain, mood swings, and apathy.

Katie Data, N.D., of Fife, Washington, first looks for intolerances or allergies to certain foods when treating patients with sleep disorders. The most common culprits in food allergies are yeast, wheat, corn, milk and other dairy products, egg whites, tomatoes, soy, shellfish, peanuts, chocolate, and food dyes and additives.

Herbert Rinkel, M.D., of the University of Oklahoma School of Medicine, is considered one of the first to bring to light the issue of food sensitivities. While still a medical student, he discovered his own intolerance to eggs and began to research the field. Dr. Rinkel found that symptoms of tension and jitteriness, common to food-sensitive individuals, are apt to manifest in restlessness and inattentiveness by day and insomnia by night. He concluded that insomnia, as well as tossing about or crying out at night, are manifestations of food intolerance. Dr. Rinkel says that fatigue is often one of the first symptoms of food intolerance and is most troublesome early in the morning upon rising. This is particularly noticeable in children with food intolerances. People suffering from food allergies are often irritable during the morning hours and may need a nap in the late afternoon. They frequently suffer from insomnia as well, according to Dr. Rinkel.[5]

Intolerance to certain foods can cause histamine (a substance produced by the body during an allergic reaction) to be released in the brain, which can disturb a person's biochemistry, and can, in some cases, lead to sleep disturbance, according to Dr. Kail. He explains that, in the brain, histamine replaces neurotransmitters, but because it does not function like other neurotransmitters, it creates a dysfunction in the biochemical pathways of the brain that are responsible for thinking, mood, and behavior. When these pathways are disrupted, the consequence is exhibited as symptoms, one of which is insomnia.

Food allergies can also disrupt blood sugar balance.[6] The body's first reaction to an allergenic food is often hypoglycemia and insulin imbalance. The physiological mechanism that regulates insulin can be thrown off balance by food allergies, as the immune system becomes stressed and overburdened by the constant response to allergenic foods. This causes too much insulin to enter the blood, precipitating hypoglycemia. The connection between sugar disorders (such as hypoglycemia) and food allergies is often ignored and so remains undiagnosed and untreated. Ralph Golan, M.D., of Seattle, Washington, author of *Optimal Wellness*, explains that allergic reactions to some foods produces symptoms identical to those of hypoglycemia.[7] As explained earlier, hypoglycemia will cause the release of cortisol and other stimulating hormones in the middle of the night, disturbing your sleep.

Drugs, Alcohol, and Nicotine

The sleeping process can be significantly disturbed by a variety of over-the-counter and prescription drugs. Drugs that may lead to insomnia include thyroid preparations, oral contraceptives, beta-blockers, and marijuana.[8] As mentioned earlier, many over-the-counter medications also contain caffeine and can increase sleep disorders through over-stimulation.

According to a recent poll, Americans who frequently use alcohol were twice as likely to wake up during the night several times a week compared to those who do not drink.[9] While alcohol may provide initial relaxation effects, the end result is interrupted, less restful sleep. Alcohol may help you fall asleep, but when its effects wear off, it disrupts the deeper sleep stages during the second half of the night, explains Sonia Ancoli-Israel, Ph.D., a sleep researcher at the University of California at San Diego.

Alcohol can reduce overall sleep time, including both REM and non-REM sleep.[10] This creates shortened, lighter, and less-restful sleep, because you will often awaken before reaching deeper, restorative sleep (stages 3 and 4) and REM sleep. If you are deprived of these stages of sleep, you will feel fatigued the following day. In one study, ten middle-aged men were given a moderate dose of alcohol six hours before scheduled bedtime. All subjects experienced reduced total sleep time, sleep efficiency, and REM sleep. In the second half of the night, they showed a two-fold increase in wakefulness.[11] Alcohol is a simple sugar and may be a factor in the development of hypoglycemia, which can disrupt sleep patterns. It can cause decreased absorption of some nutrients essential for a good night's rest, particularly the B vitamins, magnesium, and calcium.[12] Alcohol is also a diuretic, which may interrupt sleep because of the necessity of urinating several times during the night.

Smoking also inhibits sleep. Because nicotine acts as a stimulant, many smokers have insomnia and other sleep problems.[13] In a poll conducted by the National Sleep Foundation, 46% of smokers reported experiencing insomnia a few nights a week as compared to 35% of nonsmokers.[14] Nicotine is rapidly absorbed by the mucous membranes in the mouth and quickly reaches the brain. Nicotine stimulates the release of adrenaline and norepinephrine, hormones that activate the body, increase heart rate, and elevate blood pressure.[15]

Poor Diet

If you eat the typical American diet, it could be making your sleeping problems worse. Highly processed foods, containing large quantities of refined carbohydrates and simple sugars, are empty of nutritional value and overstimulate the body. There are also a number of vitamin and mineral deficiencies that affect your sleep. Deficiencies may result from poor dietary choices, digestive dysfunction, or food allergies.

■ L-tryptophan, an amino acid found in meats, cashews, and dairy products, is a precursor to melatonin, the hormone needed for sleep. Supplementing with L-tryptophan can ameliorate the symptoms of insomnia and other sleep disorders.[16]

■ The B vitamins (particularly B6) are also important for sleep as they regulate the body's use of L-tryptophan. In the absence of adequate vitamin B6 in your diet, your body cannot convert L-tryptophan into melatonin. Deficiencies in folic acid (folacin or folate; members of the B vitamin family) have been linked to insomnia and restless legs syndrome.[17]

■ Vitamin E deficiency may be a factor in restless legs syndrome.[18]

■ People suffering from insomnia may be deficient in the mineral zinc, particularly in infants with frequent nighttime waking and crying.

■ Deficiencies in copper and iron have been linked to greater difficulties in getting to sleep and decreased quality of sleep. Studies indicate that low levels of iron correlated with an increased incidence of restless legs syndrome.[19]

■ Calcium also acts as a natural sedative in the body, producing a calming effect on the central nervous system, and deficiencies have been linked to sleep problems. Sufficient amounts of magnesium (also a natural sedative) are necessary for the absorption of calcium.

In addition, many alternative practitioners recommend staying away from spicy and salty foods if you suffer from sleep disorders. These foods can cause indigestion or heartburn, which may interfere with sleep. Monosodium glutamate (MSG) and other artificial additives may disturb sleep; people who are sensitive to MSG can suffer insomnia from the stimulant effects of this food additive.

Detecting a Nutritional Deficiency

Since nutrient deficiencies may be a factor in sleep disorders, one of the first steps is to determine which nutrients may be lacking in your diet, then to design an individualized supplement program. Consult a qualified health professional trained in the intricacies of nutritional biochemistry, who can help you assess your needs and develop an effective, individualized dietary and nutritional supplement program. The following tests can be used to analyze your nutrient status, pinpoint specific deficiencies, and serve as the basis for recommending supplement dosages that best suit your needs.

For referrals to **physicians trained in nutritional and preventative medicine**, contact: American College of Advancement in Medicine (ACAM), P.O. Box 3427, Laguna Hills, CA 92654; tel: 714-583-7666.

Many mainstream physicians assess nutritional status using blood tests. These tests measure nutrient concentrations only in the blood serum—the liquid fraction of blood, and not in the blood cells (the globular or non-liquid fraction of blood). The cells are generally separated out and discarded. Unfortunately, a good deal of information about an individual's nutritional status is thrown out along with these cells.

"It's important to understand that ordinary tests on blood serum levels don't provide the correct data," says John Dommisse, M.D., a nutritional medicine specialist based in Tucson, Arizona. "What must be measured are whole blood levels." Whole blood analysis, which examines both the serum and the blood cells, is not commonly done since most mainstream physicians are looking at blood primarily to diagnose a disease, and serum testing is generally adequate for that purpose. As most mainstream physicians are oriented towards using drugs to treat symptoms, they have no interest in nutritional status and are thus not inclined to order the proper tests.

In addition to whole-blood analysis, a variety of other test procedures can help assess nutrient status. These include hair analysis, the Individualized Optimum Nutrition Panel, and the Functional Intracellular Analysis. Each of these is discussed briefly below.

Hair Analysis—Hair analysis, when correctly done, measures the body's levels of various minerals, including calcium, iron, magnesium, potassium, and zinc, among others. As the hair is considered a storage organ, it provides a biochemical record of nutritional status over a period of several months. This is why many health-care practitioners consider hair analysis to provide a better picture of underlying mineral imbalances than most blood or urine tests. Hair analysis does not assess vitamin deficiency, however, so other testing procedures are needed to supplement the findings of a hair analysis.

Individualized Optimal Nutrition (ION) Panel—The ION Panel, from MetaMetrix Medical Laboratories in Norcross, Georgia, uses a blood and a urine sample to measure 150 biochemical components. Specifically, ION checks for nutritional status in categories including vitamins, minerals, amino acids, fatty and organic acids, lipid peroxides, general blood chemistries (cholesterol, thyroid hormone, glucose), and antioxidants. Each patient's nutritional level is then compared with what is considered the healthy norm. In addition, ION can provide supplement recommendations based on the individual's test results.

Functional Intracellular Analysis—Another accurate and comprehensive technique is the Functional Intracellular Analysis (FIA) available through Spectracell Laboratories in Houston, Texas. This nutritional assay must be ordered by

For more about **hair analysis**, contact: Omegatech, 24700 Center Ridge Road, Cleveland, OH 44145; tel: 800-437-1404 or 440-835-2150; fax: 440-835-2177. For the **Functional Intracellular Analysis**, contact: Spectracell Laboratories, 515 Post Oak Blvd. Suite 830, Houston, TX 77027-9409; tel: 800-227-5227. For the **ION Panel**, contact: MetaMetrix Medical Laboratory, 5000 Peachtree Industrial Blvd., Suite 110, Norcross, GA 30071; tel: 770-446-5483 or 800-221-4640; fax: 770-441-2237.

a health-care professional, but the lab maintains a database of nutritionally oriented practitioners and will refer individuals to professionals in their area. Information is also available to consumers that they can use to educate and inform their own physicians.

Diagnosing a Food Allergy

"Accurate diagnosis of food allergies has always been the bane of allergy treatment," says Dr. Braly. The problem with diagnosing a food allergy is that reactions are often varied, inconsistent, and may take several days to develop after eating an allergy-causing food. How much or how often you eat an allergenic food or how it is cooked may be factors in whether or not you have a reaction. Or the allergy may be caused by an additive or ingredient rather than the food itself.[20] In addition, more than one food is frequently involved in causing the reaction and symptoms are often "masked" by regular consumption of the foods.

Despite the complexity surrounding the detection and diagnosis of a food allergy, mainstream medical practitioners generally take a highly simplified approach to the problem. Most rely on a procedure called the scratch or prick-puncture test, a procedure that is only about 20% accurate in detecting food allergies.[21] In truth, this test is only useful for identifying allergens that cause immediate reactions, such as those caused by pollen or dust, and is not effective in pinpointing food reactions. Another common test procedure is the RAST (Radio Allergo Sorbent Test). This blood test is useful for diagnosing allergies to pollens, dust, molds, bee venom, and other allergens. Again, this test is not very accurate in testing food allergies and can be very expensive. Most alternative medicine practitioners rarely use these tests. Instead, they recommend self-testing and laboratory procedures, such as the elimination diet, pulse test, and ELISA test, designed specifically to assess food allergies.

Do You Suffer From Food Allergies?

The following questionnaire, developed by naturopath Leon Chaitow, N.D., D.O., of London, England, can help you determine if you have a food allergy. If your answer is "no" or "never" to any question, give yourself a score of zero for that particular question; the other scores are provided with each question.

■ Do you suffer from unnatural fatigue? (Score 1 if occasionally, 2 if regularly—three times a week or more.)

■ Do you sometimes experience weight fluctuations of four or more pounds in a single day, accompanied by puffiness of the face, ankles, or fingers? (Score 1 if infrequently, 2 if frequently—more than once a month.)

■ Do you have hot flashes (apart from menopause) or find yourself sweating for no obvious reason? (Score 1 if infrequently, 2 if several times a week or more.)

■ Does your pulse race or your heart pound strongly for no obvious reason? (Score 1 if infrequently, 2 if several times a week or more.)

■ Do you have a history of food intolerance, causing any symptoms at all? (Score 2 if your answer is yes.)

■ Do you crave bread, sugary foods, milk, chocolate, coffee, or tea? (Score 2 if your answer is yes.)

■ Do you suffer from migraine or severe headaches, irritable bowel syndrome, eczema, depression, asthma, or muscle aches? (Score 2 if your answer is yes.)

The most anyone could score on this test would be 14, explains Dr. Chaitow. "If your score is five or higher, there is a strong likelihood that allergies are part of your symptom picture."

The Elimination Diet

Despite the name, this is not really a diet in the conventional sense, but a test procedure to help you identify your allergy foods. It involves three steps: 1) eliminating the potential allergenic foods from your diet for ten to 14 days; 2) carefully observing any changes in your symptoms; and 3) testing the eliminated foods by bringing them back into your diet, one by one, and noting any return of symptoms.

The foods you choose to eliminate should be from those that you eat every day or nearly every day, ones that you crave, or foods that make you feel weak. It is important to eliminate all of the suspected foods on your list, as multiple allergies are quite common and, if all are not eliminated, it could skew your testing results. Also, read the ingredients on any packaged foods very carefully to ensure you do not inadvertently consume whatever it is you are trying to eliminate (sugar, for example, or perhaps a flavor enhancer such as monosodium glutamate). Remember that delayed food allergies can take as long as 72 hours to exhibit symptoms. If you experience symptoms such as irritability, fatigue, headaches, and intense cravings during the elimination period, you may be going through withdrawal, which is a sure sign that you have been suffering from an allergy.

Keep in mind that no one food allergy test is a panacea—each method has its strengths and weaknesses and the key is to find one that works for you. Regardless of which test you use, it is best to consult a nutritional counselor or other health-care practitioner to help guide you through the process.

How to Take the Pulse Test

The pulse test is easy to self-administer and involves simply recording your pulse rate before and after meals. Stephen Langer, M.D., observes that "certain of my patients who use the pulse test have seen their heartbeat rise from 72 to as high as 180 after they have eaten an allergenic food."[23] To take the test, follow these simple instructions:

■ Find the pulse point on your wrist by placing the second finger of the opposite hand on the inside of your wrist.

■ Count the beats (pulses) for six seconds and multiply the number by ten; this is your resting pulse.

■ Record your resting pulse first thing in the morning before getting out of bed.

■ Record your pulse 30 minutes before each meal, then 30 minutes and 60 minutes after each meal.

If the difference between the morning pulse and either of the two after-meal rates is more than 12 to 16 beats, chances are you have a food allergy. Once you have identified a meal that triggers a rise in your pulse rate, you can begin testing individual foods eaten during that meal. However, in some cases, you may find that your resting pulse is higher than your after-meal pulse or that your before-meal pulse is higher than your after-meal pulse. If you observe such a pattern, it is possible that dust or some other airborne allergen is interfering with your test.[24]

The Pulse Test

This is a relatively simple test developed by Arthur Coca, M.D., a pioneer in the field of environmental medicine. Dr. Coca based his test on many years of clinical observations of patients, during which he noticed that a common symptom of many food allergies is increased heart rate. Although the pulse test can help identify food allergies, you should not conclude you are allergy-free if the foods you test do not affect your pulse rate. The problem is that not all food allergens will increase heart rate. "The weakness of this particular approach lies in the frank possibility that not every allergic reaction will necessarily produce the biochemical responses that result in a faster heartbeat," says Dr. Golan.[22] If you have no success in identifying a food allergen using the pulse test, but still suspect that you are suffering from such an allergy, you should try one of the other tests.

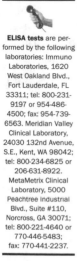

ELISA tests are performed by the following laboratories: Immuno Laboratories, 1620 West Oakland Blvd., Fort Lauderdale, FL 33311; tel: 800-231-9197 or 954-486-4500; fax: 954-739-6563. Meridian Valley Clinical Laboratory, 24030 132nd Avenue, S.E., Kent, WA 98042; tel: 800-234-6825 or 206-631-8922. MetaMetrix Clinical Laboratory, 5000 Peachtree Industrial Blvd., Suite #110, Norcross, GA 30071; tel: 800-221-4640 or 770-446-5483; fax: 770-441-2237.

The ELISA Test

The ELISA test (or enzyme-linked immunoserological assay activated-cell test) is a blood test considered by many alternative medicine practitioners to be among the most sensitive and useful in detecting food allergies. Unlike other allergy blood tests, it is able to pinpoint delayed allergic reactions. It also tests for a wide variety of substances, subjecting a patient's blood sample to 102 different food extracts. Blood samples can be sent by mail to any one of several specialized laboratories that perform this test. You can have your doctor arrange to submit a sample of your blood to the lab.

Success Story: Correcting Poor Diet Results in Better Sleep

Insomnia can arise from a combination of poor diet and work stress. Darren, 28, complained of tiredness and depression. The fatigue, he said, was due to the fact that he had been getting only 3 to 5 hours of sleep per night for the last five months. At that time, his hours at work (Darren was a chemical technician) had shifted from a standard daytime schedule to the swing shift from 4 p.m. to 12:30 p.m. His body had still not made the adjustment to the later schedule. As a result, he stayed up late and then would wake a number of times during the night.

Darren's diet was high in sugars and fatty foods, such as cheese and peanut butter. He frequently felt bloated and gassy and estimated he was 30 pounds overweight. In addition to the insomnia, lethargy, and depression, he had suffered with hay fever since the age of 17, and chronic neck pain from sitting and looking down into a microscope at work.

According to traditional Chinese medicine (TCM—SEE QUICK DEFINITION) diagnosis, Darren's tongue was flabby and wet and slightly pale with a red tip; he also had scalloped "teeth marks" on the sides of his tongue and his pulses were "slippery." All of these signs indicated Darren's spleen and stomach were deficient in energy, meaning he was not producing enough blood or digestive power. The deficiency was allowing a condition of "dampness" to build up in his body, causing the energy to stagnate in the Liver meridian (SEE QUICK DEFINITION), which was creating heat. This dampness and heat, according to TCM, was the cause of his mental restlessness and insomnia.

Darren was given an acupuncture treatment with emphasis on points along his back to strengthen the spleen, stomach, and liver functions, as well as points on the back of his neck to ease the muscle tension. On his front side, points along the Spleen, Stomach, and

For **Melakava** (available to health-care practitioners), contact: Institute for Traditional Medicine, 2017 SE Hawthorne, Portland, OR 97214; tel: 800-544-7504.

Pericardium meridians, as well as a combination of liver and large intestine points were used to release stress and mental tension. He relaxed completely during the treatment, even dozing at times. He was also given an herbal formula called Melakava, which contains melatonin, the sleep-inducing hormone that regulates the body's sleep-wake cycle, along with the Chinese herbs zizyphus and kava-kava, which have sedative and antidepressant properties.

The night of the first acupuncture treatment, Darren took two tablets of Melakava 30 minutes before bedtime. He was able to fall asleep quickly and slept through the night. He reported at the next treatment that he was averaging six hours of sleep per night and awakening refreshed for the first time in months. Darren also made significant changes to his diet, reducing his intake of dairy products, fatty foods, and sugars. He eventually eliminated cheeses completely from his diet. By the third treatment, Darren was getting an average of eight hours of sleep per night. He was less depressed and was getting enough sleep to help him cope with stresses at work. Darren was also less bothered by bloating and gas and, encouraged by his improved sleep, continued to make positive lifestyle changes by getting more exercise and eating better.

Alternative Medicine Dietary Recommendations for Better Sleep

Making better food choices can have a major influence on the quality of your sleep. By eliminating stimulants, switching to a whole foods diet, treating food allergies, and getting proper nutrient supplementation, you can help alleviate your sleep disturbances and improve your overall health as well.

Eliminate Stimulants From Your Diet

Begin by examining your diet and eliminating any foods that contain stimulating ingredients such as caffeine, sugar, or spices that can ruin your sleep. You might keep a food diary for about a week and write down everything you eat and drink, making note of the times you eat and the quality of your sleep that night. According to Peter Hauri, Ph.D., Director of the Mayo Clinic's Insomnia Program and author of *No More Sleepless Nights*, insomniacs can immediately improve their chances of getting better sleep by reducing caffeine, limiting alcohol, and eliminating smoking. "No matter what other factors might be causing your poor sleep, you can do these three things immediately and have an excellent chance of improving your sleep," says Dr. Hauri.

Caffeine—Dr. Hauri advises against consuming more than 300 mg of caffeine a day—the amount in three cups of coffee.[25] Caffeine is found in many hidden forms in commercial and processed foods; read labels to avoid ingesting additional caffeine. Some medications also contain caffeine. We have found that if someone is particularly sensitive to caffeine, even drinking a cup of coffee or tea at breakfast can affect sleep that night. Remember that the metabolic clearance of caffeine is extremely variable from person to person.

For **Caffeine Mix** (available to licensed healthcare practitioners), contact: Professional Health Products, P.O. Box 80085, 5112 S.W. Garden Home Road, Portland, OR 97280; tel: 503-245-2720 or 800-952-2219, fax: 503-452-1239.

For people who have caffeine addiction problems, we recommend an allersode, a homeopathic form of an antigen (a substance that stimulates your body to make antibodies as part of the allergic response). The allersode contains diluted forms of the allergy-producing substances along with factors that promote a resistance to their effects. Caffeine Mix is an allergy desensitization remedy containing homeopathically prepared substances from chocolate, tea, caffeine, cola, coffee, and histamine, plus components that work with the adrenal glands and liver. It will help reduce a person's sensitivity to foods containing methylxanthines, such as caffeine, which can be allergenic.

Sugar—Although pure sugar will cause the greatest insulin response in our bodies, many other foods have a similar insulinogenic (insulin stimulating) effect. To evaluate foods based on their insulin impact, a scientific rating system called the glycemic index was developed by diabetes researchers at the University of Toronto. The index offers a comparison of the insulin effect of different foods, measuring their real-life effect on blood sugar levels. Those foods with a high rating on the glycemic index cause a higher insulin response than those with a low rating. "The glycemic index ranks foods according to how fast

A Quick Guide to Dietary Changes

Leon Chaitow, N.D., D.O., of London, England, and other alternative practitioners recommend a combination of nutritional adjustments to aid sleep, including:

■ A marked reduction in alcohol consumption.

■ Avoiding caffeine in all forms (tea, coffee, cola, chocolate).

■ Taking a protein-rich snack at bedtime (yogurt is one example).

■ Eat more raw vegetables and salad greens.

■ Eat whole grains and high fiber foods and avoid simple carbohydrates such as cereals, pastries, and white flour. Whole grains contain many B vitamins, which act as natural sedatives for calming irritability and tension that may hinder deep sleep.

■ Eat more protein in the form of moderate amounts of meat, nuts, beans, and avocados. Protein is digested more slowly and doesn't cause an insulin spike, which may interfere with sleep.

■ Eat a wide variety of foods to ensure that you are getting sufficient nutrition.

■ Be aware of the fat content of foods. More important than the total fat is the kind of fat you are eating. Incorporate "healthy fats" such as olive oil and fish oils, containing omega-3 and omega-6 oils, to be certain your metabolism is running smoothly.

■ Taking one gram of niacinamide (vitamin B3) at bedtime (for those that sleep easily but awakes and cannot get back to sleep).

■ Taking 0.5 g of chlorella or other green or blue algae product at bedtime (as a source of tryptophan).

Dr. Chaitow points out that it is beneficial to follow consistent sleep ritual patterns (bath, shower, reading), and stress reduction tactics (relaxation, deep breathing).

---

they are absorbed into the blood as sugar," says Ann Louise Gittleman, M.S., C.N.S., author of *Get the Sugar Out*. "A diet based on high glycemic index foods (those absorbed most quickly) usually leads to a condition of chronic low blood sugar because you have rapid rises followed by sharp dips in blood sugar levels."[26]

Richard Podell, M.D., of Springfield, New Jersey, indicates that choosing foods with a low glycemic index is "the secret to keeping blood sugar stable and insulin low." Dr. Podell makes the following general observations:

■ Foods with a higher rating, causing a higher insulin response, include white bread, bagels, English muffins, packaged flaked cereals, instant hot cereals, low-fat frozen desserts, raisins and other dried fruits, whole milk and whole-milk cheeses, peanuts and peanut butter, hot dogs, and luncheon meats.

■ Foods with a low rating, not causing a high insulin spike, include most fresh vegetables, leafy greens, pitted fruits and melons, coarse

100% whole-grain breads and minimally processed whole-grain cereals, sweet potatoes and yams, skim milk, buttermilk, poultry, lean cuts of beef, pork, veal, shellfish, white-fleshed fish, most legumes, and most nuts.

■ Cooked foods rank higher on the index than raw foods. Similarly, fruits and vegetables that have been juiced or puréed are higher on the index than when eaten whole.[27]

Finding out whether a food product contains sugar requires more sleuthing today than it once did. Only a few manufacturers currently include the word sugar in the list of ingredients of their sugar-containing products. Instead, wanting to avoid the sugar stigma that could negatively impact sales, many food producers hide the sugars in their products behind a host of chemical synonyms. Take note that product listing any of the following ingredients really does contain sugar: corn sweetener, dextrose, dextrin, fructose, glucose, high-fructose corn syrup, fruit juice concentrates, sucrose, sorbitol, sorghum, lactose, malt, maltodextrin, maltose, mannitol, modified cornstarch, and xylitol. Although all of these are sugars, fructose does stand apart from the rest. Of all the sugars, fructose has the least severe insulin reaction.[28]

Drugs and Alcohol—Avoiding drugs and alcohol is especially important for sleep apnea. One should avoid alcohol and sleeping pills, because they slow down the respiratory drive needed during sleep and cause further relaxation of the throat muscles, which makes obstructive sleep apnea more likely to occur. Sleep laboratory tests reveal that eliminating alcohol dramatically reduces the number of sleep apnea episodes, increases the oxygen saturation levels of the blood, and leads to deeper, more restful sleep.

Eliminate Allergenic Foods

It is essential to rule out food intolerances as a cause of sleep problems. In one study of infants, sleeplessness was eliminated by removing cow's milk from the diet and then reproduced by its reintroduction.[29] Once you have identified the foods you are allergic to, the next step is to eliminate them from your diet. Initially, you should completely refrain from eating all allergenic foods for 60 to 90 days. After this period, you can begin to slowly reintroduce them into your diet. You should also vary the foods that you eat on a daily basis to avoid developing new allergies. You are likely to find that as you reintroduce the foods to which you were once sensitive, your old symptoms will not reappear. This is because most food allergies are temporary and can be cured

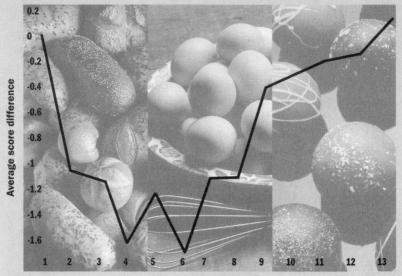

HOW TO STOP YOUR FOOD ALLERGIES FAST—The graph shows the rapid decline in reactions to suspected allergenic foods when patients completely avoided them for about two months, in a study sponsored by Immuno Laboratories. Maximum freedom from food allergy-related symptoms was achieved between the third and sixth weeks. Among foods most commonly identified as allergenic are wheat, eggs, and chocolate (pictured above), as well as milk and corn.

through abstinence. Dr. Braly estimates that only about 5% of delayed food allergies are permanent.

Remember that eliminating an allergenic food can cause withdrawal reactions. "The majority of people who give up foods they're allergic to go through a mild to moderate withdrawal phase, lasting one to five days, while the body detoxifies itself," says Dr. Braly. Allergic symptoms may get worse during this period and cravings can be intense. If the allergy foods were also your comfort foods, you may experience emotional feelings of loss and distress. Dr. Braly explains that "once the withdrawal phase has passed, the cravings also abate, and the allergy sufferer is free of dependence on that food, free of both the physiological and psychological desire to consume it so frequently, and in such great quantities."[30]

Eat a Whole Foods Diet
Diet can make a major difference for the person with a sleep disorder.

The following steps can help ensure that your diet is not working against you and your ability to sleep. Consider streamlining your diet so that it can support your body as it heals. A whole foods diet, based on whole grains, organic vegetables, skim dairy products, and free-range fish, meats, and poultry, will provide you with the variety and necessary vitamins and minerals to reestablish regular, restorative sleep.

Both alternative and conventional medicine agree that Americans should consume far less fat, animal protein, and processed foods, and eat more complex carbohydrates, especially whole grains rich in fiber, and at least five servings daily of fruits and vegetables. Buck Levin, Ph.D., R.D., Assistant Professor of Nutrition at Bastyr University in Seattle, Washington, offers a simple prescription for a healthy diet—one of natural, whole foods. "By whole foods we mean consuming a diet that is high in foods as whole as possible, with the least amount of processed, adulterated, fried, or sweetened additives," says Dr. Levin.

A whole foods, whole grain, high–complex carbohydrate, low-fat, high-fiber diet is recommended by Timothy Birdsall, N.D., of Sandpoint, Idaho. He suggests a maximum of 25% of the daily food intake be in the form of fat. In general, this amounts to 45-50 grams per day, which represents about 450 calories. He believes lowering dietary fat and increasing exercise are the two key factors to weight loss. A whole foods diet is generously filled with a wide variety of different colored vegetables, fruits, and grains; raw seeds and nuts and their butters; beans; and fermented milk products such as yogurt and kefir; and fish, poultry, and bean products like tofu. It should also be lower in animal meats, fats, and cheeses as opposed to low-fat milk products. Eating well-balanced meals at regular times during the day (four to five hours apart) will also help stabilize your blood sugar.

Dr. Rifkin advises patients to add more protein to their diets. For example, people can eat a protein snack such as turkey at night before bed. The protein helps keep the person's blood sugar level stable during the night, and turkey also contains L-tryptophan, an amino acid that has sleep-inducing properties. In addition to the bedtime snack, Dr. Rifkin will have the patient eat five small protein meals a day plus two snacks, in order to stabilize the blood sugar.

Roger Fritz, Ph.D., author of *Sleep Disorders: America's Hidden Nightmare*, says there are other ways to alter the diet to include more L-tryptophan. Since L-tryptophan must be taken without the other amino acids in order to cross the blood-brain barrier, an evening meal of carbohydrates such as potatoes, pasta, corn, and bread can be help-

Avoid These Foods	Use These Foods Instead
Refined sugars: white sugar (sucrose), fructose, corn syrup, sorbitol, mannitol. Synthetic sugars: NutraSweet™ and saccharin.	Natural sweeteners: fruit juice, raw honey, organic maple syrup, molasses, barley malt, sucanat (organic sugar cane). Avoid if diabetic or sugar intolerant.
Refined flours: white, unbleached, bleached, enriched flour and products containing these flours.	Organic whole grains: best are heirloom (genetically unaltered) grains such as kamut, quinoa, amaranth, and spelt. Grain-intolerant people may do well on heirlooms.
Synthetic fats: margarine, hydrogenated or partially hydrogenated oils, vegetable shortening, Mocha Mix™, Olestra™.	Unsaturated oils (olive, flaxseed, safflower); butter, preferably raw and organic.
High levels of saturated fats (from meats, butter, palm and coconut oils).	Use unsaturated oils such as cold-pressed grapeseed, olive, corn, canola, and safflower oils. Oils must be fresh and cold-pressed; rancid oils can be harmful.
Homogenized, pasteurized, nonfat or acidophilus milk, and processed cheese.	Raw, whole milk (contains vitamin A), cultured milk products (kefir, yogurt, buttermilk), and goat's milk; unprocessed cheese. Use in moderation if you are lactose intolerant.
Nuts and seeds: commercial, oiled, sugared, and salted. Beware of aflatoxin mold on peanuts.	Preferably organic nuts and seeds. Must be soaked (6 hrs) or blanched or roasted to destroy enzyme inhibitors.
All commercial red meat and poultry.	Lamb or organic beef, organic free-range poultry. Fish is fine if it is not from polluted waters.
Commercial eggs or egg substitutes.	Organic eggs (no chemicals, drugs, or hormones) from free-range chickens or ducks.

Avoid These Foods	Use These Foods Instead
Canned, pre-cooked, microwaved, or processed fast foods, and junk foods.	Buy fresh, organic foods first, fresh nonorganic second, frozen third, and canned if that is the only food available.
Drinks: commercial, sugared fruit juices, juice drinks, and soft drinks (both diet and regular).	Raw juices: juice your own or buy 100% juice, preferably raw and organic. Natural spritzers containing only fruit and carbonated water.
Canned coffee and commercial decaffeinated coffee.	Grind your own beans, preferably organic. Use only Swiss water-processed decaffeinated beans. Don't exceed three cups daily. Try organic black or herbal teas.

ful, as can a glass of milk before bed (milk contains L-tryptophan). People can eat high protein meals during the day to stay alert and avoid the drowsiness from carbohydrate-heavy meals. However, Dr. Fritz advises against eating sugar before bed, because it will have the opposite effect: a boost of energy and then a "sugar dip" in energy during the night (which can alarm the adrenals to produce more cortisol and wake you up).[31]

Katharine Albert, Ph.D., M.D., director of the sleep laboratory at New York Hospital-Cornell Medical Center, says nutritional deficiencies and digestive problems can aggravate insomnia, but they can be eased by watching your diet. She advises against dairy and other fatty foods before bedtime—including the L-tryptophan-containing glass of warm milk—because they can be difficult to digest. Instead, she recommends eating other, non-dairy sources of calcium throughout the day. Those include cauliflower, broccoli, and soybeans. If you still want a glass of milk, make it organic, skim milk, which is not as hard on the digestion, Dr. Albert says. She also advises people to eat foods rich in B-vitamins, including fish, whole grains, nuts, bananas, and sunflower seeds. Drink eight glasses of water throughout the day to flush toxins from the body and thus ease the work of the liver and digestive system at night.

Another dietary rule of thumb is to avoid substances that contain tyramine, a breakdown product of the amino acid tyrosine. Tyramine increases the release of the stress hormone norepinephrine. Tyramine-containing foods include caffeine, alcohol, sugar, tobacco, cheese, chocolate, sauerkraut, wine, bacon, ham, sausage, eggplant, potatoes, spinach, and tomatoes.[32]

Benefits of a Whole Foods Diet—A whole foods diet promotes health by decreasing fat and sugar intake and increasing fiber and nutrient intake. Ideally, it means more satisfaction and less overeating.

More Fiber: Most animal products, like meat, cheese, milk, eggs, and butter contain no fiber, compared to brown rice, broccoli, oatmeal, or almonds, which have 6-15 g per serving. Low fiber intake has been associated with weight gain, due to fiber's effect on insulin levels and its ability to promote satiety.[33] Fiber is also the transport system of the digestive tract, moving food wastes out of the body before they have a chance to form potentially cancer-causing and mutagenic chemicals. These toxic chemicals can cause colon cancer or pass through the gastrointestinal membrane into the bloodstream and damage other cells.

Less Fat: On a percentage-of-calories basis, most vegetables contain less than 10% fat and most grains contain from 16%-20% fat. By comparison, whole milk and cheese contain 74% fat. A rib roast is 75% fat, and eggs are 64% fat. Low-fat milk or a skinned, baked chicken breast still has 38% fat. Not only do animal foods have more fat, but most of these fats are saturated fats. In addition, a lower fat, whole foods diet means fewer calories, since an ounce of fat contains twice as many calories as an ounce of complex carbohydrates. Studies have shown that a diet containing fewer calories can increase health and extend life.[34]

Decreased Sugar Consumption: Eating a diet high in natural complex carbohydrates tends to be more filling and decreases the desire to consume processed sugars. Lower sugar consumption also decreases overall food intake. As with fat, sugar is a hidden and unwelcome ingredient in many processed foods. "When you eat sugar, your body uses up whatever vitamins and minerals it has to burn these foods off," says Linda Lizotte, R.D., C.D.N., a registered dietitian from Trumbull, Connecticut.[35]

More Nutrients: Plant foods are richer sources of nutrients than their animal counterparts. Compare wheat germ to round steak: ounce for ounce, wheat germ contains twice the vitamin B2, vitamin K, potassium, iron, and copper; three times the vitamin B6, molybdenum, and selenium; 15 times as much magnesium; and over 20 times the vitamin B1, folate, and inositol. The steak only has three nutrients in greater amounts—B12, chromium, and zinc.

Increased Variation: A greater variety of vegetables also exposes the consumer to, literally, more colorful foods—red beets, chard, yellow squash, red peppers, cabbage. "This is more important than you may have imagined," says nutritionist Lindsey Berkson, M.A., D.C. "Variations in color are due to various minerals, vitamins, and other nutrients that perform important health-promoting functions in the human body." The color variations in vegetables are due to carotenes, naturally occurring pigments that are converted into vitamin A in the body. Carotenes act as antioxidants and may be helpful for cancer prevention.

More Food Satisfaction and Less Over-Eating: Foods such as vegetables, whole grains, and beans that are dense in nutrients and fiber require more eating (chewing) time and result in consumption of fewer calories. Eating whole foods makes a person satisfied more quickly which means he or she eats less. Eating less is associated with longevity and optimal health.[36]

Timing Your Meals—Dr. Hauri also recommends that you avoid eating a heavy dinner as your body will be working overtime to digest it and this may further disrupt your sleep. He recommends a "triangle" plan—a large breakfast to start the day, a lighter lunch, and an even lighter meal for dinner—to ensure that you are not trying to digest a large meal right before you go to bed. Snacking is not discouraged, but eat proteins that are easy to digest. This will keep your blood sugar levels even and not create the energy dips that leave you reaching for sugar.

Supplementation for Better Sleep

Aside from making certain that you are consuming a balanced whole foods diet, you may want to consider supplementation with vitamins, minerals, and herbs that have been shown to help improve and restore your sleep. The following information highlights specific nutritional supplements known to aid sleep:

Vitamins

■ Vitamin B Complex—The B vitamins (collectively known as B complex) nutritionally support the brain, eyes, intestines, liver, muscles, and skin. They act as a team to help maintain healthy energy metabolism and are important for sleep. The B vitamins are known to have a sedative effect on the nerves and regulate the body's use of L-tryptophan. Stress levels, diet, and lifestyle can cause the body to use B vitamins relatively quickly.

Vitamin B1 (thiamin) and vitamin B2 (riboflavin) primarily serve in the maintenance of mucous membranes, formation of red blood cells, and metabolism of carbohydrates. Deficiencies of vitamin B1 may lead to blood sugar imbalances. Food sources: brewer's yeast is an excellent source of both of these vitamins. Supplements: B1 and B2 are commonly found in B-complex supplements.

Vitamin B3 (niacin) is necessary for oxygen transport in the blood, and fatty acid and nucleic acid formation. Niacinamide, or niacin, has been shown to prolong REM sleep and to be helpful to people with sleep maintenance insomnia, who wake up in the middle of the night and can't fall back to sleep. Low levels of B3 can cause muscle weakness, fatigue, irritability, and depression. Eating a diet high in refined sugar as well as prolonged use of antibiotics will deplete B3 reserves in the body. Food sources: meat, chicken, fish, peanuts, wheat germ, brewer's yeast and whole grains, particularly rice. Supplements: niacin is the natural form of vitamin B3 available in supplement form. When taken in dosages of over 100 milligrams, niacin can cause a very distinctive flushing, tingling, and redness that begins in the lower part of the body and moves up to the face, hands and head.[37] Niacinamide causes no flushing and is the form found in many modern supplements.[38] Typical therapeutic dose: 50-100 mg per day. Precautions: Liver enzymes may be affected when utilizing high levels of B3 or niacinamide. Use of inositol hexoniacinate has shown no toxicity and may be the best choice for this supplement.

Vitamin B5 (pantothenic acid) is vital for synthesis of hormones and support of the adrenal glands. Pantothenic acid deficiency can cause fatigue, insomnia, and depression.[39] Food sources: liver, meat, chicken, whole grains, and legumes. Eating a variety of foods can ensure adequate levels of vitamin B5. Typical therapeutic dose: 10 mg to 2,000 mg.

Vitamin B6 (pyroxidine) strongly influences the immune and nervous systems. Vitamin B6 is needed by the body for the conversion of the amino acid tryptophan to the neurotransmitter serotonin, which helps to control sleep. Deficiencies occur as a result of eating a diet high in fats and low in fruits and vegetables. Food sources: brewer's yeast, whole grains, legumes, nuts, and seeds. Supplements: there are two forms of B6, pyridoxine hydrochloride and pyridoxal-5-phosphate (the most active form). For efficient absorption of pyridoxal by the body, sufficient levels of riboflavin and magnesium should be present.[40] Typical recommended dose: 50-100 mg daily can help to prevent insomnia. Precautions: High levels of pyridoxine can cause toxic side effects.[41]

Vitamin B12 (cobalamin) is virtually absent in vegetable food sources, which means vegetarians are likely to be deficient in this vitamin. B12 is essential for normal formation of red blood cells and the maintenance of the nervous system. Food sources: meats, most fish (especially trout, mackerel, and herring), egg yolks, and yogurt. Supplements: B12 can be given in injectable form or as an oral supplement. Typical recommended dosage: 25 mg daily.

Folic acid (folacin, folate; members of the B vitamin family) is important for red blood cell formation, breakdown and utilization of proteins, and proper cell division. It is also useful for anemia, atherosclerosis, fatigue, immune weakness, infection, and osteoporosis. Food sources: green leafy vegetables such as spinach and kale, asparagus, broccoli, lima beans, green peas, sweet potatoes, bean sprouts, whole wheat, cantaloupe, strawberries, and brewer's yeast. Supplements: the folic acid content in foods can be depleted by cooking, so supplementation may be necessary. Typical recommended dose: 400 mcg daily.

■ Vitamin E (alpha tocopherol)—Vitamin E has been shown effective in treating restless legs syndrome, which may be caused by decreased circulation to the legs. In one study concerning vitamin E and restless legs syndrome, a 78-year-old female with a history of restless and "jumpy" legs found that after two months of 300 IU daily, she was completely cured.[42] In another study, a 37-year-old female with a ten-year history of severe nightly "restless legs" was placed on 300 IU daily for six weeks and 200 IU daily for the following four weeks, leading to complete relief.[43] Food sources: cold-pressed polyunsaturated vegetable oils (such as sunflower and safflower), leafy green vegetables, avocados, nuts, seeds, and whole grains. Supplements: vitamin E is actually a group of compounds called tocopherols. When purchasing supplements of vitamin E, avoid products that contain vitamin E in the DL-alpha tocopherol acetate form—this means that it is a petroleum-based synthetic form of the vitamin. The natural form of vitamin E will be designated with the letter "D". Typical recommended dose: 30 IU daily; for those suffering from restless legs syndrome, 800-1,200 IU of vitamin E should be taken per day.

Minerals

■ Calcium—Calcium and magnesium nourish the nervous system and act as natural relaxants. Many people have systems that are too acidic and need to be more alkaline and they benefit from taking these mineral supplements, which are both alkaline and a sedative. Low levels of calcium and magnesium have been associated with muscle cramping, which can disrupt sleep.[44] Calcium absorption into the cells can be compromised by whole grains and cereals, spinach, and by tannins in tea, a diet high in protein, commercial soda, refined sugar, and antacids that contain aluminum.[45] Food sources: broccoli, cabbage, almonds, hazelnuts, oats, lentils, beans, figs, currants and raisins, Brussels sprouts, cauliflower, kelp, and green leafy vegetables especially kale. Kale is very high in an easily absorbed form of calcium.[46] Supplements: bone meal, dolomite, and oyster shell calcium have been found to have the highest levels of lead and should not be used as a supplement.[47] Calcium citrate and calcium gluconate have a much better absorption level.[48] One of the best forms of absorbable calcium is microcrystalline hydroxyapatite. Typical dose: 600 mg of liquid calcium can have a relaxing effect (take calcium in a 2-to-1 ratio to magnesium). Precautions: Excessive intake of calcium oxalate may cause the formation of kidneys stones, but this risk can be decreased by using the calcium citrate and calcium gluconate forms. High calcium intake can interfere with iron absorption, cause chronic constipation, and may also increase blood pressure.[49]

■ Magnesium—Magnesium is second only to potassium as the most concentrated mineral within the cells. Magnesium helps form bones, relax muscle spasms, and decrease the pain involved in arthritis. It activates cellular enzymes and plays a large role in nerve and muscle function as well as helping to regulate the acid-alkaline balance.[50] Magnesium deficiency can cause anxiety, muscle tremors, confusion, irritability, and pain. Processed food or foods cooked at high temperatures can be depleted of their magnesium content. Food sources: tofu, nuts and seeds, and green leafy vegetables, especially kale, seaweed, and chlorophyll. Supplements: magnesium is absorbed well when taken as an oral supplement and will increase the measurable levels inside red and white blood cells.[51] We recommend using magnesium glycinate, fumerate, or citrate, which are usually better absorbed with less of a laxative effect.[52] Epsom salts (magnesium sulfate), an old-fashioned remedy, is an excellent addition to a bath, but has a strong laxative effect if taken as an oral supplement. Typical dose: 250 mg. Precautions: Very high doses of magnesium may be dangerous if kidney disease is present.

■ Chromium—Chromium is a mineral essential for regulating the production of the hormone insulin, which is responsible for stabilizing blood sugar levels. Although the body requires only small amounts of this important mineral, Americans are more likely to be deficient in chromium than any other micronutrient. Chromium is found in the outer bran portion of grains, but much of it is lost in the milling and processing of white flour (the staple ingredient in most refined bread and pasta products). The chromium that we do draw from food sources can be depleted in our bodies by various means, including a high-carbohydrate diet, infections, and physical and emotional stress. The urinary excretion of chromium can increase as much as fifty-fold under stress.[53] A high intake of white sugar also tends to deplete the body of chromium, as the mineral is used up in removing these sugars from the blood.[54]

Food sources: an excellent source of chromium is brewer's yeast (available in powder form or in tablets), wheat germ, beef and chicken, liver, whole grains, potatoes, eggs, apples, bananas, and spinach. Supplements: chromium and other minerals are better absorbed in the body when bound in a "transporter" molecule, called a chelate. Chelated minerals are better protected from damage in the digestive system. Glucose tolerance factor chelate (GTF chromium) tends to be a more bioavailable form of chromium than chromium salts, such as chromium chloride.[55] Chromium polynicotinate is another chelated variety that is chemically bound to niacin, a B-complex vitamin. According to some researchers, this form of chromium is superior to either chromium chloride or chromium picolinate. Typical recommended dosage: 250-500 mcg twice a day.

■ Copper—Copper is important for normal function of the central nervous system. Deficiencies in copper have been linked to greater difficulties in getting to sleep and decreased quality of sleep. It may also help alleviate allergic reactions, particularly the levels of histamine. The body's absorption of copper is blocked by a diet high in refined foods or from taking high levels of vitamin C, zinc,[56] and iron. Food sources: beans, lentils, shellfish (especially oysters), liver, nuts, and green leafy vegetables. Supplements: there are various forms of supplemental copper, such as copper sulfate, copper gluconate, copper picolinate, and others. Typical therapeutic dose: 2-5 mg. Precautions: Copper toxicity is seen more often than is copper deficiency. Use only after copper levels are measured through hair or urine analysis.

■ Iron—Iron is essential to red blood cell synthesis, oxygen transport, and energy production. A diet low in iron causes anemia, which has also been found to cause hypothyroidism.[57] Supplementing with iron has produced significant relief of symptoms in restless legs syndrome.[58] Food sources: kelp, organ meats, egg yolk, blackstrap molasses, lecithin, certain nuts and seeds, millet, and parsley. Supplements: the form of iron (heme) found in desiccated liver or a liquid liver extract is most easily absorbed and has fewer side effects.

Of the non-heme forms of iron, ferrous fumerate and ferrous succinate are recommended. Typical recommended dosage: 30 mg daily between meals. Precautions: Ferrous sulfate, commonly used in conventional supplements, can cause the production of free radicals and should not be used. Elevated levels of iron in the blood are associated with an increased risk for heart attacks and other cardiovascular problems, as well as low immunity.[59] Women who are menopausal and those who experience a heavy menstrual flow should consult their physicians. Overdose in infants can be serious or even fatal, so be sure that your iron supplements are out of the reach of children.

■ Zinc—Zinc may be deficient in people suffering from insomnia, particularly infants. Zinc is often lacking in a vegetarian diet, because beans, legumes, and grains—the staples of a vegetarian diet—are high in a substance known as phylate; phylates cause the elimination of zinc from the body.[60] Vegetarians forego one of the best sources of this mineral—meat. Food sources: whole grains, nuts, seeds, oysters, shellfish, and pumpkin seeds. Supplements: zinc sulfate, found in many multivitamin/multimineral preparations, is not easily absorbed by the body. Other forms of zinc that are more readily absorbed are zinc picolinate, zinc citrate, and zinc monomethionine. Typical recommended dose: 25 mg of zinc per day, along with 3 mg of copper (zinc tends to deplete copper reserves). Precautions: With medical supervision, the dosage of zinc could be increased if necessary. However, dosages should be increased with caution, as too much zinc can interfere with the functioning of the immune system. Toxicity of zinc is rarely reported; however, prolonged use of over 150 mg a day can cause anemia.

Amino Acids

Amino acids are the building blocks of proteins; in fact, proteins are actually chains of amino acids linked together, each one having a specific function. Proteins are, in turn, the building blocks of the body. Twenty-two amino acids are vital to the body's growth, development, and maintenance. Some are manufactured in the body while others, called essential amino acids, must be obtained from the diet or nutritional supplements. Semi-essential amino acids can be made by the body in amounts that are adequate to maintain basic protein requirements, however, additional dietary sources are required during times of growth or stress. Amino acid deficiency may be an underlying factor, often undetected, for sleep disorders. Vegetarians and vegans (vegetarians who eat no dairy products) often have difficulty meeting dietary protein requirements, and should take an amino acid complex supplement.

■ Tryptophan and 5-HTP—L-tryptophan is considered the best amino acid for sleeping problems. L-tryptophan is a precursor to serotonin, which is then converted into melatonin. The presence of melatonin allows the body to drop off into slumber. Tryptophan occurs naturally in certain foods, including turkey and other meats, milk and cheese, and legumes. Other tryptophan-containing foods include cashews, spinach, bananas, figs, dates, yogurt, tuna, and whole grain crackers. Research shows that tryptophan helps about half of all insomnia sufferers.[61] Unfortunately, L-tryptophan supplements are no longer readily available. During the 1980s, L-tryptophan was sold as a natural, non-habit-forming sleeping aid, until a "bad batch" manufactured in Japan caused more than a thousand people to become ill; it was subsequently banned by the U.S. Food and Drug Administration.

For information on **5-HTP**, contact: NutriCology, 400 Preda Street, San Leandro, CA 94577; tel: 800-545-9960 or 510-639-4572; fax: 510-635-6730. Life Enhancement Products, Inc., P.O. Box 751390, Petaluma, CA 94975; tel: 800-543-3873 or 707-762-6144; fax: 707-769-8016. BioSynergy Health Alternatives, 106 N. 6th Street, Suite 200, Boise, ID 83702; tel: 800-554-7145; fax: 208-342-0880.

There is, however, a substitute called 5-HTP, or 5-hydroxytryptophan, which is a form of tryptophan that is a step closer in the conversion process to serotonin. Tryptophan is usually converted in the brain into 5-HTP, which is then turned into serotonin. It has been shown to be effective in treating depression, fibromyalgia, headaches, and insomnia.[62] A Norwegian study showed that 5-HTP had an effect on sleep patterns by increasing the levels of serotonin. The researchers injected cats with 5-HTP (40 mg/kg body weight) or L-tryptophan and found that both substances had a "general deactivating effect on the waking state" and produced deep sleep.[63] The typical recommended dosage of 5-HTP is 25-50 mg daily. Higher dosages (over 100 mg) could cause some side effects, including mild nausea. Vitamin B6 should also be taken on the same day as 5-HTP, because it is necessary for converting 5-HTP into serotonin.

■ Phosphatidylserine, an amino acid that helps the hypothalamus regulate the amount of cortisol produced by the adrenals, is helpful for those who cannot sleep because of high cortisol levels, usually induced by stress. Cortisol is usually at high levels in the morning, for wakefulness, but in stressed individuals it may be high at night and prevent sleeping.

■ Jonathan Wright, M.D., Director of the Tahoma Clinic in Kent, Washington, has had success in treating insomnia using supplements of essential amino acids. He reports the case of a man who had been suffering from insomnia most of his adult life. Over the previous eighteen years, doctors had prescribed fourteen different drugs, starting

A Guide to Taking Supplements

In addition to knowing what supplements to take, it is also important to know how to take them. Jeffrey Bland, Ph.D., and Lindsey Berkson, D.C., offer the following recommendations and advisories:

■ Nutritional supplements should be taken with meals to promote increased absorption. Fat-soluble vitamins (such as vitamins A and E, beta carotene, and the essential fatty acids linoleic and alpha-linolenic acid) should be taken during the day with the meal that contains the most fat.

■ Amino acid supplements should be taken on an empty stomach at least an hour before or after a meal, and taken with fruit juice to help promote absorption. When taking an increased dosage of an isolated amino acid, be sure to supplement with an amino acid blend.

■ If you become nauseated when you take tablet supplements, consider taking a liquid form, diluted in a beverage.

■ If you become nauseated or ill within an hour after taking nutritional supplements, consider the need for a bowel cleanse or rejuvenation program prior to beginning a course of nutritional supplementation.

■ If you are taking high doses, do not take all the supplements at one time, but divide them into smaller doses throughout the day.

■ Take digestive enzymes with meals to assist digestion. If you are taking pancreatic enzymes for other therapeutic reasons, be sure to take them on an empty stomach between meals.

■ Do not take mineral supplements with high-fiber meals, as fiber can decrease mineral absorption.

■ When taking an increased dosage of an isolated B vitamin, be sure to supplement with B complex.

■ When taking nutrients, be sure to drink adequate amounts of liquid to mix with digestive juices and prevent side effects.

with sleeping pills and progressing to antidepressants. The sleeping pills left him feeling groggy while the antidepressants resulted in nightmares and, in the case of two drugs, heart trouble. He had also tried supplements of the amino acid L-tryptophan, but his insomnia did not improve. A blood test determined that the patient was deficient in five of the eight essential amino acids (his tryptophan levels were normal). Using a computer to calculate the proper proportions, Dr. Wright prescribed an amino acid blend to be taken (stirred into applesauce) twice a day. After three weeks, the patient's condition had improved markedly and, within three months, his insomnia had cleared up completely.

Supplements: The preferred amino acid supplements are labeled USP pharmaceutical grade, L-crystalline, free-form amino acids. The term *USP* means that the product meets the standards of purity and potency set by the United States Pharmacopeia. The term *free-form* refers to the highest level of purity of the amino acid. The *L* refers to one of the two forms in which most amino acids come, designated D- and L- (as in D-lysine or L-lysine). The L-form amino acids are proper for human biochemistry, as proteins in the human body are made from this form. Generally, it is not recommended for people to take individual amino acids for extended or indefinite periods as this can create an imbalance of other amino acids in

See *The Supplement Shopper* (Future Medicine Publishing, 1999; ISBN 1-887299-17-3); to order, call 800-333-HEAL.

the body and possibly cause other health conditions. If individual amino acids are going to be used to support specific health conditions, follow this course of treatment with a complex of free-form amino acids to ensure balanced amino acid nutrition. Please consult a qualified health-care professional before beginning such therapies. Individual amino acids often come with warnings or precautions for women who are pregnant or for people with certain health conditions.

Other Supplements

■ We also prescribe a homeopathic remedy called Serotonin Dopamine Liquescence that stimulates the uptake of the brain chemicals serotonin and dopamine, which will increase the availability of melatonin and help people sleep better. Serotonin is a neurotransmitter that promotes sleep, regulates pain, and influences mood. Dopamine regulates physical movements and muscular control and also influences mood, sex drive, and memory retrieval.

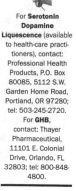

For **Serotonin Dopamine Liquescence** (available to health-care practitioners), contact: Professional Health Products, P.O. Box 80085, 5112 S.W. Garden Home Road, Portland, OR 97280; tel: 503-245-2720.
For **GHB**, contact: Thayer Pharmaceutical, 11101 E. Colonial Drive, Orlando, FL 32803; tel: 800-848-4800.

■ GHB (gammahydroxybutyric acid) is a naturally occurring neurotransmitter produced by the brain that helps to regulate sleep and energy. Dr. Rifkin, who uses GHB in treating patients with sleep disorders, says the substance has been around for many years, but has only recently gained attention. GHB, which is only available by prescription, has been used in the past in hospitals to calm restless patients. GHB comes in capsules and the typical dosage is 50 mg per kilogram of body weight, taken before bed.

CHAPTER

4 Detoxify Your Body

ALTERNATIVE PHYSICIANS working with sleep disorders know that removing toxins from the body is an essential phase in restoring their patients to health and vitality. Each year, people are exposed to thousands of toxic chemicals and pollutants in air, water, food, and soil. People carry within their bodies a "chemical cocktail" made up of industrial chemicals, pesticides, food additives, heavy metals, general anesthetics, and the residues of conventional pharmaceuticals, as well as of legal (alcohol, tobacco, caffeine) and illegal drugs (heroin, cocaine, marijuana).

Today, people are exposed to chemicals in far greater concentrations than were previous generations. For example, over 70 million Americans live in areas that exceed smog standards; most municipal drinking water contains over 700 chemicals, including excessive levels of lead. Some 3,000 chemicals are added to the food supply; and as many as 10,000 chemicals in the form of solvents, emulsifiers, and preservatives are used in food processing and storage, and can remain in the body for years.[1]

To make matters worse, food and product labels do not always list every ingredient. When people consume these foods—especially seafood, meat, and poultry—they ingest all the chemicals and pesticides that have remained as accumulated contaminants in the food chain. These pollutants lodge in the body—loading it up with poisons—

In This Chapter

- The Loading Theory of Toxicity
- The Detoxification Defense System
- Sources of Toxins
- Toxic Overload and Its Impact on Sleep
- Testing for Your Detoxification Capabilities
- Success Story: Correcting *Candida* Cures Insomnia
- Alternative Medicine Approach to Detoxification

and manifest in a variety of symptoms, including decreased immune function, nerve cell toxicity, hormonal dysfunction, psychological disturbances, and sleep disorders.

The Loading Theory of Toxicity

Alternative Medicine Approach to Detoxification

- Colon-Cleansing Programs
- Liver-Cleansing Programs
- Eliminating Yeast and Parasites

The "loading theory" of toxicity, according to its formulator, Serafina Corsello, M.D., director of the Corsello Centers for Nutritional Complementary Medicine in New York City and Huntington, New York, states that no single factor causes a disease. Rather, the cumulative load of multiple poisons creates an illness like insomnia.

This is compounded of layers of toxicity, malnutrition, and dysfunction. People don't get a disease—they develop it, Dr. Corsello explains. Over time, multiple factors weigh down the immune system and eventually throw it out of balance. Among the typical stressors there are toxic metals (mercury leaching from fillings, aluminum), petrochemical residues (pesticides and fertilizers), chemical pollutants (in the water and air), electromagnetic pollution (power lines), undiagnosed food allergies, nutritional deficiencies, biochemical imbalances, insufficient exercise, and emotional stress (family, job, and personal).

All these factors impinge on the immune system's natural vitality to resist the downhill slide into illness, says Dr. Corsello. "These factors interact and compound each other to break down the immune system. In fact, these stressors may be accumulating for years, over a lifetime, before they send the system into disregulation."

Increasingly, toxicity is being identified as the predisposing factor in a long list of acute and chronic illnesses, including sleep disorders, environmental illness and chronic fatigue, degenerative diseases, and cancer.[2] "The current level of chemicals in the food and water supply and the indoor and outdoor environment has lowered our threshold of resistance to disease and has altered our body's metabolism, causing enzyme dysfunction, nutritional deficiencies, and hormonal imbalances," says Marshall Mandell, M.D., a pioneer of environmental medicine based in Norwalk, Connecticut.

Detoxifying the body is another important component in promoting the health of the immune system and addressing other factors that may be contributing to your sleep disorder. As our environment and food are increasingly saturated with chemicals, the body's mechanisms for elimination of toxins cannot keep up with the chemical deluge. The constant circulation of toxins in the body taxes the immune system, which must continually strive to destroy them. It is advisable to take measures to remove the toxins stored in the body.

Detoxification Defense System

The detoxification system has two lines of defense—specific organs prevent toxins from entering the body and others neutralize and excrete the poisonous compounds that get through this initial line of defense. When functioning properly, the body's defenses protect healthy tissues from damage by harmful free radicals or circulating toxins. Key components of the detoxification system include:

- Gastrointestinal barrier, including the small and large intestines
- Liver
- Lymphatic system, which transports waste products from the cells to the major organs of detoxification
- Kidneys, bladder, and other components of the urinary system
- Skin, including sweat and sebaceous glands
- Lungs

The gastrointestinal system is typically the first line of defense against toxins and, when compromised, the first place to harbor seeds of disease. "The digestive system is one of the first screening systems against the daily load of contact with bacteria, viruses, and parasites, that, if left unchecked, would constitute a grave threat to our entire immune system," says Dr. Corsello. A healthy intestine is immunologically vigilant against undesirable pathogens and toxins. One that is overburdened and compromised fails to perform its immune defensive role and may start contributing to the emergence of chronic disease. "A large onslaught of infective agents can overcome the immune vigilance of most people, even in the presence of so-called 'normal' immune systems." The intestines consist of a complex and delicately balanced population of mixed microflora in which the friendly, beneficial bacteria should outnumber the harmful ones. But this ecology is easily upset, says Dr. Corsello, leading to a condition of imbalance called dysbiosis.

Within the 25 feet of the intestinal lining are many hiding places for disease-causing agents, which then break through the intestinal membrane and gain access to the bloodstream. This is one facet of how sleep disorders begin—once the bowel is toxic, the entire body soon follows. If the intestines are letting toxins through, then the liver, lymph, kidneys, skin, and other organs involved in detoxification become overwhelmed.

The liver bears most of the burden for eliminating toxins. The liver, located beneath the right lower part of the rib cage, is the largest and one of the most complicated organs in the body, rivaled only by the brain. The liver collects and removes foreign particles and chemicals from the blood and detoxifies these poisons through three systems: (1) the Kupffer cells; (2) Phase I and Phase II systems, involving over 75 enzymes; and (3) the production of bile. Each system feeds into the other, and all three need to be operating at full efficiency for proper detoxification.

Approximately 1,500 milliliters of blood pass through the liver each minute for filtering. The major players in this filtering project are the Kupffer cells, a type of white blood cell that engulfs foreign matter in the blood before it passes through the rest of the liver. When the liver is damaged, toxic, congested, or

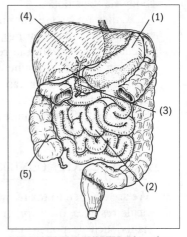

THE DIGESTIVE SYSTEM. Digestion begins in the mouth, then food travels to the stomach (1), where it is further broken down by gastric juices. Next, the partially digested food goes to the small intestine (2) where enzymes from the pancreas (3) and bile produced by the liver (4) act upon the food to extract nutrients for absorption into blood and lymph cells. The unusable food materials are sent to the large intestine (5) for evacuation from the body.

sluggish, the filtration system breaks down, allowing increased levels of antigens, foreign proteins, bowel microorganisms, and dietary waste products to pass through the liver and enter the general circulatory system.

When a toxic chemical like alcohol enters the liver, reactions begin which attempt to break down these chemicals into harmless substances. Phase I is the oxidation phase, in which enzymes "burn" or oxidize chemicals into intermediate substances. Phase II enzymes act to combine these decomposed substances with other molecules (such as sulfur, glutathione, and glycine) to make them more water-soluble and easier for the body to excrete.[3] Bile (excreted by the liver, stored in the gallbladder, and pumped into the small intestine as needed) makes intestinal contents less acidic and prevents putrefaction of intestinal contents. The goal of the liver's detoxification systems is to convert toxins into a water-soluble form for easy elimination from the body via the stool.

Other toxins are eliminated through the lymphatic system, kidneys, the skin (by sweating), and respiratory system. When imbalances occur in this system, the result can be poor digestion, constipation, bloating and gas, immune dysfunction, reduced liver function, and a host of degenerative diseases, including sleep disorders. Detoxification can reduce or eliminate the body's "toxic load," restore the proper functioning of the immune and other systems, and help alleviate your sleep problems.

Sources of Toxins

We are exposed to toxins every day of our lives, in chemicals and pesticide residues, mercury amalgam dental fillings, biological contaminants such as pollen and parasites, and genetically altered foods, among other sources. Even our own bodies can produce toxins, called endobiotics, which can prove harmful to us if not properly controlled.

Environmental Pollution

Toxins emanate from a variety of noxious sources, but chiefly from environmental pollution. Unavoidably, many of us carry around an internal "chemical cocktail" derived from absorbing industrial by-products (coal tar or fuel exhaust), pesticides, herbicides, household contaminants (found in cleaners, paints, plastics, and solvents), and biological contaminants (pollens, molds, dust mites, and parasites). We are also exposed to toxins from processed or genetically altered foods, alcohol or tap water (which usually contains heavy metals), and even the newspaper (from the inks used in printing).

Since the 1980s, physicians began using the term *sick building syndrome* (SBS) to refer to a host of symptoms produced by low-grade toxic environmental conditions found in living or office spaces. SBS symptoms include respiratory, eye, and skin diseases, headaches, memory loss, fatigue, lethargy, temporary weight loss, infections, irritability, and impaired balance. All of these suppress the immune system, rendering the individual susceptible to long-term chronic illness.

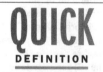

QUICK

DEFINITION

Environmental estrogens are foreign compounds and/or chemical toxins that mimic the effects of estrogen in the body. Environmental estrogens, also called xenobiotics or xenoestrogens, are present primarily in man-made chemicals ("greenhouse gases," herbicides, and pesticides such as DDT) and industrial by-products (from manufacture of plastics and paper, as well as from the incineration of hazardous wastes).

Endocrine glands, including the testicles, ovaries, pancreas, adrenals, thyroid, parathyroid, and pituitary, are central to the regulation and normalization of all the body's complex, interconnected systems, from metabolism and heat production to spermatogenesis and uterine preparations for pregnancy.

Xenobiotics or environmental estrogens (SEE QUICK DEFINITION) have been linked to endocrine disruption and to severe breakdown of the integrity of the digestive system. Each year, an estimated 1,000 new synthetic chemicals enter the world market, swelling the planetary total to well over 100,000. All of these are completely foreign and potentially harmful to the function of the digestive system and endocrine glands (SEE QUICK DEFINITION). Evidence is accumulating that these chemicals, even at very low concentrations and exposures, cause "hormone havoc"—autoimmune diseases, clinical depression, and reproductive system disorders, among others.

Toxins can also enter the body in ways other than through breathing or swallowing—in particular, through the skin's pores. (Those same pores, of course, also facilitate the elimination of toxic chemicals). Approximately 70% of the toxins from tap water enter the body through the skin; the remaining 20% of the toxins enter via ingestion. Tap water in the United States contains chlorine, aluminum, pesticides, lead, copper, and other toxic substances.[4]

Harmful Metals and Chemicals

Conventional dental amalgams or "silver" fillings are actually made of tin, copper, silver, nickel, zinc, and the toxic metal mercury. These fillings disintegrate over time, and have been shown in some instances to release these toxic metals into the body, affecting the bones and the central nervous system and brain. Evidence now shows that mercury amalgams are the major source of mercury exposure for the general public, at rates six times higher than those found in fish and seafood.[5] One of the symptoms of mercury toxicity is disturbed sleep.

Copper-lined pipes in plumbing systems can be another source of toxicity. A greenish-brown ring around the tub, sink, or toilet can indicate that your water is contaminated with copper, which is toxic at high levels. According to Paul C. Eck, Ph.D., and Larry Wilson, M.D., of the Eck Institute of Applied Nutrition and Bioenergetics in Phoenix, Arizona, many of the most prevalent metabolic dysfunctions of our time are in some way related to a copper imbalance and/or copper toxicity. Copper toxicity can cause liver problems, adrenal fatigue, allergies, and osteoarthritis.[6] Other sources of copper include birth control pills and intrauterine devices, and fungicides and pesticides—all of which contain copper as a main ingredient. A thorough analysis from a health-care practitioner, including nutritional and heavy-metal assessment, can determine whether copper detoxification or supplementation is needed.

Symptom Analysis of Patients Who Eliminated Mercury-Containing Dental Fillings

The following represents a summary of 1,569 patients in six different studies evaluating the health effects of replacing mercury-containing dental fillings with non-mercury fillings. The data was derived from the following sources: 762 Patient Adverse Reaction Reports submitted to the FDA by patients, and 807 patient reports from Sweden, Denmark, Canada, and the United States.[8]

% of Total Reporting	Symptom	Number Reporting	Number Improved or Cured	% of Cure or Improvement
14	Allergy	221	196	89
5	Anxiety	86	80	93
5	Bad temper	81	68	84
6	Bloating	88	70	80
6	Blood pressure problems	99	53	54
5	Chest pains	79	69	87
22	Depression	347	315	91
22	Dizziness	343	301	88
45	Fatigue	705	603	86
15	Intestinal problems	231	192	83
8	Gum problems	129	121	94
34	Headaches	531	460	87
12	Insomnia	187	146	78
10	Irregular heartbeat	159	139	87
8	Irritability	132	119	90
17	Lack of concentration	270	216	80
6	Lack of energy	91	88	97
17	Memory loss	265	193	73
17	Metallic taste	260	247	95
7	Multiple sclerosis	113	86	76
8	Muscle tremor	126	104	82

Chemicals found in dry-cleaning fluids (trichloroethylene), paint solvents (toluene), municipal water supplies (phenol and chlorine), carpets and flooring (formaldehyde), and some imported produce (DDT pesticide residues) are also potentially harmful, depending on your level of susceptibility. Studies have proven that these chemicals can interfere with proper nerve and muscle function, cause skeletal and muscular changes, and alter mental functioning.[7]

Inner Toxins

Environmental toxins are only one layer of the toxic load that our bodies must process. Endobiotics—toxins produced within the body—are also present and are potentially dangerous if not efficiently eliminated. Endobiotics include uric and lactic acid, homocysteine, nitric oxide, intestinal toxins, and cellular debris from dead microorganisms. These are normal by-products of metabolic processes that are typically broken down by the liver and excreted from the body. But in someone with a compromised immune system, they tend to accumulate in the blood where they burden the detoxification pathways or initiate an allergic reaction.

The Yeast Connection

A yeast is a type of single-celled organism found throughout nature—in the soil, on vegetables and fruits, and in the human body. *Candida albicans* is a very common variety of yeast, frequently present in small quantities in the intestines and in a woman's vagina. It is not harmful under normal conditions (that is, when its numbers are few), but it can cause considerable damage when its colonies grow and multiply. *Candida* then becomes pathogenic, transforming from a simple yeast into an aggressive fungus. This potential for mutating from a benign organism to a pathogenic one is why William Crook, M.D., describes *Candida* as a kind of microbiological "Dr. Jekyll and Mr. Hyde." Candidiasis causes a lengthy and

Toxins That Can Poison the Liver

- Pesticides, herbicides, and fungicides
- Antibiotics and growth hormones used in agriculture
- Vaccinations
- Food additives and preservatives
- Prescription drugs
- Auto exhaust
- Fluoride
- Household cleaning fluids
- Mercury amalgam fillings
- Recreational drugs
- Electromagnetic fields
- X rays
- Alcohol
- Tobacco
- Coffee
- Hydrogenated fats
- Fried foods
- Cosmetics[9]

diverse list of allergic reactions which makes it particularly difficult to diagnose. The symptoms can range from sleep disturbances, fatigue, and digestive difficulties to joint pains, food cravings, and emotional problems.[10] *Candida* can also cause a person to develop food allergies, according to James Braly, M.D., medical director of Immuno Labs in Fort Lauderdale, Florida, by burrowing into and damaging the intestinal lining.[11] This may cause breaches in the lining, allowing food particles to seep out of the intestines and into the bloodstream (a condition known as leaky gut syndrome).

The Parasite Connection

Parasite infections are often overlooked because they can cause a wide variety of health problems that mimic other diseases. Among the conditions that can be caused by parasites are fatigue, hypoglycemia, skin problems, sleep disorders, depression, upper respiratory tract infections, environmental illness, PMS, and gastrointestinal problems. Hermann Bueno, M.D., of New York City, an international authority on parasitic disease, says that parasites neutralize the action of hormones. "Parasites block the 'entryway' [the receptor site] where these hormones penetrate and interact with the cells of the target organ," he says. This blocking at the cellular level prevents hormones from stimulating the body's organs, which, in turn, can cause a myriad of illnesses. Several of these illnesses, such as hypoglycemia (low blood sugar) and hypothyroidism (an underactive thyroid), are known to cause sleep disorders. The parasites themselves may also invade the bloodstream, causing the immune system to channel much of its energy and resources to subduing them. Such an immune response can cause widespread, allergy-like symptoms that contribute to sleep disturbances.

Toxic Overload and Its Impact on Sleep

When our bodies become overloaded with toxins and our detoxification pathways are overwhelmed, one result is disturbed sleep. While it may not seem readily apparent, the role of the liver and colon are important for establishing and maintaining regular, restful sleep. If either system is not working properly, the body can become dangerously toxic. One of the main causes of sleeplessness—especially sleep-maintenance insomnia, in which people wake up in the middle of the night—is trouble in the liver and the gastrointestinal tract.

We treated a woman named Laurie, a professional hair colorist. She came to our clinic in desperation because of her insomnia. Laurie would wake up after two hours of sleep and rarely be able to fall asleep again. Conventional medicine hadn't helped her and antibiotics made her sinus infections and skin conditions even worse. We suspected that the coloring chemicals she worked with and the antibiotics had made her liver toxic. The functional liver test confirmed our diagnosis. At our suggestion, Laurie took a month off from work and we put her on a liver detoxification program. In addition, we taught her breathing techniques, self-hypnosis, and acupressure as stress reduction tools to help her sleep. After three weeks on this program, Laurie began to sleep through the night and she continues to do well. She was not able to change her profession, so every month she repeats the liver detoxification. That, along with the adjustments she's made in her lifestyle, keeps her sleeping soundly.

■ Heavy Metal–Induced Reactions—We have found that poisoning from toxic metals such as mercury, lead, copper, thallium, and arsenic can lead to insomnia, fatigue, and lethargy. Mercury (from amalgam fillings) in particular causes a number of reactions that can disturb sleep. It interferes with the transmission of nerve impulses from the brain to the rest of the body, producing tremors, tingling sensations, and numbness. Mercury also interferes with hormone function and can deactivate minerals such as calcium and magnesium that are important for sound sleep.[12] A recent study found that patients with dental amalgams had a significantly higher incidence of insomnia (as well as anger, depression, and anxiety) than those without amalgams, because mercury affected neurotransmitters in the brain.[13]

■ Allergies—*Candida* infection can directly alter sleep patterns, according to a study with animals.[14] Yeast infections can also cause food allergies to develop. Food allergies can trigger the overproduction of insulin, the hormone that controls blood sugar levels; a blood sugar imbalance (hypoglycemia) can potentially result in sleep problems. Chloride and fluoride in water, along with pesticides that leach out of the soil and into our food and water supply, are the most commonly targeted toxic exposures. People who are sensitive to these chemicals can have allergic responses that include insomnia. In those who are environmentally sensitive, breathing car fumes and other toxic substances can trigger a cascade of internal biochemical events that disturb sleep.

■ Blood Sugar Imbalances—Parasites can cause hypoglycemia or low blood sugar. Nighttime hypoglycemia releases adrenaline, cortisol, and other hormones to stimulate the brain and indicate that it is time to eat. This can awaken you or prevent you from entering a deep sleep state.

■ Slow Metabolism—If the liver is toxic, it will not be able to adequately process toxins out of the body. This may mean that caffeine, medications, and other stimulants remain in the body and disrupt your sleep.

■ Nutrient Deficiencies—It is also important to remember that exposure to environmental toxins depletes certain vitamins and minerals from our bodies and can lower our immune system's ability to fight off infections. "When nutrients such as the B vitamins, iron, antioxidants and specific trace minerals are depleted in the diet, the liver's ability to function effectively as a detoxification organ is impaired. This impairment causes the individual to become more vulnerable to the environment," Dr. Bland says.[15] These nutrients are also critical for the formation of neurotransmitters and hormones such as melatonin necessary for sleep.

Testing Your Detoxification Capabilities

Determining how efficiently the body can detoxify itself is especially useful for those with sleep disorders. Here are two laboratory tests that can help.

Functional Liver Detoxification Profile—If your liver is unable to adequately detoxify your body's store of toxins and waste products, this situation may contribute significantly to the emergence and continuation of your arthritis. Excess free radicals and by-products of incomplete metabolism resulting from poor detoxification can create problems in the cells. Specifically, they can interfere with the movement of substances across the cell membrane and induce damage to the mitochondria, the cells' "energy factories." The Detoxification Profile helps to identify places where your system is impaired in its ability to detoxify. Specifically, it looks at the liver's ability to convert potentially dangerous toxins into harmless substances that can then be eliminated by the body, in the two major chemical reactions, Phase I and Phase II. The Detoxification Profile determines the presence of enzymes needed to start the conversion process and the rate at which Phase I and II are operating.

For information about the **Functional Liver Detoxification Profile and Oxidative Stress Profile**, contact: Great Smokies Diagnostic Laboratory, 63 Zillicoa Street, Asheville, NC 28801; tel: 704-253-0621 or 800-522-4762; fax: 704-252-9303.

Oxidative Stress Profile—When your ability to detoxify is impaired and/or you are deficient in antioxidants, free radicals run unchallenged throughout the body, damaging cells. They tend to affect the immune, endocrine, and nervous systems, damaging mitochondria, interrupting communication among cells, and depleting key nutrients and antioxidants. This is called oxidative stress. The Oxidative Stress Profile assesses the degree of free-radical damage in the body and it measures the body's levels of glutathione, an amino acid–complex central to detoxification.

Diagnosing Candidiasis

Candidiasis causes systemic illnesses that produce a wide variety of symptoms. This makes candidiasis difficult to accurately diagnose, since it shares symptoms with so many other conditions. Leon Chaitow, N.D., D.O., of London, England, notes that when symptoms are chronic rather than acute or sudden, he generally suspects a yeast infection. Another clue is if specific symptoms have been previously treated without success, then the diagnosis usually suggests candidiasis. Some physicians rely on laboratory test results to diagnose the condition. However, while these tests are helpful, it is important not to depend on them exclusively. For example, blood tests can be used to pinpoint *Candida* antibodies. But since most people normally have *Candida* organisms in their systems, the tests may show antibodies even if the patient is not suffering from candidiasis. The truth is there is no single diagnostic test. Stephen Langer, M.D., indicates that "the clincher to any diagnosis is not so much what is happening in the laboratory as what is happening in the patient." The combination of an individual's complete medical history and examination, the patient's response to treatment, and information culled from laboratory tests is the key to a correct diagnosis.[16]

Dr. Chaitow describes the likely candidate for *Candida* overgrowth as someone whose medical history includes steroid hormone medications (cortisone or corticosteroids, often prescribed for skin conditions such as rashes, eczema, or psoriasis), prolonged or repeated use of antibiotics, medications for treating ulcers, or oral contraceptives. Certain illnesses, such as diabetes, cancer, and AIDS, can also increase susceptibility to *Candida* overgrowth.

"All too often more than one influence is operating," says Dr. Chaitow. "Over a few years, a patient may have had antibiotics for a variety of conditions, while using steroids as well, perhaps in the form of the contraceptive pill. If the patient also happens to be living on a diet rich in sugars, then the *Candida* is very likely to have spread beyond its usual borders into new territory."[17]

A qualified practitioner should take your complete medical history to determine if you have a *Candida* infection, but here are a few questions to ask yourself to see if you are at risk (the more questions that you answer affirmatively, the greater your risk):

■ Have you taken repeated courses of antibiotics or steroids (e.g., cortisone)?

■ Have you used birth-control pills?

■ Have you had repeated fungal infections ("jock itch," athlete's foot, ringworm)?

■ Do you regularly have any of these symptoms—bloating, headaches, depression, fatigue, memory problems, impotence or lack of interest in sex, muscle aches with no apparent cause, brain fogginess?

■ Do you experience symptoms of PMS (pre-menstrual syndrome)?

■ Do you have cravings for sweets, products containing white flour, or alcoholic beverages?

■ Do you repeatedly experience any of these health difficulties— inappropriate drowsiness, mood swings, rashes, bad breath, dry mouth, post-nasal drip or nasal congestion, heartburn, urinary frequency or urgency?[18]

Blood Tests—Blood tests can look for *Candida* antibodies (SEE QUICK DEFINITION) in the body. When *Candida* assumes its fungal form, the immune system responds by producing special antibodies to fight off the infection. Consequently, if a large concentration of these antibodies are found in the blood, you may be experiencing a *Candida* outbreak. Dr. Langer notes that "if the yeast antibodies are elevated and the test is positive, the yeast infection is active and threatening."[19] However, the antibody test may be misleading, because most individuals normally have *Candida* organisms in their bodies. The Anti-Candida Antibodies Panel, from Great Smokies Diagnostic Laboratory, in Asheville, North Carolina, is a blood test measures the levels of antibodies (specifically, the immunoglobulins IgG and IgM) against *Candida*. The IgG levels indicate both past and ongoing infection, while the IgM level may be a truer reflection of present infection.

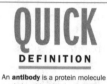

QUICK
DEFINITION

An **antibody** is a protein molecule made by white blood cells in the lymph tissue and activated by the immune system against specific foreign proteins (antigens). An antibody, also referred to as an immunoglobulin, binds to the antigen as a preliminary for destroying it.

Darkfield Microscopy—The blood can also be examined visually using a darkfield microscope to detect the presence of the *Candida* fungus. Darkfield microscopy is a way of studying living whole blood cells under a specially adapted microscope that projects the image (magnified 1,400 times) onto a video screen. The skilled physician can detect early signs of illness in the form of microorganisms in the blood known to produce disease. Specifically, darkfield microscopy reveals distortions of red blood cells (which indicates nutritional status), possible undesirable bacterial or fungal life forms (like *Candida*), and other blood ecology patterns indicative of health or illness.[20]

Stool Analysis—Another test used to diagnose candidiasis is a stool analysis, which can help assess digestive function through laboratory examination of a stool sample. The Great Smokies Comprehensive Digestive Stool Analysis (CDSA) can measure how much yeast is actually present in the intestines. If the stool contains abnormally large amounts of *Candida*, this may indicate candidiasis. The CDSA can also look at levels of beneficial bacteria in the intestines as well as other digestive markers for determining *Candida* levels. Another stool analysis test, the Yeast Screen-Candascan, from Diagnos-Techs, Inc., measures levels of all types of yeast, including *Candida*.

For information about the **Anti-Candida Antibodies Panel and Comprehensive Digestive Stool Analysis**, contact: Great Smokies Diagnostic Laboratory, 63 Zillicoa Street, Asheville, NC 28801; tel: 800-522-4762 or 704-253-0621; fax: 704-252-9303. For the **Yeast Screen-Candascan**, contact: Diagnos-Techs, Inc., 6620 South 192nd Place, J-104, Kent, WA 98032; tel: 800-878-3787 or 425-251-0596; fax: 425-251-0637.

Diagnosing a Parasite Infection

Symptoms and personal history are the first two things a physician should check when diagnosing a possible parasite infection. "I always begin with a detailed picture of the symptoms and then gather a complete history that will indicate if exposure to parasites should be factored in," says Leo Galland, M.D., author of *The Four Pillars of Healing*. "Red flags are things like a recent trip out of the country, extensive use of antibiotics which weaken the immune system, or having a child in day care, where it's estimated 30% of staff are infected."

After determining whether a parasite infection may exist from a patient's symptoms and history, physicians generally then confirm the diagnosis with various testing procedures. Different parasites require different formulations to kill them, so an accurate diagnosis is an important step in any treatment program. A number of diagnostic tools can be useful in determining if you have parasites, including a purged stool test and mucus and blood tests.

Purged Stool Test—Ann Louise Gittleman, M.S., recommends using a purged stool test for parasites. This method differs from standard stool analysis—the patient ingests 1 1/2 ounces of a high-sodium solution on an empty stomach to

A purged stool test is not recommended for individuals with high blood pressure as the high-sodium solution may exacerbate their problem, according to Gittleman. Pregnant women and those suffering from an intestinal obstruction or appendicitis should not take this test.

Assessing Parasite Exposure

A medical history assessing the patient's potential exposure to parasites is crucial to getting an accurate diagnosis. Dr. Bueno and other alternative medicine practitioners typically ask patients the following questions to assess the likelihood of a parasite exposure:

■ What is your travel history (inside and outside the U.S.)?

■ What is the source of your drinking water? Have you ever drunk water from streams or rivers while camping?

■ Do you have pets in your household or are you in close contact with animals?

■ Do you frequently eat out, particularly at ethnic restaurants, sushi bars, or salad bars?

■ Do you like to eat raw fruits and vegetables?

■ Do you like raw or undercooked meat or fish?

■ Do you work in a hospital, day care center, sanitation department, around animals, or garden?

■ Do you engage in oral or anal sex?

■ Do you have some or all of these symptoms—dark circles under your eyes, distended abdomen, bluish lips, allergies, diarrhea or constipation, anemia, skin eruptions, anal itching, chronic fatigue, loss of appetite, insomnia, depression, or sugar cravings?[21]

encourage more frequent and powerful bowel movements. These induced stool samples have higher levels of mucus, which provide higher numbers of organisms. Parasites generally begin to appear after the fourth bowel movement, but sometimes it may take as many as 12 bowel movements to dislodge them. The purged stool test may be more accurate than conventional stool analysis for diagnosing a parasite infection. The problem with a random stool sample is that parasites cling to the wall of the intestines and simply may not be present in the feces.[22]

Uni Key Health Systems of Bozeman, Montana, makes a do-it-yourself purged stool test kit endorsed by Gittleman. You can do this test at home and send the sample to a parasitology laboratory for analysis. The test can detect 15 types of worms, more than a dozen types of protozoa, and yeasts like *Candida albicans*. The test results are sent to Gittleman's office and she will offer advice on treatment options.

Bueno-Parrish Test—Another test procedure recommended by alternative care practitioners is the Bueno-Parrish test. This test, developed by Dr. Bueno, involves the use of a rectal mucus swab to identify parasites. The procedure, technically called an anoscopy, involves taking a sample of mucus from inside the rectum with a cotton swab. A stain that makes even fragments of parasites visible is then applied to the swab material and examined with the help of a

For information on **stool analysis**, contact: Uni Key Health Systems, P.O. Box 7168, Bozeman, MT 59771; tel: 406-586-9424 or 800-888-4353. Great Smokies Diagnostic Laboratory, 63 Zillicoa Street, Asheville, NC 28801; tel: 828-253-0621 or 800-522-4762; fax: 828-252-9303. Meridian Valley Clinical Laboratory, 515 West Harrison Street, Suite 9, Kent, WA 98032; tel: 800-234-6825 or 253-859-8700; fax: 253-859-1135. For the **Bueno-Parrish test**, contact: Lexington Professional Center, 133 E 73rd Street, New York, NY 10021; tel: 212-988-4800. For more on **blood tests**, contact: Parasitic Disease Consultants Laboratory, 2177-J Flintstone Drive, Tucker, GA 30084; tel: 404-496-1370.

microscope. This procedure has helped identify parasite infections in patients who had previously been misdiagnosed.[23]

Blood Tests—Blood tests may be useful for diagnosing some parasitic infections. Elevated levels of a special white blood cell called an eosinophil may indicate a parasite infection. Blood tests can also measure levels of antibodies to some parasites. Abnormal blood levels of some nutrients may indicate parasites. For example, low levels of iron, folic acid, and calcium may indicate the presence of *Giardia*.[24]

Success Story: Correcting *Candida* Cures Insomnia

"If only I could sleep, I know I would be better," said Sally, a school teacher in her 30s, who had a *Candida* infection and chronic fatigue syndrome. She had been unable to work for the past year because of her severe tiredness. She often spent the day in bed, but barely slept at all. In addition, she suffered from bloating after eating, chronic constipation, and emotional swings. Sometimes, she would force herself to exercise and, the next day, she would be worse.

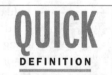

DEFINITION

Intestinal dysbiosis refers to an imbalance between intestinal flora. Specifically, these flora are friendly, beneficial bacteria, called probiotics, such as *Lactobacillus acidophilus* and *Bifidobacterium bifidum*, and unfriendly bacteria in the intestines such as *Escherichia coli* and *Clostridum perfringens*. In dysbiosis, the unfriendly bacteria predominate; they begin fermentation, producing toxic by-products that interfere with the normal elimination cycle. Dysbiosis is considered a primary cause or major cofactor in the development of many health problems, such as acne, yeast overgrowth, chronic fatigue, depression, digestive disorders, bloating, food allergies, PMS, rheumatoid arthritis, and cancer.

During the exam, Sally said that she had suffered from teen-age acne. In order to cure the acne, she underwent a year of antibiotic therapy. In addition, she had a series of upper respiratory infections in her early 20s, for which she was given more antibiotics. Heavy doses of antibiotics can destroy healthy bacteria in the intestines, resulting in digestive problems and also setting the ground for *Candida* to develop. The results of a stool test on Sally showed that had indeed occurred: Sally suffered from dysbiosis (SEE QUICK DEFINITION), malabsorption (the nutrients from her food were

QUICK
DEFINITION

Craniosacral therapy refers to correcting imbalances in the relationship among breathing, the sacrum (the base of the backbone attached to the pelvis) and the bones of the skull (cranium), especially the occiput. The sacrum acts as a pump to propel cerebrospinal fluid up the spine to the brain; the cranial bones contract and pump it back down. Health depends on a smoothly functioning sacro-occipital pump. Craniosacral therapy, as delivered by a chiropractor or other trained practitioner, is a light-touch adjustment that restores the sacrum to full motion and balance with respect to the cranial bones.

For more on **craniosacral therapy and other physical therapies**, see Chapter 9: Correcting Structural Imbalances, pp. 224-247.

CAUTION

Any detoxification effort should always be planned and executed under professional supervision. Those recovering from substance abuse, alcoholics, diabetics, people with eating disorders, and those who are underweight or physically weak or who have an underactive thyroid or hypoglycemic condition are urged not to detoxify without consulting a licensed health-care professional.

not being absorbed properly) and liver toxicity (the liver becomes sluggish and loses its efficiency in eliminating toxins).

Sally was placed on a yeast-free diet and given garlic and grapefruit seed extract to detoxify and rehabilitate her intestinal tract and liver. She also received various physical treatments, including acupuncture, craniosacral work (SEE QUICK DEFINITION), and applied kinesiology.

After one month on the program, Sally began to sleep through the night. As her energy and strength began returning, she started on a very minimal exercise program to tone her muscles. She also received hypnotherapy for attitudinal changes, relaxation exercises to do at home, and recipes for herbal baths to prepare for herself before bed. After three months on the program, Sally was able to return to her teaching job.

Alternative Medicine Approach to Detoxification

A detoxification program should be tailored to the individual's specific condition, including disease state, toxic burden, and the functional capacity of their major detoxifying organs (intestines, liver, and lymphatic system, among others). The process must progress at a rate that the body can handle without causing greater injury. During detoxification, many people experience a "healing crisis" or brief worsening of symptoms immediately followed by significant improvement. Although the healing crisis is uncomfortable, it usually indicates that toxins are being effectively removed from the body. However, a health-care professional should be alerted when symptoms worsen during detoxification to avoid complications or unintended injury. Efforts must be made to increase the production of antioxidants prior to any detoxification program to avert or diminish a healing crisis.

Below, we outline a number of detoxification strategies for cleansing the colon and liver and for eliminating parasites and yeast infections.

Colon-Cleansing Programs

Increased interest in colon health has led to a surge in the development of colon-cleansing programs. Most of these programs utilize a cleansing supplement in addition to recommending a basic dietary program. The supplements generally contain a combination of herbs, nutrients, enzymes, and toxin-absorbers designed to help remove the false lining in the colon and enhance digestion and absorption of food. Many of these supplements include ingredients that also cleanse the liver, gallbladder, and lymph.

A.M./P.M. Ultimate Cleanse™

A.M./P.M. Ultimate Cleanse is a cleansing program designed by Lindsey Duncan, C.N., of Santa Monica, California. The program includes two herbal and fiber formulas called Multi-Herb™ and Multi-Fiber™. The formulas are made from 29 cleansing herbs, amino acids, antioxidants, digestive enzymes, vitamins, and minerals, and five kinds of fiber. Both the Multi-Herb and Multi-Fiber formulas are taken in the morning and evening, in gradually increasing dosages for several weeks. The key to the effectiveness of the formula, Duncan explains, is that of timing: the morning formula stimulates while the evening formula relaxes. Duncan's formulas target not only the bowel, but the liver, lungs, skin, and lymph. "The goal is to stimulate, feed, and detoxify the complete internal body, not just the bowel," states Duncan. At the end of the program, a person should be having two to three bowel movements every day.

Nature's Pure Body Program™

Nature's Pure Body Program is made by the Pure Body Institute of Beverly Hills, California. The program relies on an herbal supplement that is a blend of 27 herbs specifically chosen for their ability to flush toxins out of the organs and old fecal matter from the intestines. The program consists of two sets of pills: colon and whole-body blends. Users start with one colon pill and three whole-body pills taken twice daily with water, 30 minutes before breakfast and 30 minutes before dinner. The colon pills can be increased to three pills twice daily (or more) until the bowels move twice daily. The whole-body pills are increased from three up to 4-7 taken two times daily. Users also need to increase their intake of pure water (at least 64 ounces daily), take one day off from the pills every

For information about **A.M./P.M. Ultimate Cleanse™**, contact: Nature's Secret, 4 Health Inc., 5485 Conestoga Court, Boulder, CO 80301; tel: 303-546-6306; fax: 303-546-6416. For **Nature's Pure Body Program™**, contact: Pure Body Institute of Beverly Hills, 423 East Ojai Avenue #107, Ojai, CA 93023; tel: 800-952-7873 or 805-653-5448; fax: 805-653-0373.

week, and take a daily multivitamin. The program is designed to last about 30 days. First-time users may find that three courses of the program are required for complete inner cleansing and detoxification.

Cleanse Thyself™: The Arise & Shine Program—Naturopath Richard Anderson, N.D., N.M.D., of Mt. Shasta, California, introduced the Cleanse Thyself colon-cleansing program in 1986. This four-phased program enables users to "clean your entire alimentary canal from your tongue to your stomach, to your organs, all the way down to your colon," says Dr. Anderson. Dr. Anderson recommends that the prospective user first test both saliva and urine for pH balance, using pH tester papers included in the kit. pH is the degree of acidity and alkalinity of a solution, measured on a scale of 1 (acidic) to 14 (alkaline).

The results of the pH test determine what level of the Cleanse Thyself program should be used, from the Mildest Phase to the Master Phase. The Mildest Phase of the Cleanse Thyself Program is designed for those whose bodies are weaker, chronically or severely ill, or elderly enough that they need a very gentle approach to cleansing, Dr. Anderson explains. "Persons who use the Mildest Phase generally show a severely over-acid condition (which can also appear as over-alkalinity) prior to preparing for cleansing. For such a person, the first step before beginning to cleanse must be to begin to alkalinize so that the body has enough resources to handle cleansing in a positive manner."

Those on the Mildest Phase start with a breakfast of fresh fruit, while their lunch and dinner should emphasize alkaline-forming foods, such as salad greens, raw vegetables, potatoes, and more fresh fruits. The user on this phase also consumes two Cleanse Thyself Shakes, consisting of liquid bentonite (a purifying clay), psyllium husk powder, and pure water. The Master Phase involves fasting from solid foods while taking the supplements along with fresh juices. "The Master Phase should only be attempted by persons whose bodies have already attained an adequate reservoir of electrolytes and strength to handle this powerful level of cleansing," says Dr. Anderson.

To soften and break up toxic waste material while detoxifying, the program provides two customized elements called Chomper and Herbal Nutrition. Chomper is an herbal laxative (in tablet form) containing plantain, *Cascara sagrada*, barberry, peppermint, sheep sorrel, fennel seed, ginger root, myrrh gum, red raspberry, rhubarb root, golden seal, and lobelia. Herbal Nutrition is a vitamin supplement (containing alfalfa, dandelion, shavegrass, chickweed, marshmallow root, yellow dock, rosehips,

For information about the **Cleanse Thyself™ program**, contact: Arise & Shine, 401 Berry Street, P.O. Box 1439, Mt. Shasta, CA 96067; tel: 916-926-0891 or 800-688-2444; fax: 916-926-8866.

hawthorne, licorice root, Irish moss, kelp, amylase, and cellulase) that helps strengthen and nourish the body during the detoxification process. Both Chomper and Herbal Nutrition are taken daily, says Dr. Anderson.

Each successive stage in the Cleanse Thyself program involves stricter dietary controls and a higher intake of program supplements and a correspondingly deeper cleansing. Typically, the overall cleansing program takes four weeks, in which three are devoted to the Pre-Cleanse, and one week for the Power or Master Phase. "What took months, years, or a lifetime to create cannot be cleaned up in a week's time," says Dr. Anderson.

It is common to have physical reactions to the colon cleansing process. These reactions may include headaches, vomiting, diarrhea, fatigue or dizziness. For all the discomfort, this is actually a sign that the process is working and that you are eliminating toxins from your body. If these symptoms occur, you may need to temporarily cutback on your cleansing procedure.

Enemas and Colonic Irrigations—Some health-care practitioners recommend using either an enema or colonic irrigation to augment a colon-cleansing program. Colon hydrotherapist Joyce Koleno of Cleveland, Ohio, says that colonics should be used at the very beginning of any colon cleansing program. An enema involves injecting water into the colon via a small plastic tube inserted into the rectum. The tube is attached to a compressible sack called an enema bag and generally about one cup to one quart of warm water is used. The water flushes out the lower portion of the colon. Because of the body's natural evacuation reflex, the fluids injected can't remain there very long—the bowel demands to be emptied promptly.

A colonic irrigation, also called a colonic or a "high enema," follows a similar procedure; however, it goes further and accomplishes more. A colonic irrigation moves water slowly through the entire length of the colon, so that the waste matter lining the walls of the intestine will soften and detach. To administer a colonic, therapists generally have their patients lie on a treatment table and a specially designed funnel, called a speculum, is inserted into the rectum. Several gallons of water flow in and out of the colon through the speculum and the attached tubing during the irrigation. The therapist monitors the temperature and pressure of the water and also massages the abdomen. A single treatment can take anywhere from 20-45 minutes.

For referrals to **trained colon therapists**, contact: International Association for Colon Hydrotherapy (I-ACT), 2204 N.W. Loop 410, San Antonio, TX 78230; tel: 210-266-2888. For information on **colema boards**, contact: Colema Boards of California, P.O. Box 1879, Cottonwood, CA 96022; tel: 916-347-5868 or 800-544-8147

The number and frequency of irrigation or enema treatments needed will vary, depending on the condition of the colon and the nature of the overall cleansing program. It's not unusual for some people to require anywhere from

6-18 treatments, which can be given daily or weekly. Your colon therapist should be a trained, licensed professional, though they need not be a doctor.

You can administer your own colonic irrigation, using a home colonic unit called a Colema Board. The principle and procedure is basically the same as that employed in a clinic, but the device is less high-tech, using a gravity-feed system to supply water rather than a mechanical pump; the unit is designed to fit over a standard toilet. To ensure that your irrigations are proceeding safely, it's always best to obtain guidance from a trained health-care professional.

Dietary Support for Your Colon—The foundation of any colon cleansing program must begin with a healthy diet and adequate intake of fiber and water. Your diet during a colon cleanse should be very high in fiber and fresh raw vegetables and fruits, and low in acid-forming foods that stimulate the intestines to secrete mucus. During the cleansing period, it is preferable to completely stop eating all milk products and all refined white flour products, such as pastas, breads, and baked goods, and eliminate all sugar. You should also reduce your intake of eggs, meat, chicken, most fish, nuts, seeds, and unsprouted beans and grains.

Fiber acts like a sponge, absorbing water as it goes through the stomach and the small intestine, and arrives in the colon full of moisture. Diets low in fiber cause fecal material to become dry and hard to expel, whereas a diet high in fiber will greatly reduce transit time. Fiber consists of the cell walls of plants and certain indigestible food residues. There are two basic types of fiber: soluble and insoluble. The insoluble fibers are found in wheat and corn bran, whole grains, nuts, legumes, and some vegetables; they increase fecal size and weight and promote regular bowel movements. However, insoluble fibers can also irritate the bowel, especially if it is already sensitive or inflamed. Soluble fibers are not irritating to the bowel. They are found in fruits and vegetables, oat bran, barley, beans, and peas. Ingesting foods containing these fibers stimulates bowel movements, decreases appetite, and leads to weight loss. One excellent source of fiber is powdered psyllium husk. This form of fiber is most often used for intestinal cleansing because of its superior ability to absorb moisture, lubricate the intestines, and "mop up" contaminants. Other good forms of fiber are flax seed, guar gum, and apple pectin.

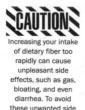

Increasing your intake of dietary fiber too rapidly can cause unpleasant side effects, such as gas, bloating, and even diarrhea. To avoid these unwanted side effects, increase fiber consumption gradually.

Soluble fiber requires copious amounts of water to carry it to the colon. Without sufficient water, the colon tries to extract every possible drop from the food we eat, which contributes to fecal matter becoming extremely dry and compacted. Adults need at least 8-10 cups of water daily, but few people drink that much. Other liquids, such as milk, coffee, tea, juice, and soda, are not substitutes for pure water. Even if your drink plenty of these other liquids, you need to consume 60-80 ounces of purified water daily.

Liver-Cleansing Programs
Appropriate cleansing treatments for the liver vary depending on the extent of the toxic overload. In general, mild toxicity can be corrected by consuming ample quantities of fresh fruit, vegetables, whole grains, and a limited amount of high-quality proteins. It is important to stop eating and drinking harmful substances, such as alcohol, caffeine, and unsaturated fats. Periodic liver-cleansing treatments can also help prevent an excess buildup of liver toxins. One of the hallmarks of natural medicine is attention to the condition of the internal organs, especially the liver and gallbladder. It is surprisingly easy to use herbs and nutrients to safely and effectively cleanse these organs. Many holistic practitioners, in fact, recommend such an organ cleansing on a yearly basis as a disease prevention and health maintenance strategy.

Flushing the Liver—"Liver flushes are used to stimulate the elimination of wastes from the body, to open and cool the liver, to increase bile flow, and to improve overall liver function," says Christopher Hobbs, L.Ac., herbalist and author of *Foundation of Health*. Here are his instructions for preparing and administering a liver flush·

1. Squeeze enough fresh lemons or limes to produce one cup of juice. Dilute with a small amount of distilled or spring water, if desired, but the more sour, the better it will perform as a liver cleanser. Orange and grapefruit juice may also be used, provided they are blended with some lemon or lime juice.

2. Add the juice of 1-2 cloves of garlic and a small amount of raw grated ginger juice. Grate the ginger on a cheese or vegetable grater and then press the shreds into a garlic press to get juice, or put a 1-2 inch piece of ginger root through the juicer.

3. Add one tablespoon of high quality, organic, extra virgin olive oil to the juice. Blend or shake all ingredients.

4. Take the drink in the morning and do not eat any food for one hour afterward.

5. After an hour has elapsed, drink two cups of an herbal blend that Dr. Hobbs calls "Polari Tea." To prepare Polari Tea, combine these dry herbs and simmer for 20 minutes: fennel (one part), flax (one part),

How to Administer the Coffee Enema

Here is the regimen generally recommended by health researcher Etienne Callebout, M.D., of London, England, for administering the coffee enema:

1) Add three tablespoons of ground organic coffee (not instant or decaffeinated) to two pints of distilled water. Boil for five minutes (uncovered) to burn off oils; then cover, lower heat, and simmer for an additional 15 minutes.

2) Strain and cool to body temperature. Lubricate rectal enema tube with K-Y Jelly or other lubricant. Hang enema bag above you, but not more than two feet from your body; the best level is approximately six inches above the intestines. Lying on your right side, draw both legs close to the abdomen.

3) Insert the tube several inches into rectum. Open the stopcock and allow fluid to run in very slowly to avoid cramping.

Breathe deeply and try to relax. Retain the solution for 12-15 minutes. If you have trouble retaining or taking the full amount, lower the bag; if you feel spasms, lower the bag to the floor to relieve the pressure. After about 20 seconds, slowly start raising the bucket toward the original level. You can also pinch the tube to control the flow.

4) With symptoms of toxicity, such as headaches, fever, nausea, intestinal spasm, and drowsiness, one may increase the frequency of enemas. Take in one to two pints each time for these conditions.

5) Upon waking the next morning, if you experience headaches and drowsiness, an additional enema is recommended that night. Eat a piece of fruit before the first coffee enema of the day to activate the upper digestive tract. Keep all equipment clean.

burdock ($\frac{1}{4}$ part), fenugreek (one part), and licorice ($\frac{1}{4}$ part). Then, add peppermint (one part) and steep for an additional ten minutes. For convenience, several quarts of Polari tea may be prepared in advance and refrigerated.

6. Do the flush for ten days, discontinue for three days, then resume for ten days—this is one cycle. Repeat for another cycle. Dr. Hobbs suggests doing the liver flush (two full cycles) twice yearly.

The Coffee Enema—The coffee enema, a therapy easily done at home, helps to purge the liver of accumulated toxins, dead cells, and waste products. The enema is prepared by brewing organic caffeinated coffee through a natural brown filter, letting it cool to body temperature, and delivering it via an enema bag. Coffee contains choleretics, substances which increase the flow of bile from the gallbladder.[25] Early research by Max Gerson, M.D., founder of the Gerson Institute, in Bonita, California, and originator of the Gerson Diet Therapy, established that a coffee enema is effective in stimulating the complex system of liver detoxification.[26]

Castor Oil Packs—Castor oil comes from the bean of the castor plant, *Oleum ricini*. The plant itself is quite poisonous, but the oil pressed out of the bean is safe to use, since the toxic constituents remain in the seeds. The Egyptians used castor oil as a laxative for cleansing the bowels and as a scalp rub to make hair grow and shine. Castor oil packs have been used for many conditions, including liver problems, constipation, and other ailments involving elimination, as well as non-malignant ovarian fibroid cysts and headaches.[27] The oil helps to draw out toxins, release tension, and improve blood circulation, especially in the lower abdomen.

Support During Liver Detoxification—Certain dietary recommendations will help support the liver during the detoxification process. Try to avoid fats from animal sources (meats and dairy) and limit the overall amount of animal foods you eat. Incorporate more chlorophyll-rich foods (particularly dark leafy greens) and raw vegetables into your diet. Artichokes, asparagus, celery, radishes, and beets are vegetables considered to have liver-cleansing properties. When the liver becomes toxic, more water is required to help flush impurities from the liver out through the kidneys. You should drink eight large glasses of pure water daily to bring your liver back to health; the best source for drinking water is distilled water.

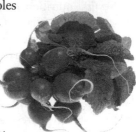

Certain herbs have a mild detoxifying effect on the liver. Taken regularly, these herbs can be used to prevent liver disease and maintain the health of this vital organ. Milk thistle (*Silybum marianum*) grows primarily in Europe, where it is often prescribed to treat and protect the liver. As far back as the 17th

Castor Oil Pack Instructions

1) Fold flannel sheet into three sections to fit over your whole abdomen.
2) Cut a piece of plastic one to two inches larger than flannel sheet.
3) Soak flannel sheet in gently heated castor oil. Fold it over and squeeze until some of the liquid oozes out. Unfold.
4) Prepare the surface where you will be lying. Place a large plastic sheet and an old towel over the surface to prevent staining.
5) Lie down on the towel and place the oil-soaked flannel sheet over your abdomen. Place fitted plastic piece over the flannel sheet. Apply a hot water bottle over the area.
6) Wrap towel under and around your torso.
7) Rest for one to two hours.
8) Wash your body with a solution of three tablespoons baking soda to one quart water to rinse off the oil.
9) Repeat as instructed by a physician.

For **herbal liver formulas** (available only to health-care professionals), contact: Apple-A-Day, 4201 Bee Caves Road, Suite C-212, Austin, TX 78746-6458; tel: 512-328-3996; fax: 512-328-0812.

century, this herb was known as "a friend to liver and blood." The active ingredient in milk thistle is silymarin, a substance that prevents inflammation and protects against the harmful effects of free radicals. It also stimulates liver cell growth and the production of bile. Milk thistle seeds can be used to make a tea or powdered seeds can be taken in capsule form. To make a tea, steep one teaspoon of seeds in $1/2$ cup of water; drink one to $1^1/2$ cups of tea daily. For the powdered form of milk thistle, take one capsule (approximately one teaspoon) with water five times per day.

"Dandelion root (*Taraxacum officinale*) is regarded as one of the finest liver remedies, both as food and as medicine," according to naturopaths Michael Murray, N.D., and Joseph Pizzorno, Jr., N.D., authors of *A Textbook of Natural Medicine*. The common dandelion has been used for centuries as a liver remedy and weight-loss aid. Its ability to stimulate the production and secretion of bile was first noted by researchers in 1875. Dandelion is also a potent diuretic, meaning it promotes the excretion of urine, which helps flush toxins from the body. Drs. Murray and Pizzorno typically suggest taking four grams of dried root (available in capsule form) or 4-8 ml of dandelion extract, three times daily.

Oregon grape root (*Berberis aquifolium*) is considered a gentle stimulant for the liver and gallbladder. It helps improve overall liver function as well as its detoxification processes. Because of its bitter taste, Oregon grape root is generally taken as a tea: mix one part Oregon grape root with one part dandelion root and $1/4$ part fennel seed.

Eliminating Yeast

Several nutritional supplements have been shown to be effective in treating candidiasis. Garlic, a well-known folk remedy, is now formulated as an odorless extract called allicin. Allicin is the active ingredient in garlic, and has been found to be more potent than many other anti-fungal agents; a typical recommended dose is 4,000 mcg daily (equal to about one clove of fresh garlic). As an alternative to the garlic extract, you can also take either liquid garlic (available at health food stores) or fresh garlic cloves.

Caprylic acid is a naturally occurring fatty acid found in coconut oil that has been shown to be an effective anti-fungal agent. In one study, patients taking 3,600 mg of caprylic acid daily for two weeks completely eliminated their *Candida*. Dr. Murray typically recommends a dosage of 1,000-2,000 mg daily, taken with meals. Since caprylic acid is readily absorbed into the system, it should be taken in an enteric-coated or sustained-release form so that it is absorbed in the small intestines rather than the stomach. Other fatty acids derived from olives (oleic acid) and castor beans have also been found to be useful for treating candidiasis.

Chlorophyll is an excellent liver purifier and healer that is also effective in reducing *Candida*. Naturopath Bernard Jensen, Ph.D., author of *Chlorella, Jewel of the Far East*, considers chlorella (a food algae) as the best source of chlorophyll. He indicates that chlorella can heal a toxic, mineral-deficient liver and soothe bowel tissue and stimulate bowel function; a typical dose is 100 mg of chlorella daily. Other sources of chlorophyll are barley juice, wheat grass juice, and spirulina (available at most health food stores).

Herbs are often used by alternative medicine practitioners to kill harmful yeasts and enhance immune function. They can be taken in teas, dried in capsules or tablets, or in suppository form. Dr. Murray recommends an anti-fungal agent consisting of a preparation of oregano, thyme, peppermint, and rosemary oils (0.2-0.4 ml twice daily between meals). Dr. Murray

> **⚠CAUTION⚠**
> Berberine-containing plants are generally non-toxic at recommended dosages, but high doses can interfere with vita-min-B metabolism. They are not recommended for use by pregnant women.

also recommends taking barberry (*Berberis vulgaris*) or Oregon grape (*Berberis aquifolium*). These herbs contain berberine, a natural antibiotic which acts against *Candida* overgrowth, normalizes intestinal flora, helps digestive problems, has antidiarrheal properties, and stimulates the immune system by increasing blood supply to the spleen. He usually recommends taking these herbs three times daily as a tea (2-4 g), tincture (6-12 ml), fluid extract (2-4 ml), or powdered solid (250-500 mg).

James Braly, M.D., recommends goldenseal root extract, standardized to 5% or more of its active ingredient (hydrastine), at a dose of 250 mg twice daily. In a recent study, goldenseal worked better in killing off *Candida* than other common anti-*Candida* therapies, according to Dr. Braly. Pau d'arco is another herb that has long been used to treat infections and intestinal complaints and is reportedly an analgesic, antiviral, diuretic, and fungicide. This South American herb, also known as taheebo, is often prepared as a tea. Other anti-fungal and antibacterial herbs used to treat candidiasis include German

---

For information about **SuperGarlic 3X** (an allicin formula), contact: Metagenics, Inc., 971 Calle Negocio, San Clemente, CA 92673; tel: 800-877-1703; fax: 949-366-0818. For **Caprylate Complex** (caprylic acid), contact: Progressive Labs, 1907 N. Britain Road, Irving, TX 75061; tel: 800-527-9512. For information on **Candimycin** (oregano, thyme, peppermint, and rosemary oils), contact: PhytoPharmica, P.O. Box 1745, Green Bay,WI54305; tel: 800-376-7889 or 920-469-9099; fax: 920-469-4418. For **ADP** (another preparation of oregano, thyme, peppermint, and rosemary oils), contact: Biotics Research, P.O. Box 36888, Houston, TX 77236; tel: 800-231-5777; fax: 281-240-2304. For **Triple Yeast Defense,** a formula containing pau d'arco and grapefruit seed extract, contact:Imhotep, Inc., P.O. Box 183, Main Street, Ruby, NY 12475; tel: 800-677-8577; fax: 914-336-5446.

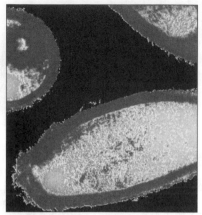

Friendly bacteria, or probiotics, refer to beneficial microbes inhabiting the human gastrointestinal tract where they are essential for proper nutrient assimilation. The human body contains an estimated several trillion beneficial bacteria comprising over 400 species, all necessary for health. Among the more well-known of these are *Lactobacillus acidophilus* (pictured here) and *Bifidobacterium bifidum*. Overly acidic bodily conditions, chronic constipation or diarrhea, dietary imbalances, consumption of highly processed foods, and the excessive use of antibiotics and hormonal drugs can interfere with probiotic function and even reduce the number of these microbes, setting up conditions for illness.

For more information about **FOS and NutraFlora**, contact: Nutrition Company, 1400 W. 122nd Avenue, Suite 110, Westminster, CO 80234; tel: 303-254-8012; fax: 303-254-8201. For **UltraFlora Plus and Probioplex**, two FOS supplements distributed by Metagenics APN, 4403 Vineland Road, Suite B10, Orlando, FL 32811; tel: 800-647-6100.

chamomile, ginger, cinnamon, rosemary, licorice, and gentian.

Probiotics—A healthy growth of "friendly" bacteria in the intestines—particularly *L. acidophilus* and *B. bifidum*—is the best defense against yeast infections. Cabbage is one of the best food sources of friendly bacteria; eat it raw or juice it daily. Other foods that can help revitalize the colon and encourage the growth of normal bacteria include rice protein, chicory, onions, garlic, asparagus, and bananas. *B. bifidum* is also found in yogurt and kefir (a fermented milk drink). Another way to repopulate the intestines with friendly bacteria is to take a probiotic supplement, particularly one containing *L. acidophilus* and *B. bifidum*.

Another useful supplement is FOS (fructo-oligosaccharide), a sugar that specifically encourages friendly bacteria to multiply. FOS acts like an intestinal "fertilizer," selectively feeding the healthy microflora in the large intestine so that their numbers can usefully increase. FOS is found in small amounts in garlic, honey, Jerusalem artichokes, soybeans, burdock, chicory root, asparagus, banana, rye, barley, tomato, onions, and triticale. NutraFlora®, a FOS supplement found in most health food stores, contains 95% pure FOS to be used as a dietary supplement.

Ayurvedic Medicine—Ayurvedic medicine considers candidiasis to be a condition caused by *ama*, the improper digestion of foods, according to Virender Sodhi, M.D.

Virender Sodhi, M.D., N.D.: 2115 112th Avenue NE, Bellevue, WA 98004; tel: 425-453-8022; fax: 425-451-2670.

(Ayurveda), N.D., of Bellevue, Washington. As do other alternative physicians, Dr. Sodhi attributes this malfunction, and thus candidiasis, to the widespread use of antibiotics, birth-control pills and hormones, environmental stress, and society's addiction to sugar in the diet. "Ayurvedic medicine believes that these stresses on the system cause carbohydrates to be digested improperly," he says. "Furthermore, the immune system in the gut becomes worn down."

To address the *Candida* overgrowth and bolster immunity, Dr. Sodhi uses grapefruit seed oil and tannic acid, which act as anti-fungals and antibiotics, while *L. acidophilus* helps restore the balance of friendly bacteria in the intestines. Long pepper, ginger, cayenne, and the Ayurvedic herbs trikatu and neem taken 30 minutes before meals increase immune and digestive functions. He further recommends that his patients cleanse toxins from their systems using the *panchakarma* program, which involves herbs and dietary modification (see "Ayurvedic Detoxification," p. 113). With Dr. Sodhi's approach, candidiasis can usually be eliminated in four to six months.

Eradicating Parasites

Like other toxins, parasites can make it harder for the liver, kidneys, and intestines to detoxify and eliminate wastes from the body. If testing

Ayurvedic Detoxification

Ayurveda is the traditional medicine of India, based on many centuries of empirical use. Its name means "end of the Vedas" (which were India's sacred texts), implying that a holistic medicine may be founded on spiritual principles. Ayurveda describes three metabolic, constitutional, and body types (*doshas*), in association with the basic elements of Nature in combination. These are *vata* (air and ether, rooted in intestines), *pitta* (fire and water/stomach), and *kapha* (water and earth/lungs).

An ayurvedic procedure called *panchakarma* can be used for sleeping disorders where the body is in a toxic state and in need of cleansing. *Panchakarma* is often very effective in pacifying and calming the body because it assists in cleansing the intestines, and, by transference, the mind, leading to restful sleep.

Panchakarma actually is a series of treatments that includes massage with medicated herbs (*abhyanga*) and *shirodhara*, a treatment involving dripping oil on the forehead. *Panchakarma* can be done five to seven days in a row, two or more hours a day, or every other day. In addition to the massage and warm oil drip, it can include: *nasya*, a nasal administration of herbs in which drops of medicated oils are placed in the sinuses; *basti*, herbalized oil enemas that are injected into the colon with a catheter and syringe; *swedna*, a steam treatment with herbs designed to open up and detoxify the body through sweating; and *vrechanana*, a purgation.

reveals that you have a parasitic infection, you may want to consider taking the following practical steps, recommended by William Lee Cowden, M.D., of Richardson, Texas, to rid your system of parasites.

1) Cleanse the Intestines: Parasites tend to embed themselves in the intestinal wall, but over the course of several weeks, you can flush them out by using some of these natural substances (preferably in combination): psyllium husks, agar-agar, citrus pectin, papaya extract, pumpkin seeds, flaxseeds, comfrey root, beet root, and bentonite clay (take bentonite only in combination with another substance, such as psyllium). You might also take extra vitamin C (minimum 2 g daily, but higher amounts up to individual bowel tolerance are more useful) to help flush out your intestines. Note, however, that vitamin C taken at the same time as wormwood (below) renders wormwood ineffective.

2) Do a Colon Irrigation: Irrigate the colon with 2-16 quarts of water via enema. To the water you may add black walnut tincture or extract, garlic juice, vinegar (two tablespoons per quart of water), blackstrap molasses (one tablespoon per quart of water), or organically grown coffee. Use filtered or distilled water for the enema; further sterilize it by boiling or ozonating it for 10-15 minutes before use, including before using it to prepare the coffee.

3) Prepare Your System: It is prudent to give your gallbladder and liver a week to prepare for the parasite program. To flush the gallbladder of its toxins, take lime juice in warm water or Swedish Bitters before each meal. Eliminate all refined and natural sugars, meats, and dairy products during the parasite program; even better, start cutting back on them during this preparatory week. Take barberry bark capsules, dandelion, or similar herbal extract to help cleanse the liver. The amount depends on health and the strength or composition of the specific substance or product used.

4) The Herbal Cleanout: Naturopathic physician Hulda Regehr Clark, N.D., Ph.D., recommends using a blend of three herbs to flush the parasites out of your system: black walnut hull tincture, wormwood capsules, and fresh ground cloves (to kill the parasites' eggs).

Dietary and Herbal Support—If you suspect a parasitic infection, you should eliminate all uncooked foods from your diet and cook all meats until well done; soak both organic and inorganic vegetables in salted water (one tablespoon per five cups) for a minimum of 30 minutes before cooking. It is also advisable to eliminate coffee, all sugars including fruits and honey, and all milk and dairy products, with the possible exception of raw goat's milk. Raw goat's milk contains secretory IgA and IgG immunoglobulins, types of antibodies that help strengthen the immune system. According to naturopath Steven Bailey, N.D., of Portland, Oregon, IgA and IgG are helpful in the treatment of parasites.

Gittleman says that the best diet for a parasite infection is one that "supports the host and starves the parasite." Specifically, she recommends against eating any sugar, white flour, or processed foods (such as prepackaged snack foods). Once inside the body, these foods provide ideal conditions for parasites to breed. She has found that a diet composed of 25% fat, 25% protein, and 50% complex carbohydrates (a type of starch found in vegetables and whole grains) is best for people with parasite infections. Gittleman also advises limiting your intake of raw fruits and vegetables; instead, cook both fruits and vegetables. Sufficient levels of vitamin A are particularly important for preventing parasites, as this vitamin seems to increase resistance to penetration by larvae. Good dietary sources of vitamin A include properly cooked carrots, sweet potatoes, squash, and salad greens. A combination formula of digestive enzymes, taken between meals, may also be helpful for eliminating parasite larvae or eggs in the intestines.

Certain foods are anti-parasitic, according to Gittleman, and you should incorporate more of these foods in your diet. These include pineapple and papaya, either as fresh juice or in supplement form, eaten in combination with pepsin (a stomach enzyme) and betaine hydrochloric acid (a supplement form of stomach acid). Avoid all meats and dairy products for at least one week at the beginning of therapy. You can also use pomegranate juice (four 8-ounce glasses daily), papaya seeds, fresh figs, finely ground pumpkin seeds ($^1/_4$ cup to $^1/_2$ cup daily), or two cloves of raw garlic daily. Because pomegranate juice can irritate the intestines, you should not drink it for more than four to five days at a time. Other anti-parasitic foods include onions, kelp, blackberries, raw cabbage, and ground almonds.

Herbal remedies have been used effectively for centuries for the treatment of parasitic infections. These remedies can

For more on **herbal parasite formulas**, contact: Uni Key Health Systems, P.O. Box 7168, Bozeman, MT 59771; tel: 406-586-9424 or 800-888-4353. Allergy Research Group, 400 Preda Street, San Leandro, CA 94577; tel: 800-545-9960 or 510-639-4572; fax: 510-635-6730. Thorne Research, Inc., P.O. Box 25, Dover, ID 83825; tel: 800-228-1966 or 208-263-1337; fax: 208-265-2488. Tyler Encapsulations, 2204-8 N.W. Birdsdale, Gresham, OR 97030; tel: 800-869-9705 or 503-661-5401; fax: 503-666-4913.

How Chinese Medicine Views Insomnia

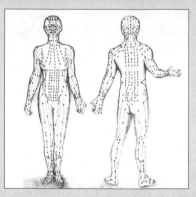

In conventional Western medicine, two insomniacs who come to a physician with the same complaint—restless sleep—in all likelihood would leave the physician's office with the same prescription for the same sleeping pills. In traditional Chinese medicine, however, the practitioner might look at one person and determine her restless sleep is caused by a deficiency of heart yin energy, for example. For that person, the practitioner would prescribe heart- and yin-strengthening herbs and heart- and yin-tonifying acupuncture points as well as lifestyle changes such as improved diet, exercises, and meditation. For another person, the practitioner might see his restless sleep is caused by an excess in liver yang energy, and would prescribe herbs and points that calm the liver as well as the lifestyle changes tailored for his overactive stress level.

While that type of customized diagnosis may be complex, the basic premise of Chinese medicine is very simple. The underlying cause of an illness or condition is always the same: an imbalance in the person's energy field. It's the practitioner's job to determine what part of the energy field is out of balance and which organ systems are affected. Roger Jahnke, O.M.D., an acupuncturist and herbalist in Santa Barbara, California, says the concept of the human being as an energy field is essential to an understanding of how Chinese medicine works.

Once a Chinese medicine practitioner has determined where a person's energy is out of balance, they can suggest acupuncture treatments. Acupuncture and herbal therapy are the main tools Chinese medicine practitioners have been using for more than 5,000 years. The procedure involves the insertion of slender, sterilized, solid needles into the body at specific points on 12 different energy pathways called meridians or channels. The channels are associated with organ systems of the body, such as the kidney channel, liver channel or stomach channel. Chinese scientists have also found acupuncture can affect blood sugar

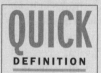

DEFINITION

Traditional Chinese medicine (TCM) originated in China over 5,000 years ago and is a comprehensive system of medical practice that heals the body according to the principles of nature and balance. A Chinese medicine physician considers the flow of vital energy (*qi*) in a patient through close examination of the patient's pulses, tongue, body odor, voice tone and strength, and general demeanor, among other elements. Underlying imbalances and disharmony in the body are described in terminology analogous to the natural world (heat, cold, dryness, or dampness). The concept of balance, or the interrelationship of organs, is central to TCM.

and cholesterol levels, gastrointestinal function, and immune system activity. American researchers have found evidence that acupuncture releases the body's own anti-inflammatory agents, as well as sending pain-blocking signals to the spinal cord.

Specific treatments for insomnia will vary greatly, depending on both the patient and on the practitioner. The acupuncturist will want to know, for example, if you have trouble falling asleep or staying asleep. People who can't fall asleep may be deficient in blood energy, whereas the person who wakes up during the night could be deficient in yin energy. Another common question is what time you wake up during the night. Chinese medicine recognizes an organ time clock—two-hour time periods in which certain organ systems are more active. If you always wake up at 1:30 a.m., for example, you're in liver time (1 a.m. to 3 a.m.), which could mean you have an

To **locate a TCM practitioner**, contact: National Certification Commission for Acupuncture and Oriental Medicine (NCCAOM), 11 Canal Center Plaza, Suite 300, Alexandria, VA 22314; tel: 703-548-9004; fax: 703-548-9079. American Association of Acupuncture and Oriental Medicine, 4101 Lake Boone Trail, Suite 201, Raleigh, NC 27607; tel: 919-787-5181.

imbalance in your Liver channel.

Acupuncturist Giovanni Maciocia, a noted author of several textbooks on Chinese medicine, says there are at least four main excess, or full, patterns of insomnia and at least five main deficient, or empty, patterns. In the excess patterns, one of the body's energy systems, such as liver fire (fire is a yang energy) or heart fire, is overactive. In the deficient patterns, one or more of the energy systems, such as spleen, blood, kidney, heart, or liver yin, is weak and not doing its job. Each of those nine main patterns requires a different set of acupuncture points and a different herbal formula.[28]

Dr. Jahnke tends to look at insomnia as mainly a deficiency of yin— whether in the kidneys, the liver, or the heart. Most of the insomnia cases Dr. Jahnke sees are from yin deficiencies, although he does see some people with insomnia caused by digestive problems.

also help prevent a parasitic infection when water or food conditions are questionable. According to Dr. Galland, it is advisable to continue any treatment regimen until at least two parasite tests, performed one month apart on purged stool specimens, are negative.

■ Citrus Seed Extract—Citrus seed extract is highly active against protozoa, bacteria, and yeast, and has long been used in the treatment of parasitic infections. It is not absorbed into the tissue, is nontoxic and generally hypoallergenic, and can be administered for up to several months, a length of time which may be required to eliminate *Giardia* and the candidiasis that often accompanies it.

■ *Artemisia annua*—This is an herbal remedy of Chinese origin. Its antiprotozoal activity is especially effective against *Giardia*, but some caution is advisable—it can initially cause a worsening of symptoms, allergic reactions, and some intestinal irritation. *Artemisia annua* is often prescribed by Dr. Galland, along with citrus seed extract. It may be used with additional herbs known for their antiparasitic activity and can also be used in conjunction with conventional drug therapy.

■ *Artemisia absinthium*—This is one of the oldest European medicinal plants. Known as "wormwood," it was highly prized by Hippocrates and is similar to the *Artemisia annua* of Chinese herbal tradition. *Artemisia absinthium* taken alone can be toxic, though, and therefore should be used in combination with other herbs to nullify its toxicity.

Traditional Chinese Medicine—In traditional Chinese medicine, Chinese herbs are the primary treatment for parasites and the type used depends on the location of the parasites in the body, according to Maoshing Ni, D.O.M., Ph.D., L.Ac., of Yo San University of Traditional Chinese Medicine, in Santa Monica, California. For intestinal parasites purgative herbs are usually used. Pumpkin and quisqualis seeds are two common remedies. The pumpkin seeds are eaten raw, while the quisqualis seeds are usually roasted. Both are taken every morning on an empty stomach, approximately 10-12 seeds of each, for about two weeks. "Quisqualis and pumpkin seeds are mild and safe enough for adults and children to take daily as a preventative measure as well," says Dr. Ni.

Meliae seeds are much stronger than either pumpkin or quisqualis and should only be taken in more severe cases. The meliae seeds paralyze the parasites for approximately eight hours, allowing the body to eliminate them through the bowels. Betel nut is another typical treatment for intestinal parasites. The nut is chewed raw like chewing tobacco. "It can give a certain sense of euphoria, too, because it is slightly toxic," says Dr. Ni. "This is negligible, but some people might get diarrhea." Depending on the type of parasite, they may be able to get through the intestinal walls and into the bloodstream. "In situations like this you have to use some very strong antibiotic-like herbs," says Dr. Ni, "such as goldenseal and coptidis which are antiparasitic as well." While eliminating the parasites with herbs, Dr. Ni also strengthens the immune system in order to get at the underlying cause of the parasitic infestation. He reports that nutrition and herbs such as ginseng, ligustri berries, and schisandra berries can accomplish this. He has good success with his three-month treatment program addressing both components.

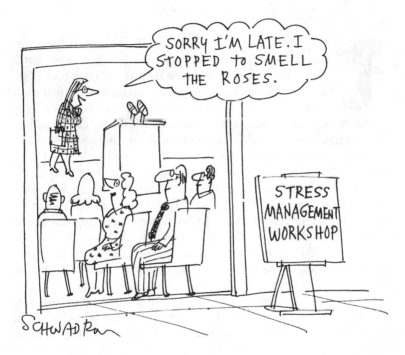

5 Resetting the Body Clock

THE BODY CLOCK and circadian rhythms primarily determine our sleep/wake patterns. When the body's pacemaker and sleep cycle are thrown off course—by factors both in and out of your control—sleep problems ensue. Sleep-onset insomnia, advanced and delayed sleep phase syndromes, and even REM behavior disorder can be caused by disrupted circadian rhythms and melatonin imbalances. While not a sleep problem per se, seasonal affective disorder (SAD), or the "winter blues," is also an outgrowth of a confused body clock.

Trappings of our modern lives generally cause sleep-wake rhythm disruptions. Shift work and traveling across time zones set up the body for sleep problems. Other factors, including inadequate exposure to light, improper diet, pharmaceutical drugs, electromagnetic fields, and stress, can impair the pineal gland's ability to produce the sleep-inducing hormone melatonin, drastically altering sleep patterns.

Circadian sleep problems are reversible if you take steps to reset, or entrain, your body clock to follow a new schedule. Light therapy, chronotherapy, and magnet therapy are proven alternative therapies for circadian disruption. Melatonin supplementation, diet modification, exercise, stress management, and good sleep hygiene can also alleviate many sleep disorders. While avoidance of the practices that disturb the body clock is the best way to prevent recurrence of sleep problems, even shift workers and frequent flyers can use these therapies to their advantage and may enjoy deep, restorative sleep.

In This Chapter

- Free-Running and Entrained Circadian Rhythms

- Factors That Disrupt Sleep/Wake Rhythms

- Alternative Theraples to Reset Your Body Clock

- Beating the Winter Blues

Free-Running and Entrained Circadian Rhythms

To comprehend how disruptions in circadian rhythms can cause sleep disorders, it's important to understand how our body clocks keep time. As described in Chapter 1, bundles of nerves in the hypothalamus called the suprachiasmatic nuclei (SCN) measure the passage of time. The SCN also transmits light signals from the optic nerves to various organs along the nervous system, including the pineal gland. Light signals suppress the pineal gland's secretion of the sleep-inducing hormone melatonin into the bloodstream; darkness activates the process. Melatonin receptors have been found on SCN cells, leading researchers to speculate that the SCN's functions are to some degree regulated by melatonin. Together, melatonin and the SCN appear to guide our circadian rhythms, natural cycles governing fluctuations in body temperature, hormone release, and sleep/wake patterns (see "The Circadian Rhythms of the Body," p. 122).

Alternative Therapies to Reset Your Body Clock

- Lifestyle Modifications
- Light Therapy
- Chronotherapy
- Magnet Therapy
- Melatonin Supplements

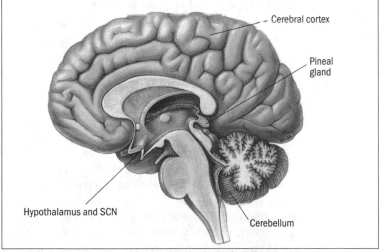

Cerebral cortex

Pineal gland

Hypothalamus and SCN

Cerebellum

Parts of the brain involved in the body clock or circadian rhythms.

The Circadian Rhythms of the Body

Sleep/wake patterns are not the only type of bodily function recurring according to circadian rhythms. Body temperature and hormone levels also fluctuate throughout the day and, for the most part, correspond directly or indirectly to sleep/wake patterns. For instance, during the daytime wakeful period, the blood levels of the hormone melatonin are low while body temperature is high; during sleep phases, melatonin is high—spiking at around 3 a.m. then declining rapidly—but body temperature is low, down approximately 1.5° F from daytime peak levels. Human growth hormone levels are very low during the waking hours, but rise during sleep, spiking usually in the first two hours. It's important to note that reducing body temperature will not induce secretion of melatonin or sleep.[1] On the contrary, raising the body temperature is correlated with an increase in melatonin and may provide therapeutic benefits for people with sleep problems (see "Take a Hot Bath for a Good Night's Sleep," p. 134).

Cortisol, a naturally occurring adrenal hormone also produced during the stress response, has a different cycle. Levels of this hormone start off very high in the morning waking hours, declining over the course of the day, reaching a low midway through sleep, and then spiking around 5 a.m. or approximately an hour before awakening. When stress disrupts cortisol's circadian rhythms, especially at night, cortisol levels become elevated when they are normally low. This shift can have profound effects on sleep/wake patterns and potentially cause sleep disturbances.

Circadian means "around a day," and indeed humans' circadian rhythms repeat approximately every 24 hours. But our body clocks do not naturally follow the sun's 24-hour day. Several experiments have been conducted to test the innate length of circadian rhythms. In these tests, the lab environments (ranging from caves in the Swiss Alps to a hospital in the Bronx) were strictly controlled so that all time cues (*zeitgeber*, or "time-giver" in German)—the sun's rising and setting, clocks, TVs and radios, men's five-o'clock shadows and, in some studies, electromagnetic fields—were eradicated. Researchers discovered that, freed from the constraints of 24-hour time cues, the human biological clock runs according to a 25-hour day. At the beginning of the Bronx test, subjects were sent to bed at 11 p.m. and awakened around 8 a.m. for 20 days. At the end of this time, the subjects were allowed to decide their own sleeping schedules. At first the subjects voluntarily went to sleep at 11 p.m. and arose at 8 a.m., but as the days progressed, they started sleeping an hour later each subsequent night, awakening an hour later each morning (midnight and 9 a.m.; 1 a.m. and 10 a.m., etc.). Weeks into the *zeitgeber*-deprived test, subjects were falling asleep at 4 p.m. and waking up at midnight, ready for breakfast.[2]

These findings proved that the free-running (without time cues) biological clock measures 25-hour days and that the sleep/wake circadian rhythms likewise follow 25-hour cycles. A recently discovered gene called the "Clock gene" may be responsible for the free-running instinct. It's believed that this genetic predisposition makes us more adaptable to seasonal changes (although some of us do suffer from physiological and psychological problems during seasonal changes—see "Beating the Winter Blues," p. 143).

These and other studies elucidate the power and function of *zeitgebers*—showing how we use light and other environmental cues to live and sleep by the sun's 24-hour cycle. At the same time, our circadian adaptability makes us extremely susceptible to *zeitgebers*. Normally time and light cues reset, or entrain, our body clocks to run by the sun's 24-hour cycle, an adjustment that our clocks and circadian rhythms generally adapt to easily. In fact, our body clocks and circadian rhythms can be reset about two hours each day—allowing us to perform normally on 23-hour or 27-hour schedules.

However, when we drastically change work schedules, travel across time zones, or are chronically exposed to inadequate light, electromagnetic fields, and other factors, our normal temporal cues vanish or become erratic, confusing our body clocks. This situation is called *internal desynchronization*. Internal desynchronization ultimately disrupts the timing and duration of melatonin secretion, leading to sleep/wake rhythm disturbances such as insomnia, advanced or delayed sleep phase syndromes, and REM behavior disorders, as well as seasonal affective disorder.

Factors That Disrupt Sleep/Wake Rhythms

As discussed above, traveling across time zones and shift work can disrupt circadian sleep/wake rhythms, but so can other factors that alter our levels of melatonin. Improper exposure to light—whether too little in the day or too much at night—is a predominate cause of melatonin imbalances. Extremely low frequency electromagnetic fields, emotional stress, some medications, and poor diet can also impair melatonin secretion.

Traveling Across Time Zones

If you've ever traveled by plane across time zones—for instance, from San Francisco to New York or New York to Paris—more than likely you've experienced jet lag. This condition is characterized by fatigue, irritability, difficulty in concentration, and an inability to sleep at the local bedtime. Flying across times zones can drastically disorient your circadian rhythms, because the temporal cues (light/dark) of the destination are not synchronized with your own.

Jet lag only occurs following airplane travel, and only when traveling east–west or west–east. Were you to walk or even drive from San Francisco to New York, the transit time would be slow enough for you to gradually adjust to new time zones and *zeitgebers*. And should you fly from New York City to Lima, Peru, you may be uncomfortable or restless during the long flight, but your sleep rhythms would be unaffected because you'd remain in the same time zone.

West–east travel affects sleep more adversely than east–west, and the more eastern time zones you cross, the more difficult it will be to adjust to the local time and sleep patterns. Suppose you leave San Francisco at 7 a.m. on a nonstop flight bound for New York. The flight takes approximately five hours and you land at noon, which is 3 p.m. in New York. During the course of the day, you will likely feel more alert than New Yorkers, but by local bedtime of 10 p.m., your body clock will think it's 7 p.m. Try as you may, you will likely have a difficult time falling asleep this early in your sleep/wake rhythms— even though darkness has fallen and other environmental cues indicate it's bedtime. You will probably also have trouble awakening at local morning time of 7 a.m., even though it's light outside, as it will feel like 4 a.m.—when your circadian rhythms are at their deepest sleep phase.

Research shows that, without intervention, it takes a little less than a day for each time zone crossed to entrain your body clock to the new time schedule.[3] Therefore, it will take approximately two days to adapt to New York time. Flying from New York to Paris, a ten-hour flight, will entail crossing five time zones. Thus, your circadian rhythms will act as if it's 5 p.m. when it is 10 p.m. local time. And it will take about four days before you feel comfortable with the Parisian time and sleep patterns. Meanwhile, mental function will be impaired due to sleep deprivations—and safety is a special concern for airline pilots and others adversely affected by jet lag.

East–west travel usually presents fewer disruptions to sleep/wake patterns. If you leave from New York at 7 a.m. local time on a five-hour nonstop flight, you'll arrive to San Francisco at noon New York time, which is 9 a.m. in San Francisco. You may feel more tired that night and go to bed earlier than your San Francisco counterparts, and awaken earlier the next morning, but in general your sleep will be only minimally and briefly affected, because synchronizing to the new time and light cues won't require advancing your circadian rhythms. As our internal clocks are genetically predisposed to 25-hour days, delays in phase shift are easier to accommodate than are abbreviations.

Shift Work

Approximately 25 million Americans work regular or rotating hours outside the 9-to-5 daytime schedule.[4] These include hospital employees, industrial plant workers, and security personnel. As our society demands more around-the-clock services, financial institutions, photocopy shops, supermarkets, and communications companies have also established round-the-clock shifts. Sleep researchers, ironically, also are among this population. While nonstop work increases productivity and provides conveniences for the rest of us, shift work is a burden for circadian rhythms. Studies indicate that 62% of shift workers suffer from sleep/wake disturbances, compared with 20% of daytime workers.[5] Sleep deprivation can have numerous detrimental consequences to personal health and safety, including poor mental performance, tension, fatigue, and gastrointestinal and cardiovascular problems. An estimated 15% of newly hired shift workers develop gastrointestinal problems.[6]

In the 1880s, the invention of the light bulb allowed factories to operate 24 hours a day, seven days a week. Until that time, the duration of daylight determined work schedules—approximately 14 hours during the summer and 11 during the winter. But with the advent of artificial light, industrial plants imposed shift work, in which two or three sets of workers would rotate around the clock, keeping production at a consistent pace. Today, three shifts are common—day (8 a.m. to 5 p.m.), swing (4 p.m. to 1 a.m.), and graveyard (midnight to 9 a.m.). Some shift workers maintain a regular schedule, while others may rotate, going from several days or weeks of day shift, for instance, to a period of evening shift, then a period of graveyard shift, with days off interspersed.

The fundamental problem with shift work is that it requires the individual to disregard circadian rhythms and temporal cues. Whereas in cases of jet lag, travelers can ultimately reset their body clocks to synchronize with the local sunrise and sunset, night- and rotating-shift workers are expected to function contrary to natural cycles. For instance, up to ten million Americans are at work between 3 a.m. and 5 a.m.[7] This is the sleepiest time for most people, when melatonin levels are high, muscles are relaxed, and body temperature is low—the body clock is urging you to sleep. This is also the time of night when many accidents occur on the job.

When night workers go home in the morning, the sunlight suppresses melatonin production and the circadian rhythms enter the alert phase. As a result, many night-shift workers suffer from sleep-onset and sleep-maintenance insomnia. In fact, most night workers sleep only five or six hours a day, and are chronically sleep-deprived.[8]

Rotating-shift workers may experience even more frequent and severe sleep and associated health problems. The most debilitating rotation schedules are those that run counterclockwise—for example, night then evening then day, or day then night then evening, with days off in between. These schedules require the person to constantly advance their sleep/wake phases. Since we innately run on a longer, 25-hour time schedule, advancing phases by up to eight hours during any given week causes serious circadian disturbances. Animal studies have found that weekly drastic (12-hour) changes in light/dark patterns (the equivalent of weekly rotating day and night shifts) reduces life span by 11%.[9] Human studies indicate that counterclockwise shift rotation increases the likelihood of coronary heart disease. Less disruptive rotation schedules are those that run clockwise (day, evening, night).

All of these problems are further exacerbated by the fact that on weekends or days off, shift workers tend to re-synchronize their sleep/wake rhythms with *zeitgebers*, sleeping at night and rising in the morning. Resuming shift schedules often intensifies the sleep/wake disturbances.

Light—Too Little or Too Much

As we've seen in the case of night-shift workers, light plays a crucial role in determining our sleep/wake patterns. This is due to the interplay between ambient light and the pineal gland. In Chapter 1, we described how the suprachiasmatic nuclei—the circadian pacemaker in the hypothalamus—send outside light signals via the nervous system to the pineal gland, the primary producer of the hormone melatonin (the gastrointestinal system also secretes some melatonin). The pineal gland needs darkness to produce melatonin, because light deactivates certain enzymes necessary for converting serotonin into melatonin.[10] Several studies have shown that melatonin production significantly drops or is completely inhibited by inadequate exposure to natural bright light during the day and also by excessive exposure to artificial bright light at night. Both factors can cause sleep-onset insomnia as well as seasonal affective disorder.

To review **how the pineal gland produces melatonin**, see Chapter 1, The Basics of Sleep, pp. 14-33.

Americans spend the vast majority of their time indoors, usually in windowless cubicles and energy-efficient homes under low-intensity artificial lights. A 1994 study found that middle-class, middle-aged adults in San Diego, California, spend 4% of their time outdoors—most of that time in their cars.[11] It's likely that people who live in less sunny climates spend more time indoors. Night-shift workers are worse off, spending only 2.6% of their time outdoors.[12] It's estimated that the majority of people are exposed to light levels of less than 100 lux (a measurement of light intensity) for much of the day.[13] One hundred lux is the amount of light that would enter your eyes if you were looking at a 100-watt bulb from a distance of five feet in an otherwise dark room. Ordinary fluorescent lights may emit 400 lux, while a room lit by sunlight can be up to 3,000 lux. On a clear summer day, the light outside can be up to 100,000 lux; even on gloomy, stormy days, outdoor light is rarely below 500 lux.[14]

The lack of exposure to bright sunlight—or at least high-intensity artificial (full spectrum) lights—is associated with diminished nocturnal melatonin production. This may be due to the reduced daytime levels of serotonin. Studies indicate that people subject to typical amounts of indoor light have lower serotonin levels than those exposed to bright sunlight.[15] It appears that the enzymatic process of converting the amino acid tryptophan into serotonin requires light, just as the conversion from serotonin into melatonin requires darkness. Less serotonin produced during the day means less melatonin made at night. This correlates with sleep-onset insomnia. In one study, night-shift workers who were not exposed to sunlight or full-spectrum light between 600 lux and 900 lux experienced lower melatonin secretion levels and a longer sleep latency time than those who were exposed to bright light.[16] Interestingly, 90% of blind people frequently suffer from insomnia, probably due to their inability to receive light signals.[17]

Testing for Melatonin Levels

In diagnosing and reviewing your sleep problems, your doctor may test for melatonin levels at different times of the day. This is usually done by analyzing urine or blood samples with a radioimmunoassay (RIA). This test measures the minute amounts of melatonin excreted in the urine or circulating in the blood. Melatonin is present in the body in picograms, or trillionths of a gram. Since each person's levels of melatonin vary, it's difficult to assess "normal" values. However, if your melatonin levels are significantly lower than expected during the sleep phases, this can indicate that various lifestyle or dietary factors may be impairing the pineal gland's ability to convert melatonin. In this case, your doctor may recommend melatonin supplementation and other therapies.

Light, Melatonin, and the Elderly

For reasons still being researched, the elderly produce very low levels of melatonin, and suffer a corresponding increase in insomnia, advanced sleep phase syndrome, and other sleep disorders. Some sleep researchers speculate that this is caused by neurochemical alterations of the suprachiasmatic nuclei (SCN) that occur during the aging process.[23] Other researchers believe pineal gland calcification or a more sedentary lifestyle leads to disruptions in sleep/wake patterns. However, recent studies suggest that a deficiency of sunlight contributes to depleted melatonin levels in older people.

One study compared melatonin levels of elderly subjects who lived independently and were exposed to more bright sunlight to the melatonin levels of elderly patients who lived in nursing homes and were less likely to have outdoor activity. Based on these findings, the researchers suggest that a lack of exposure to bright light may lead to reduction of melatonin secretion in old age.[24] In another study, researchers concluded that sunlight deprivation is a significant factor in disturbed sleep patterns in institutionalized elderly patients. They recommend that older people with sleep problems be exposed to sunlight for at least two hours each day to boost nighttime melatonin production.[25]

Conversely, exposure to light at night—even for five minutes—is detrimental to melatonin production.[18] In one study, six men exposed to bright artificial light (greater than 3,000 lux) from sunset to 2 a.m. on one night experienced inhibition of melatonin urine excretion (indicative of delayed pineal secretion) during the light exposure. The subsequent night, when the subjects resumed normal exposure to light and darkness, melatonin excretion was still delayed, this time by one hour.[19] Even nighttime exposure of as little as 100 lux can inhibit nocturnal production of melatonin in some people.[20] The effect of nighttime light on sleepers varies greatly—500 lux of light has been shown to impair melatonin production by 8% in some people, but by 98% in others,[21] and delaying sleep onset for 30 minutes.[22] Common practices such as leaving bright lights on before going to bed or even sleeping with a nightlight on can negatively impact your melatonin production and lead to sleep disturbances.

Magnetic and Electromagnetic Fields

Light—whether natural or artificial—isn't the only environmental phenomenon proven to affect and potentially impair the pineal gland's ability to secrete melatonin. Numerous recent studies show that electromagnetic fields (EMFs)—both natural and artificial—can also cause sleep/wake disturbances by inhibiting melatonin production.

The pineal gland is not only a photosensitive (light sensitive) structure, it is also receptive of magnetic fields. This makes sense when you consider that visible light is actually a very high frequency electromagnetic field (SEE QUICK DEFINITION), oscillating 1,015 hertz (Hz), or 1,000,000,000,000,000 times per second. In comparison, human brain waves in deep sleep oscillate at about 2-4 Hz. In studies on migratory birds, scientists discovered that the pineal gland, in conjunction with the hormone melatonin, functions as the brain's navigating system. This "master gland" is able to detect variations of the earth's magnetic field and use that information to locate geographical directions (north, south, east, west) and determine seasonal cues (the earth's magnetic fields changes daily and seasonally).[26]

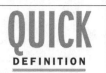

DEFINITION

Electromagnetic fields are measured for two properties—electrical current (in units of hertz, or cycles per second) and magnetic strength (in units of gauss). The best way to comprehend gauss (G) is to compare it to the earth's magnetic field, which is 0.5 gauss. A refrigerator magnet is approximately 10 gauss. Ten thousand gauss comprise one tesla (T). One microtesla (muT) is equal to 10 milligauss (mG—one thousandth of a gauss). The intensity of electromagnetic devices such as computer monitors and electric ranges are often described in terms of milligauss and sometimes hertz. Studies have shown that EMFs of less than 300 hertz and more than 2 milligauss can disrupt melatonin production.

In one study, researchers removed the pineal glands of pied flycatchers, a type of migratory bird. A subset of the birds received melatonin supplementation while the other did not. The researchers observed that the birds lacking pineal glands and melatonin supplementation did not migrate during the expected season (autumn) and were unable to orient themselves to the migratory patterns (southwest). Birds that received melatonin supplementation,

For more about **electromagnetic fields**, see Chapter 7: Protection from a Toxic Environment, pp. 174-199.

however, chose the correct season and direction in which to migrate.[27] Other studies have found that the pineal glands of several animal species have magnetically sensitive cells.[28] While no conclusive evidence proves that human pineal gland cells are likewise receptive to magnetic fields, human studies confirm that drops in the earth's magnetic field—which occur during various solar and lunar events—cause a significant decline in melatonin levels.[29]

Geomagnetic fields are obviously not the only magnetic phenomena in our lives. Indeed, we're exposed to numerous artificial magnetic and electromagnetic (magnetism generated by electricity) fields every day, in varying frequencies—radio waves, artificial-light waves, microwaves, EMFs emitted by refrigerators, TVs, computer monitors, and many other common appliances. Numerous animal and human studies show that chronic exposure to extremely low frequency EMFs (electrical currents of less than 300 Hz) suppresses nighttime melatonin secretions.[30] In one study, 12 men were exposed for three weeks to extremely low frequency EMFs (29 milligauss or 40 Hz) either in the morning or afternoon. All test subjects showed significant drops in nocturnal melatonin secretion regardless of time of EMF exposure.[31] Another study showed that work-related exposure to 16.7 Hz magnetic fields, ranging from 10 mG to 200 mG, significantly decreased nighttime melatonin excretion levels; levels rebounded on the test subjects' days off.[32] The nighttime use of electric blankets, which have extremely low frequency EMFs, is also linked to suppressed melatonin secretion.[33]

It's also worth noting that extremely low frequency EMFs have been repeatedly linked to the development of breast cancer. Melatonin has been shown to reduce the growth of mammary tumor cells in cows.[34] There are thousands of melatonin receptor sites in a woman's reproductive system. Melatonin enhances intercellular communications and lower levels may cause a less efficient reproductive physiology and a greater vulnerability to breast cancer. Extremely low frequency EMFs may not only suppress melatonin secretion—they may also impair the body's ability to fight cancer cells. The proliferation of electronic devices in our lives parallels the increase in the incidence of breast cancer over the same years.

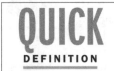

DEFINITION

Cortisol is a hormone secreted by the adrenal glands, which are located atop the kidneys. Cortisol secretion (as well as the adrenal gland's other hormones, DHEA, adrenaline, and aldosterone) occurs in daily cycles, peaking in the morning and having the lowest values at night. Cortisol promotes protein building, regulates insulin and glycogen synthesis, and helps produce prostaglandins. Under conditions of stress, high amounts of cortisol are released; chronic excess secretion is associated with obesity and suppressed thyroid function. Imbalances in cortisol secretion are linked with low energy, muscle dysfunction, impaired bone repair, thyroid dysfunction, immune system depression, sleep disorders, poor skin regeneration, and decreased growth hormone uptake.

Physical and Emotional Stress

Stress can have a detrimental effect on nocturnal melatonin production, often causing insomnia and other sleep/wake rhythm disturbances. For the purposes of this chapter, we'll define stress by the presence of high blood levels of cortisol (SEE QUICK DEFINITION). Intense physical exercise and emotional problems often trigger the stress response, resulting in a large release of cortisol.

As with melatonin, cortisol release is regulated by circadian rhythms, with levels the highest in the dawn hours—the same time that melatonin levels begin to dramatically decline. Research indicates that cortisol helps our body make the transition from deep sleep (which is prompted by melatonin) to light sleep and wakefulness.[35] Scientists believe that cortisol is able to reverse deep sleep by reducing the brain's uptake of serotonin, thereby suppressing production of melatonin.[36]

When large amounts of this hormone are released at nighttime—as a result of physical exercise or emotional upsets—people will likely experience difficulty falling or staying asleep. In one study, nighttime physical stress and the associated high cortisol levels produced a one- to two-hour phase delay of nocturnal melatonin release in men.[37] These findings prompted the study's researchers to claim that stress may act similarly to light in shifting human circadian rhythms—in other words, causing sleep/wake pattern disturbances.

For more on **how stress causes sleep problems**, see Chapter 6: Resolve Emotional Issues, pp. 146-173.

Medications

Several commonly used medications can suppress melatonin production, leading to sleep/wake disturbances. Short-term use of over-the-counter (OTC) pain relievers, heart medications, anti-anxiety drugs, even sleeping pills, has been shown to interfere with the nocturnal secretion of melatonin. Avoiding these medications is the only definite way to reverse their effects on melatonin; taking the drugs earlier in the day may minimize their impact on sleep. Statistics regarding sleep deprivation in older people rarely take into account the use of multiple medications and their effects on sleep patterns.

Nonsteroidal, anti-inflammatory drugs (NSAIDs), which include the widely used OTC pain-killing drugs ibuprofen, aspirin, and indomethacin, greatly reduce melatonin secretion at night and even disturb the amount of restorative deep sleep. This is due to their inhibitory effect on the synthesis of prostaglandins, hormone-like substances necessary in the production of melatonin.[38] In one study, subjects administered standard dosages of aspirin or ibuprofen twice in one day suffered significantly higher rates of delayed sleep onset and repeated nighttime awakenings than did the control subjects. Additionally, subjects who took ibuprofen also experienced delayed onset of the deep stages of sleep.[39] In another study, one standard dosage of indomethacin (given at 6 p.m.) completely suppressed normal nocturnal secretion of melatonin.[40] Acetaminophen, a non-NSAID pain-killer, does not appear to significantly interfere with melatonin production, but research finds that it does have a slight adverse effect on sleep.[41]

Two commonly prescribed types of heart drugs—beta-blockers and calcium-channel blockers—also impair melatonin production. Beta-blockers are often used to treat heart problems such as high blood pressure, angina, and arrhythmias (abnormal heart rhythms). They function by interfering with specific cell receptors called beta-adrenergic receptors, which results in relaxed heart rate, lowered blood pressure, and suspension of normal nighttime melatonin production. The beta-blockers propranolol and atenolol are particularly damaging to melatonin levels. Calcium-channel blockers also seriously impair nighttime melatonin levels. As their name suggests, calcium-channel blockers impede the flow of calcium to cardiovascular cells, thus relaxing the arteries and reducing the amount of oxygen needed by the heart. These drugs can also suppress the flow of calcium to pineal cells, which need calcium to make melatonin.[42]

Benzodiazepines are tranquilizing drugs frequently prescribed for anxiety and insomnia. However, several studies show that benzodiazepines, including diazepam (Valium®), alprazolam (Xanax®), and flunitrazepam, may impair the central nervous system's ability to relay light information to the pineal gland.[43] In one test, six healthy subjects were given diazepam and their nocturnal melatonin levels were then measured. In all subjects, melatonin levels were suppressed throughout the night.[44] Other studies have found that another benzodiazepine, alprazolam, also diminished nighttime melatonin levels, resulting in less time spent in deep sleep stages.[45] Benzodiazepines may also lead to melatonin rebound during the day, in which melatonin production nearly reaches regular nighttime levels during the day, causing excessive daytime sleepiness.[46]

Poor Diet

Caffeine and alcohol are the usual suspects in sleep problems—and indeed, they've been shown to impair melatonin production. One study showed that 200 mg of caffeine (the amount found in two cups of brewed coffee) significantly reduced nighttime melatonin levels, most likely by suppressing the neuromodulator adenosine that is crucial to melatonin synthesis.[47] Alcohol (ethanol) has been found to depress nocturnal melatonin secretion, due to its inhibitory effect on the adrenal hormone norepinephrine, which promotes the pineal cells' production of melatonin.[48]

Imbalances of certain vitamins and minerals may also disrupt the normal levels of melatonin. Vitamin B12 deficiencies have been shown in several studies to suppress melatonin production.[49] For this reason, B12 is effective in conjunction with light therapy for sleep phase syndromes. Also, deficiencies of magnesium and vitamins B1 and B6 may reduce melatonin levels, since these nutrients are essential in activating the enzymes that facilitate production of serotonin and melatonin.[50]

For more information on **how poor diet causes sleep disorders**, see Chapter 3: Improve Your Diet, pp. 56-85.

Alternative Therapies to Reset Your Body Clock

Alternative medicine offers a broad range of therapies to reset your body clock and resolve sleep/wake rhythm disturbances. Some are simple, no-cost steps—avoid caffeine and alcohol, exercise, spend more time outdoors. Other therapies require special purchases, such as light boxes or magnets, and are best administered under the guidance of a health-care practitioner. Melatonin supplements are effective and widely available. However, most alternative medicine physicians recommend integrating lifestyle changes (such as diet modification and light therapy) before turning to melatonin supplementation, because given the proper nourishment and light/dark cycles, our bodies can naturally produce sufficient amounts of this hormone.

Lifestyle Modifications

Making a few adjustments to your daily routine can get you snoozing again. One of the most important steps to improving your sleep is avoiding caffeine and alcohol. If you decide to continue consuming caffeine-containing beverages and foods, do so earlier in the day. Drink coffee no later than 10 a.m. Alcohol consumption whould be discontinued completely. Also, steer clear of NSAIDs and other melatonin-suppressing drugs at night. Try taking them earlier in the day—talk to your physician about altering your dosage schedule for prescription medications.

Next, eat foods that will boost natural melatonin production. Foods such as oats, corn, rice, and tomatoes contain high amounts of naturally occurring melatonin. Eating these shortly before bedtime will promote higher nocturnal melatonin secretion. Additionally, foods rich in tryptophan, such as spirulina, soy nuts, cottage cheese, turkey, and tofu, provide the building blocks to melatonin. Russel J. Reiter, Ph.D., author of *Melatonin: Your Body's Wonder Drug*, also recommends supplementing with calcium (1,000 mg), magnesium (500 mg), and niacinamide (100 mg) before bed, since these minerals are essential in converting tryptophan into serotonin and then melatonin.[51] Also, take a vitamin B6 supplement (25-50 mg) in the morning to facilitate serotonin production during the day.

Starting to exercise is an important way to manage stress. Additionally, it will help elevate your body temperature,

To learn more about **how dietary modifications and nutrient supplementation can eliminate sleep disorders**, see Chapter 3: Improve Your Diet, pp. 56-85.

Take a Hot Bath for a Good Night's Sleep

A hot bath isn't just a relaxing experience, it's also a natural sleep aid. In the National Sleep Foundation's 1999 sleep survey, 65% of adults reported that they fell asleep more quickly and slept better than usual after soaking in a hot bath, and research substantiates these claims. In one study, researchers found that after taking a hot bath, subjects' body temperature rose about 2° F and melatonin levels also increased.[53] Apparently, the pineal gland responds to a sudden rise in body temperature by producing melatonin, which decreases and normalizes body temperature. A pleasant side effect is that you are lulled to sleep.

For other tips on **how to reduce stress and improve sleep**, see Chapter 6: Resolve Emotional Issues, pp. 146-173. For more on **using exercise to improve sleep**, see Chapter 9: Correcting Structural Imbalances, pp. 224-247.

which will be followed by a drop in temperature and improved sleep four to six hours later.[52] Proper timing is crucial: the best time to exercise to improve your sleep is during the late afternoon (5 p.m. or earlier). As discussed above, physical exertion at nighttime can incite a stress response, resulting in high levels of cortisol.

Light Therapy

Light therapy relies on the body's natural ability to reset its sleep/wake rhythms according to the *zeitgeber* of light. As we discussed earlier, the presence of external light inhibits melatonin secretion; darkness promotes it. The premise behind light therapy is simple—get more light exposure during the day and less at night. Dimming the lights at night probably won't be a hardship, but making sure that you receive adequate amounts of bright light during the day can be difficult.

One way you can increase exposure to bright light is by going outdoors more often, for an hour or more each day. Make it a habit to get outdoors first thing in the morning to expose yourself to natural sunlight. Alternately, you can sit by a large, east-facing window while you eat breakfast or spend your lunch break outdoors. As we know, the sun's ultraviolet rays can damage our skin and eyes, leading to various health problems, so be sure to wear UV-protective sunglasses (with minimal tint so the light can enter the retinas) and sunscreen.

We realize that many things may prevent you from spending prolonged periods outdoors—cold weather, illness, work, and other obligations. To enjoy the benefits of natural sunlight indoors, install full-spectrum light bulbs in your house and office. Full-spectrum light is a balanced blend of all colors in the visible spectrum, closely resembling what we get from sunlight. Conventional incandescent light bulbs illuminate more intensely on the yellow part of the color spectrum. Lee Hartley, Ed.D., a researcher on light therapy, suggests mounting a row of four to six full-spectrum fluorescent bulbs in a vanity fixture over your bathroom sink. "This is an excellent method for maximum impact," she says, "because the body receives the same effect as natural sunlight in the morning. You wake up quicker and with less morning shock."

Additionally, you may consider using light boxes, specially designed devices consisting of full-spectrum fluorescent lights that simulate early-morning sunlight. Light boxes typically cost $300-$1,000 and are widely available in a various sizes and styles (wall units, desk lamps, light visors). They usually come in values of 2,500 lux and 10,000 lux. Most standard therapy protocols recommend two hours of exposure to 2,500 lux daily; some doctors recommend using 10,000-lux boxes for only 30 minutes daily. You can perform the light therapy first thing in the morning, sitting before the light box with your eyes open but not staring directly into the light, either at work (assuming you work at a desk or in some manner of stationary pursuit) or at home. (Research has found that external light is sensed by other organs than the eyes—one study, in fact, found that light exposure to the back of the knee suppressed melatonin production. The therapeutic applications of these findings are not assessed at this time.)

Some doctors may also recommend vitamin B12 supplements in conjunction with light therapy, as this vitamin appears to enhance a person's photosensitivity. Researchers have found three hours of light therapy (2,500-3,000 lux) accompanied by intravenous vitamin B12 (5-6 mg daily) reset the circadian rhythms of melatonin secretion and can be effective in rectifying delayed sleep phase syndromes and other sleep/wake disturbances.[54]

Generally, it takes about 14 days of light therapy to see if you're getting benefits. Individuals should never stare into the light during therapy and should be careful to choose light sources that screen out ultraviolet rays. People with eye problems such as diabetic retinopathy or macular degeneration should not employ light therapy without their doctor's consent.

For more information on **light therapy**, contact: Society for Light Treatment and Biological Rhythms, Inc., 10200 West 44th Avenue, Suite 304, Wheat Ridge, CO 80033-2840; tel: 303-422-7905; fax: 303-422-8894. For sources of **full-spectrum lighting and light boxes**, contact: Seventh Generation, One Mill Street, Box A-26, Burlington, VT 05401-1530; tel: 800-456-1191 or 802-658-3773; fax: 802-658-1771. Verilux, Inc., 9 Viaduct Road, Stamford, CT 06907; tel: 800-786-6850 or 203-921-2430; fax: 203-921-2427; website: www.ergo-light.com. Ott-Lite Systems Inc., 28 Parker Way, Santa Barbara, CA 93101; tel: 800-234-3724 or 805-564-3467; fax: 805-564-2147. Environmental Lighting Concepts, Inc., 1214 West Cass Street, Tampa, FL 33606; tel: 800-842-8848 or 813-621-0058; fax: 813-626-8790.

Chronotherapy

The majority of people suffering from sleep/wake rhythm disturbances will find relief through increased daytime exposure to sunlight or light boxes. However, for those who experience extreme delayed sleep phase syndrome, chronotherapy ("time" therapy) may be the appropriate therapy. Chronotherapy is based on the theory that by delaying bedtime for several days, it is possible to move the sleeping time to a more conventional timeframe, such as 9 p.m. to 6 a.m. In practical terms, if you do not get to sleep until 2 a.m. and rise at 10 a.m., you can begin by delaying your bedtime until 5 a.m. the first night. Each successive day, add another three-hour delay until you have moved around the clock. In this example, the second day you go to bed at 8 a.m. and rise at 4 p.m. This method is best done during vacation or other times when you are not committed to a regular work schedule or other obligations.

Magnet Therapy

Magnetic fields exist everywhere: they emanate from the earth, from changes in the weather, and even from the human body. The use of magnetic devices to generate controlled magnetic fields has proven to be an effective diagnostic tool (MRI, magnetic resonance imaging) and therapy for rheumatoid disease, inflammation, cancer, circulatory problems, and other illnesses. Magnetic therapy can influence the flow of varying electrical currents (normally present in all organisms) that govern the nervous system and other biological systems. Controlled use of magnetic fields can benefit sleep disorder sufferers by reversing the detrimental effects of extremely low frequency electromagnetic fields on the pineal gland.

For sleep disorders arising out of disruptions to melatonin production, alternative medicine doctors recommend therapy with negative-pole magnets. Magnet therapy may offer permanent relief to those suffering from various sleep/wake disturbances, including insomnia and even sleep apnea. Though the use of magnets has been shown to improve cases of multiple sclerosis and Parkinson's disease, very few studies have tested the efficacy of magnets on sleep disorders. One recent study, however, showed that three weeks of magnet therapy permanently eliminated a chronic case of sleep paralysis in a multiple sclerosis patient. This report suggests that magnet therapy promoted melatonin secretion, since REM sleep disorders such as sleep paralysis have been linked to melatonin deficiency.[56] In treating sleep disorders, magnets are used in various placements—on the abdomen (some amount of melatonin is secreted by the intestines), on the eyes, and in specially designed mattress pads.

A Quick Review of Magnet Basics

All magnets have two poles: positive (or "S" for south, usually marked in red) and negative (or "N" for north, usually marked in green). Negative magnetic energy normalizes and calms systems of the human body, while positive magnetic energy overstimulates or disrupts the biological system. For this reason, negative poles are most frequently directed towards the body. Do not apply positive magnetic poles directly to the body unless under medical supervision.

The strength of a magnet is measured in gauss units (which measures the intensity of magnetic flux). Every magnetic device has a manufacturer's gauss rating; however, the actual strength of the magnet at the skin surface is often much less than this number. For example, a 4,000-gauss magnet transmits about 1,200 gauss to the patient. Magnets placed in pillow or bed pads will render even lower amounts of field strength at the skin surface, because a magnet's strength quickly decreases with the distance from the subject. The strength of the magnet also depends on its size and thickness. Therapeutic magnets use from 200 gauss to 1,500 gauss (only a fraction of what an MRI machine emits), while a common refrigerator magnet emits 10 gauss.[55]

The most common types of magnets used in magnetic therapy are ceramic and neodymium (a rare earth chemical). These elements are mixed with iron to increase the magnet's strength or the duration of magnetic charge. The most powerful (and expensive) magnets are neodymium, while ceramic magnets are less expensive but still keep their charge for many years. These types of magnetic materials are incorporated into various types of products available at health food stores or through mail-order catalogs. Ceramic and neodymium magnets are available as plastiform strips that attach to the skin by an elastic adhesive, wrist and back supports, seat pads, and strips worn inside shoes; magnetic blankets and beds are also available for promoting sleep and reducing stress.

Commercially available, negatively poled mattress pads are the easiest way of using magnet therapy. You simply place the pad, with a quilt covering, on top of the mattress (for maximum strength) or between the mattress and box spring. However, mattress pads can be costly and your doctor may determine that magnet placement on your eyes or abdomen will be more effective for your condition. In most cases, you can discontinue magnet therapy once your condition has improved, or you can continue to use magnets as a preventive measure.

An alternative to magnetized mattress pads requires a 5" x 6" multi-magnet flexible mat. This mat is composed of strips of plastiform magnets, which are placed sufficiently close together to make a solid field, but far enough apart for flexibility. In bed before going to

For more on **minimizing the effects of electromagnetic fields on sleep patterns**, see Chapter 7: Protection from a Toxic Environment, pp. 174-199.

For information on **using and purchasing therapeutic magnets and mattress pads**, contact: Philpott Medical Services, 17171 Southeast 29th Street, Choctaw, OK 73020; tel: 405-390-3009. American Health Service, 531 Bank Lane, Highwood, IL 60040; tel: 800-544-7521. To learn more about **magnet therapy**, contact: Bio-Electro-Magnetics Institute, 2490 West Moana Lane, Reno, NV 89509-3936; tel: 702-827-9099.

sleep, place the smaller side of the mat from the forehead down to the tip of the nose. This covers the eyes, sinuses, and nose. Directly on top of this mat and over the eyes, place 1" x $\frac{1}{2}$" neodymium disc magnets, which magnetically adhere to the mat. Also place four 4" x 6" x 1" ceramic magnets at the headboard. Sleep with these magnets in place throughout the night. Be sure to keep the bedroom dark. To increase the depth of sleep, place a 5" x 12" multimagnet flexible mat across your abdomen before going to sleep. For additional magnetic reinforcement, center on the mat a 4" x 6" x $\frac{1}{2}$" ceramic magnet, positioned lengthwise on the body. Instead of the mat, you can use a 4" x 12" x $\frac{1}{8}$" plastiform magnet strip across the abdomen.

Precautions: There are conflicting methods of naming the magnetic poles. To be effective, magnets need to be marked correctly, so be sure to use magnets marked according to the Davis/Rawls system (developed by Dr. Albert Roy Davis in 1936). Avoid touching the sides of thick, therapeutic magnets and never use magnets with holes in the middle. Keep magnets one to two feet away from tape cassettes and computer diskettes. People with cancer or any infection (including *Candida*, viruses, and bacteria) should avoid exposure to bipolar magnets. Do not use magnets on your chest if you have a pacemaker and a pregnant woman should not use magnets on her abdomen. Do not use magnetic beds for longer than 8-10 hours a day. For long-term results, use magnets at night and supplement with magnets during the day. It is best to be under the guidance and supervision of a health-care professional if you want to use magnet therapy. Don't combine melatonin supplementation with magnet therapy without first consulting your doctor.

Melatonin Supplementation

Melatonin is popularly regarded as a wonder drug for its immune-boosting, age-defying, and, of course, its sleep-enhancing properties—and rightly so. Research repeatedly confirms the benefits of melatonin supplementation for various sleep/wake rhythm disturbances. Further studies have found that melatonin supplements are non-toxic and very safe for short-term use, with only mild side effects such as headaches and abdominal cramps in test subjects administered extremely large doses of melatonin (3,000 mg to 6,600 mg).

Melatonin effectively relieves insomnia (including cases associated with jet lag and shift work), sleep phase syndromes, and REM behavior disorders, in all age groups. Melatonin has been shown to decrease sleep-onset latency in Stages 1 and 2 (light sleep), a helpful boost for those suffering from sleep-onset insomnia.[57] Melatonin has also been found to significantly increase deep sleep, REM sleep, and sleep efficiency (time spent in sound asleep), without the "hangover" or stupor effects common with other over-the-counter and prescription sleeping pills. It has also been shown to dramatically improve the sleep/wake cycle in blind people, who often suffer from problems with free-running circadian rhythms due to their inability to detect light.[58] Melatonin pills work quickly—people usually fall asleep within 30 minutes of taking the supplements.

If melatonin does have a down side, it is on two counts. First, researchers have not discovered the optimal dose of melatonin supplementation. Thus, people taking this hormone generally need to experiment with different dosages before finding the right one for their needs. Second, the long-term effects of melatonin supplementation are unknown. As with any hormone replacement therapy, there is a chance the pineal gland could stop producing its own melatonin if you are supplying it from an external source; this could cause the gland to atrophy. Additionally, the melatonin in supplements is synthetically derived, varying in some molecular ways from natural melatonin and may have detrimental long-term effects.

Hence, we advise against self-dosing melatonin supplements on a long-term basis or in certain conditions, without first consulting a health-care practitioner who can monitor your levels of melatonin. Never take melatonin supplements during the day unless advised by your doctor, as this will further disrupt your circadian rhythms. Do not operate machinery or drive after taking melatonin supplements. One additional warning: Expect vivid, even bizarre dreams for up to two months upon starting melatonin supplements, as this hormone stimulates REM sleep.

For Insomnia—Numerous studies have found melatonin supplements very effective for insomnia, especially in the elderly.[63] For sleep-onset and other types of insomnia, the standard dosage of melatonin is between 0.2 mg to 10 mg, approximately 30 minutes before bedtime. As discussed above, optimal dosages vary, so begin by taking 1-2 mg and

While melatonin has been shown to be very safe in short-term use, it is advised that people with severe allergies, severe mental illness, autoimmune diseases, and immune-system cancers such as lymphoma and leukemia, avoid melatonin supplements since the hormone may exacerbate these conditions.[59] Pregnant or nursing women or should not take melatonin, as its impact on fetal and newborn development is not known. Women who are trying to conceive should avoid high doses of melatonin (10 mg or more), which has been shown to prevent ovulation.[60] Melatonin is also not recommended for healthy children (who have high levels of natural melatonin) and people taking steroid drugs such as cortisone (as melatonin may counteract their effectiveness).[61] Men taking high doses of melatonin should consider supplementing with vitamin E, as vitamin E reverses the suppressive effects of melatonin on testosterone production.[62]

For **sources of melatonin supplements**, contact: Life Extension Foundation, 995 S.W. 24th Street, Ft. Lauderdale, FL 33315; tel: 877-900-9073 or 954-766-8433; website: www.lef.org. Source Naturals, Threshold Enterprises, 23 Janis Way, Scotts Valley, CA 95066; tel: 800-777-5677 or 831-438-1144.

increasing or decreasing as necessary to reach the lowest dose that induces sleep. It's best to take melatonin at the same time each night to properly reset your body clock. The duration of supplementation depends on your sleep problem. If you suffer from chronic insomnia and other lifestyle modifications don't help, you may need to take melatonin supplements every night. On the other hand, if you experience occasional insomnia due to stress, illness, or other factors, use melatonin supplements only as needed.

For Jet Lag—In studies on people traveling by plane across time zones, those treated with melatonin supplements reported less severe symptoms of jet lag than placebo-treated subjects. They also returned more rapidly to their normal sleep patterns, experienced less daytime fatigue, and reported reaching normal energy levels more rapidly.[64]

While most doctors agree that melatonin is effective for jet lag, the best time to take melatonin is debatable. Alfred Lewy, M.D., a sleep researcher at Oregon Health Sciences University, advises that you start taking melatonin the day before travel, and early in the day to start shifting your clock forward or backward. For example, if you're traveling from the West Coast to the East Coast of the U.S., you will need to advance your body clock by three hours. So you can take a small dose of melatonin (0.5 mg, just enough to shift your body without causing excessive daytime drowsiness) at 2 p.m. the day before you travel (5 p.m. at your destination). Then take the same dose at 2 p.m. the day of travel, and at 5 p.m. the first full day on the East Coast. This will help you feel tired on Eastern time. The day before you return home, take melatonin first thing in the morning, and for the two subsequent days upon your return. This will delay your body clock so you will be able to stay up on Pacific time.

Ray Sahelian, M.D., author of *Melatonin: Nature's Sleeping Pill*, advises taking melatonin when you get to your destination in the evening of the new time zone, especially when traveling west to east. He advocates increasing the dosage by about 1 mg for every hour earlier you want to sleep. For example, if you take a day flight from Los Angeles to New York, by midnight in New York, it will be only 9 p.m. in Los Angeles, so it may be hard for you to go to sleep. Because of the three-hour difference, you take 3 mg of melatonin sometime between 10 and 11 p.m. Eastern Time.[65]

A third strategy is to start taking 0.5 mg of melatonin on the plane when it's 8:30 p.m. or 9 p.m. at your destination. Then, when you arrive, take between 0.5 mg and 5 mg (as much as needed to fall quickly asleep) the first night or two, at the local bedtime. You can also use sunlight to help your body make the shift. When traveling west to east, avoid daylight until after 10 a.m., and then get out in the sun for about a half-hour at midday. In traveling east to west, avoid daylight after 6 p.m.

For Shift Work—Dr. Reiter recommends that shift workers take 1-5 mg of melatonin at the beginning of desired sleep time, or as needed. Wearing dark wraparound sunglasses and sleeping in a dark room will help stave off the melatonin-suppressing lights. Dr. Lewy, however, discourages shift workers from self-treatment because the circadian issues at play, especially in the case of rotating-shift work, are difficult to reset. He advises that shift workers find a chronobiologist (doctor skilled in resetting body clocks) to help them—with light therapy and melatonin—to shift their body clocks to a stable rhythm.

For Sleep Phase Syndromes—Two other sleep/wake disturbances are caused by disruptions in the melatonin production cycle: advanced sleep phase syndrome (ASPS), in which people fall asleep in early evening and then wake up well before dawn, and delayed sleep phase syndrome (DSPS), in which people habitually stay up until 2 a.m. or later and sleep until 11 a.m.

Success Story: Melatonin Lets Chronic Insomniac Sleep Again

William Lee Cowden, M.D., of Dallas, Texas, has had excellent success using melatonin supplements in treating insomnia. He reports that one of his former patients, a man from Florida, had suffered from insomnia for ten years, sleeping only three hours a night. The patient had visited numerous sleep disorder centers as well as dozens of sleep specialists, and had tried virtually every prescription drug for insomnia—all to no avail. Over the years, the chronic insomnia had made the man extremely irritable and difficult to live with.

Dr. Cowden, believing the insomnia was due to an imbalance in melatonin, instructed his patient to take melatonin-boosting steps—avoid sugar and caffeine, sleep in a totally darkened room, and remove all electrical devices such as clocks, radios, and televisions. He recommended that the patient take melatonin supplements nightly, between 10 p.m. and midnight, for two weeks, then every other night for two months. Dr. Cowden also gave the patient supplements of vitamin C and omega-3 essential fatty acids, which are instrumental in producing prostaglandins, hormone-like substances that aid in melatonin synthesis. After a few nights following this regimen, the patient was sleeping seven to eight hours a night, and after two months, he reported that he was sleeping as well as he had during childhood.

Sleep Rituals

Once you have reset your circadian rhythms and find that your body is responding to natural cues for sleep, such as sunlight in the morning, you may want to consider establishing a "sleep ritual." A sleep ritual is a conscious effort to set aside adequate time to allow yourself to relax and release the day's activities. The sleep ritual reduces nighttime stress, minimizing the adverse effects cortisol on melatonin production. It can also take on the status of *zeitgeber* with your body clock, providing temporal cues that it's almost time to go to sleep. Sonia Ancoli-Israel, Ph.D., a sleep researcher at the University of California at San Diego Department of Psychiatry, recommends integrating these steps into your own sleep ritual:

Set Aside Worry Time—Many of us tend to worry about the day's or next day's events while in bed. Dr. Ancoli-Israel recommends spending time in the daytime to process your concerns. "We suggest that people find 20 minutes, half an hour, earlier in the day, when they can sit down quietly, put out the 'Do Not Disturb' sign, and worry. That's your chance to sit and think about all the things that you're concerned about. Get it out of your system so once you get into bed at night, or if you wake up in the middle of the night, you don't have to start thinking about all of it."

Clear Your Head of Thoughts—To cease the internal chatter of anxiety and other sleep-inhibiting thoughts at night, Dr. Ancoli-Israel recommends employing some sort of meditative process. She says that this can range from counting sheep to more elaborate forms of meditation. Concentrating on your breathing will help clear your mind, simply breathe deeply and count each breath.

Relax Before Bedtime—Do not engage in any stimulating activities before going to bed. Avoid working, spending time on the computer, perhaps even watching TV. Do things that are relaxing and allow your mind and body to unwind and slow down. Read, knit, or listen to soothing music.

Don't Rush the Sleep Ritual— Set aside a specific time window for the sleep ritual and give yourself adequate time to do all of these activities. It will be counterproductive to rush through your meditation or anything else and expect yourself to drop off to sleep. Any activity, whether physical or mental, that is stimulating or creates arousal, is likely to interfere with your sleep.

or noon. ASPS sufferers tend to be elderly, while people with DSPS are often in their teens or early-twenties.

Dr. Lewy has successfully treated both advanced and delayed syndromes with a combination of light boxes and low-dose melatonin supplements.[66] People with ASPS can look at bright light (2,500 lux) in the early evening, when the body is just about to start its melatonin production. The light will delay the melatonin buildup and keep them awake. Then, upon awakening in the early morning, take 0.5 mg of melatonin to promote melatonin secretion in the predawn darkness.

DSPS patients need to reverse the process: look at bright light first thing in the morning and take 0.5 mg of melatonin in early evening or seven hours after they get up. One study showed that taking 1-2 mg of melatonin two hours before desired bedtime helped patients with extreme DSPS (falling asleep at 5 a.m.) reset their body clocks in eight weeks.[67] With all cases of sleep phase syndrome, patients can discontinue melatonin supplementation once they've achieved their ideal sleep rhythms.

For REM Behavior Disorder—Melatonin has shown great promise in eliminating REM behavior disorder (RBD), a sleep problem characterized by head banging and other repetitive bodily movements during the REM stage of sleep. Melatonin is involved in immobilizing the body during REM sleep; hence, RBD indicates a melatonin deficiency, due to a desynchronization of melatonin secretion and sleep stages. In one study, six patients with RBD were administered 3 mg of melatonin 30 minutes before bedtime. Within one week, five patients experienced a dramatic reduction of RBD episodes; after six weeks, these patients slept normally.[68] In another study, a man fully recovered from RBD after five months of melatonin treatment (3 mg daily). When melatonin supplementation was discontinued, his RBD symptoms reappeared, only to vanish when the melatonin treatment was restored.[69]

Beating the Winter Blues

In recent decades, the "winter blues" have gained scientific credibility. Physicians now talk about SAD—seasonal affective disorder—the measurable negative effects that sunlight deprivation produces in some people. The symptoms of SAD's winter doldrums are no doubt familiar to many. It is estimated that more than ten million Americans experience SAD every year, and another 25 million get some milder depressive symptoms on a seasonal basis. Additionally, the more northern the latitude at which you live, the shorter your days and the more susceptible you are to SAD. In the United States, cases of SAD increase the further north you go, with estimates ranging from 1.4% of the population in Florida to 9.7% in New Hampshire.[70]

What does SAD feel like? Typically, there is chronic depression and fatigue, which may leave you bedridden; hypersomnia (increased sleep by as much as four hours or more per night) and reduced quality of sleep, leaving you feeling less refreshed; and cravings for carbohydrates and candy, which sometimes can lead to significant weight gain. Women with SAD may report that their premenstrual symptoms are aggravated. Similar seasonal behavioral changes, particularly increased sleep and variations in appetite, are seen in other mammals.

How does a shortage of sunlight cause these changes? According to naturopathic physician and educator Michael T. Murray, N.D., author of *Natural Alternatives to Prozac*, the cause may be in your hormones. "The key hormonal change may be reduced secretion of melatonin from the pineal gland and an increased secretion of cortisol by the adrenal glands." These hormones also affect your mood; studies have found decreased melatonin and increased cortisol levels in depressed patients. The lessening of lights throws off the body's internal clock and its sleep-inducing hormone. It's like a season-long case of jet lag.

Numerous studies show that therapy with natural or full-spectrum lights drastically reduces the symptoms of SAD. Spending one hour outside in the morning light can eliminate SAD in 50% of patients.[71] Of course, this isn't always an option, so light box therapy may be useful (see "Light Therapy," p. 134). Studies have shown that the efficacy of light box therapy on SAD may vary according to time of day. In one study, for instance, 10,000-lux light therapy for 30 minutes in the morning was 69% effective in reversing SAD, while evening exposure was up to 80% effective.[72] However, other studies have shown converse results. Regardless of light-therapy timing, symptoms usually begin to improve after two to four days of treatment, with full improvement evident in two weeks.[73]

Light therapy also seems to help people who are concerned about gaining weight in the winter. The carbohydrate cravings that frequently accompany SAD are associated with serotonin deficiency, a possible outgrowth of cortisol increase. Serotonin, the neurotransmitter believed to regulate appetite, is produced during light exposure.

Success Story: SAD No More with Light Therapy

Twenty years ago, Sherrie Baxter left sunny Oklahoma, her native state, for Vancouver, Washington, in the Pacific Northwest. As the years went by, Sherrie would become tired and depressed and find herself craving carbohydrates as soon as autumn, with its characteristic overcast skies and dark mornings, would arrive. She'd also stay up late and had trouble getting up in the morning. The depression and fatigue mysteriously lifted by April or May. "One of things I remember was during Christmas: I was walking through the stores and they were playing the holiday music, and I just started crying for no reason. I had no problems like that in spring or summer," she recalls.

In 1985, both Sherrie, then 28, and her mother, who had the same symptoms, signed up as research subjects for a study on seasonal affective disorder at Oregon Health Sciences University in Portland. For three weeks, the two women lived in special quarters where the amount of light was strictly controlled. Technicians took regular blood samples day and night to monitor their levels of melatonin. The researchers were testing whether the lack of light in the morning allowed melatonin to be produced later in the day, causing the women's SAD symptoms.

For information about **light boxes**, contact: Enviro-Med, 1600 S.E. 141st Avenue, Vancouver, WA 98683; tel: 800-222-3296 or 360-256-6989; website: www.bio-light.com.

The first week of the study, Sherrie and her mother were kept mostly in near-darkness except for one dim light bulb. The only break was at 2 p.m., when they were told to stay in front of 4-by-6-foot, 2,500-lux light boxes for about two hours. In the second week, the technicians began setting up the light boxes progressively earlier. The third week, the researchers woke the women at 6 a.m. to use the light boxes immediately upon awakening. By the fourth day of that regimen, Sherrie and her mother were no longer depressed and were full of energy. When they got the blood test results, they realized that the positive changes were occurring because the morning light had normalized their melatonin production cycle.

"I tend to be skeptical of things until I see proof," says Sherrie, now 43. "But we were able to see this was a physical thing happening and that was useful to me." After the study, Sherrie starting making light boxes for herself, and, several years later, started her own business, Enviro-Med, to sell them.

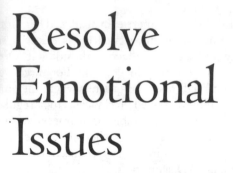

CHAPTER

6

Resolve Emotional Issues

STRESS IS A COMMON PART of everyday life, but it can become harmful to the body when it is prolonged or chronic. It affects the body in very real, physical ways by influencing the immune and hormonal systems. For those with sleep disorders, this can mean poor sleep quality and restless nights. A basic premise of mind/body medicine is that chronic stress and other emotional issues contribute to illness and that relaxation techniques and learning positive ways of coping with these issues will improve your health. In this chapter, we examine how stress, suppressed emotions, and lifestyle choices can contribute to sleep problems. We also explore a number of therapies that can help you change negative thought patterns into more healthful ones, deal with stress in a positive way, and incorporate habits for relaxation into your life.

In This Chapter

- Success Story: A Return-to-Sleep Strategy
- Stress and Your Sleep Problems
- Are You Stressed Out?
- Success Story: Homeopathy Cures Insomnia
- Mind/Body Therapies for Better Sleep

Success Story: A Return-to-Sleep Strategy

By the time Jean found her way to the Lankenau Hospital's Sleep Disorders Center in suburban Philadelphia, Pennsylvania, she had been having trouble sleeping for six years. The problems started when she went into training for a new job. The training required that Jean work the swing shift, 3-11 p.m., for several months, a change from her normal 8:30 a.m. to 4:30 p.m. work schedule. Jean was unable to get to sleep when she came home from the training and ended up staying up quite late, then sleeping until midmorning. When she resumed her normal work schedule, she was still on a disrupted sleep schedule, so she began to fall asleep at about 11 p.m. and wake up at 2:30 a.m., unable to fall back to sleep.

After two years of only getting about three hours sleep on many nights, Jean developed what psychologist Robert E. Becker, Ph.D, calls "anticipatory anxiety." The person starts to worry early in the day about how they will sleep that night. "They start thinking, 'How am I going to do tonight? What time shall I go to bed?'" he says.

In Jean's case, the anticipatory anxiety grew for the next four years until, at age 31, she was so distraught she enrolled in the hospital's sleep disorders program. By this time, Jean was losing mental concentration, was emotionally on edge, and her marriage was shaky, all due to the sleeping problems. She told Dr. Becker she did not want to take sleep medication or other drugs.

By the time they get to the Sleep Disorders Center, Jean and other clients typically have tried the full range of home remedies, from warm milk to herb tea to a glass of wine to hot baths. The ones who try the sleeping pills or other drugs find they only work for a short period of time and then the insomnia returns, he says. They've also tried listening to music, talking to their spouses, talking to themselves—strategies that work for the general population, but they don't work once people have developed anticipatory anxiety, according to Dr. Becker.

"What we need to do is to stop the anticipatory anxiety as much as we can," Dr. Becker says. "For Jean, we needed to get a return-to-sleep strategy in place, because as soon as the wakeup happens, all the body chemistry starts to come alert again." People make themselves even more alert, he says, by reading, watching television, or working at their computers when they wake up in the middle of the night. Those activities can increase mental stimulation, instead of inducing relaxation. Dr. Becker established Jean's return-to-sleep strategy as follows:

1. Have a guided imagery tape in a tape recorder and ready to play. The tape includes descriptions of floating in a balloon, walking in the

Mind/Body Therapies for Better Sleep

- Meditation
- Biofeedback
- Hypnotherapy
- Visualization/Guided Imagery
- Counseling
- Cranial Electrical Stimulation
- Herbal Therapy
- Homeopathic Remedies
- Aromatherapy
- Flower Remedies

How to Do Diaphragmatic Breathing

- Lie on your back, and place your hands on your abdomen immediately below the navel, with your middle fingertips touching.
- Breathe through your nose, inhaling slowly, and push your abdomen out as if it were a balloon expanding; your fingers should separate.
- As your abdomen expands, your diaphragm will move downward, allowing fresh air to enter the bottom of your lungs.
- As the breath continues, expand your chest. More air should now enter, filling the middle part of your lungs.
- Slightly contract your abdomen, raise your shoulders and collarbones; this will fill your upper lungs.
- Hold your breath for a few seconds (a slow count to seven) without straining.
- Slowly exhale through your nose, drawing in your abdomen; exhaling completely will expel all the stale air. After air is exhaled, hold for a count of seven.

This may take some practice or cause slight dizziness at the beginning; this is normal. The most important thing is not to strain or to force yourself to breathe slower than is comfortable.

woods, lying on the beach, or floating in a boat. This type of visualization is right-brain activity, which shuts off the left brain's worry and anxiety about not getting enough sleep.

2. Start diaphragmatic (belly) breathing. The normal resting breathing rate is 15 breaths a minute, but when people wake up and start worrying, their breathing rate goes up to about 20 breaths a minute. Diaphragmatic breathing uses your diaphragm and belly muscles instead of your intercostal, or chest, muscles; the purpose is to slow the breathing rate down. Dr. Becker taught Jean how to do diaphragmatic breathing and also gave her a video to help her practice the technique. He instructed her to use the visualization tape and start diaphragmatic breathing immediately upon awakening and continue for 30 minutes.

3. Change sleep location. If Jean did not fall back asleep in 30 minutes, she was instructed to get up and move to another bed that was already set up and waiting in another part of the house. The reason for the change is to get Jean away from any cues in her primary bedroom that signal for her to be awake. By getting into a different bed, with different textures, temperature, and smells, it breaks down the conditioned response that she had in the other bedroom.

4. If the new location does not induce sleep, then Jean was to get up and do some kind of mindless activity, such as sitting and sipping a cup of warm milk, and not thinking about anything. She could also replay the

visualization tape or have a small snack, such as a banana or some turkey or other protein. Then she was to go back to the new location.

After one week on the program, Jean was sleeping seven hours on four nights and six hours on three nights. The first two strategies—visualization tape plus diaphragmatic breathing—were successful in getting Jean back to sleep. Jean maintained the strategies and her sleep continued to improve. Her next goal was to have ten consecutive nights of solid sleep. After she achieved that, Dr. Becker allowed her to relax a bit on the strategies, but kept watch to make sure that Jean didn't slip into worrying about whether the insomnia would come back, particularly at the time of a stressful event. He monitored her closely over the next three months, and when Jean did relapse, which most people do, she went back on the return-to-sleep program.

Stress and Your Sleep Problems

Although the concept of stress—being "stressed out" or "under constant stress"—may be commonly discussed today, its role as a contributing factor in many diseases is underappreciated. Estimates suggest that as much as 70% to 80% of all visits to physicians' offices are for stress-related problems.[1] Chronic stress directly affects the immune system, and if not effectively dealt with, can seriously compromise health.

Stress is a pervasive problem among Americans, according to a 1996 poll of corporate executives. For example, 44% of employees polled said their work load is excessive compared to 37% in 1988; 43% are bothered by excessive job pressure; and 55% worry considerably about their company's future; 25% of both men and women feel stressed out at work every day, another 12% feel it almost every day, and another 38% feel it once to several days a week.[2]

Stress can be defined as a reaction (to any stimulus or interference) that upsets normal functioning and disturbs mental or physical health. It can be brought on by internal conditions such as illness, pain, emotional conflict, or psychological problems, or by external circumstances, such as bereavement, financial problems, loss of job or spouse, relocation, food allergies, and electromag-

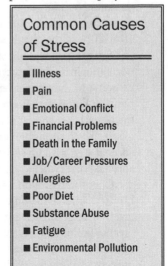

Common Causes of Stress

- Illness
- Pain
- Emotional Conflict
- Financial Problems
- Death in the Family
- Job/Career Pressures
- Allergies
- Poor Diet
- Substance Abuse
- Fatigue
- Environmental Pollution

netic fields. Stress, when it becomes chronic, is often unrecognized by the person whose body is experiencing it; one begins to accept it as a fact of life, without being aware of how it is actually compromising all bodily function and preparing the foundation for illness.

More specifically, research confirms that high levels of emotional stress increase one's susceptibility to illness. Unrelieved, chronic stress begins taxing and eventually weakening or even suppressing the immune system. Stress can also lead to hormonal imbalances which, in turn, interfere with immune function. Of all the body's systems, stress damages immune function the most. It does so by overly activating the sympathetic part of the autonomic nervous system, the part that controls the "fight-or-flight" response and initiates adrenaline and cortisol release.

Research in psychoneuroimmunology, or PNI, has shown that the immune and nervous systems are linked by extensive networks of nerve endings in the spleen, bone marrow, lymph nodes, and thymus gland (a primary source of T cells). At the same time, receptors for a variety of chemical messengers—catecholamines, prostaglandins, thyroid hormone, growth hormone, sex hormones, serotonin, and endorphins—have been found on the surfaces of white blood cells. Such connections serve to integrate the activities of the immune, hormonal, and nervous systems, enabling the mind and emotional states to influence the body's resistance to disease.[3]

Stress and the Adrenal Glands

The adrenal glands, part of the body's endocrine system, are located atop the kidneys. The glands are composed of two types of tissue: the adrenal medulla and the adrenal cortex. The adrenal medulla, comprising 10%-20% of the gland, is located in the interior portion and is responsible for the production of the hormones epinephrine (adrenaline) and norepinephrine (noradrenaline). These hormones are released in direct response to the sympathetic nervous system, which is responsible for the fight-or-flight response to stress or physical threats. The adrenal cortex, the outer layer, surrounds the medulla and accounts for 80%-90% of the gland. It is responsible for the production of corticosteroids (also called adrenal steroids). Over 30 different steroids have been isolated from the adrenal cortex, including cortisol and cortisone.

Cortisol secretion (as well as the adrenal gland's other steroids, DHEA, adrenaline, and aldosterone) occurs in daily cycles, peaking in the morning and having the lowest values at night. Cortisol promotes protein building, regulates insulin and glycogen synthesis, and helps produce prostaglandins (hormone-like fatty acids involved in inflammatory processes). Under conditions of stress, high amounts of cortisol are released. Imbalances in cortisol secretion are linked with low energy, inflammation, muscle dysfunction, impaired bone repair, thyroid dysfunction, immune system depression, sleep disorders, and poor skin regeneration.

A number of studies have found a connection between stress and disturbed sleeping patterns. In one study, comparisons between good and poor sleepers showed that stress and insufficient skills for coping with stress contributed to ongoing sleep disorders.[5] Another study indicated that, on average, 41% of insomnia cases were related to stress or other emotional factors.[6] And a recent study of 15 chronic insomniacs found that elevated levels of the stress hormones cortisol and adrenaline were positively correlated with the amount and quality of sleep.[7]

In October 1995, a panel of the National Institutes of Health announced that their review of the clinical data showed that meditation and other relaxation techniques (such as biofeedback and hypnosis) can be effective treatments for insomnia and chronic pain. The panel was made up of experts in behavior, pain and sleep medicine, nursing, psychology, and neurology.[8]

Are You Stressed Out?

If you answer "yes" to more than five of the questions below, it indicates that you have too much stress in your life. In parentheses after each question are some potential underlying causes for the problem.

Fight-or-Flight Response

Pioneering stress researcher Hans Selye, M.D., a Canadian physiologist, noted a consistent pattern of response to stress and termed these the general adaptation syndrome (GAS), commonly referred to as the "fight-or-flight" response. The GAS occurs in three stages: the alarm reaction, the stage of resistance, and the stage of exhaustion.

Initially, the body's biochemistry tends to react to stress in an orderly fashion. Stimulation of the sympathetic nervous system (part of the autonomic nervous system) activates the secretion of hormones from the endocrine glands and constricts both the blood vessels and the involuntary muscles of the body. When the endocrine glands (pancreas, thyroid, pituitary, sex glands, and particularly the adrenals) are stimulated, heart rate, glucose metabolism, and oxygen consumption increase. The parasympathetic nervous system is also stimulated, which begins a process of relaxation. The pituitary gland responds by releasing a variety of hormones throughout the body, which influence the defensive and adaptive mechanisms. Endorphins, the body's own natural painkillers, are also released.

Dr. Selye points out, however, that eventually chronic stress depletes the body's resources and its ability to adapt. If stress continues and remains unattended for a long period, coping functions will be compromised and illness will result.[4]

- Do you often grind your teeth? (digestive dysfunction, parasites)
- Is your breath shallow and irregular? (low metabolic energy, food allergies)
- Are your hands and feet cold? (hormonal imbalance, adrenal/thyroid weakness)
- Do you have trouble sleeping or tend to wake up tired? (liver dysfunction, food allergies)
- Do you often have an upset stomach? (food allergies)
- Do you get mad or irritated easily? (liver dysfunction)
- Do you feel worthless? (low metabolic energy, chronic fatigue)
- Do you constantly worry? (hormonal imbalance)
- Do you have problems concentrating and articulating your thoughts? (low metabolic energy, digestive or hormonal imbalance)
- Do you frequently fidget, chew your fingers, or bite your nails? (food allergies, digestive disturbances)
- Do you have high blood pressure? (food allergies, digestive disturbances)
- Do you eat, drink, or smoke excessively? (low metabolic energy, poor diet)
- Do you sometimes turn to recreational drugs just to get away? (low metabolic energy, poor diet)

Are Your Adrenal Glands Stressed?

The Adrenal Stress Index (ASI) evaluates how well one's adrenal glands are functioning by tracking hormone levels over a 24-hour cycle (circadian rhythm). Four saliva samples taken at intervals throughout the day are used to reconstruct the adrenal rhythm in the laboratory. Saliva has been shown to closely mirror blood levels of hormones and a saliva test is also less invasive. These samples are used to determine whether two main stress hormones (cortisol and DHEA) are being secreted in proper proportion to each other, and at the right times. Based on the results, a physician can prescribe the appropriate treatment to restore the balance of hormones and correct the circadian rhythm.

Success Story: Homeopathy Cures Insomnia

Dolores, a 38-year-old hospital desk clerk, had tried almost all the traditional and alternative cures for her insomnia. For the past five years, Dolores would either fall asleep easily and then wake up at 3 a.m. or 4 a.m., unable to fall back asleep, or, if she had trouble falling asleep, she would be up until 3 a.m. Alternatively, she would fall asleep easily but wake up every hour, starting around 1 a.m., and then by early morning be awake for good. By the time she came to Thomas Kruzel, N.D., of Gresham, Oregon, Dolores had tried enrolling in a hospital sleep clinic, sampled several sleep drugs, taken the herb valerian, and tried taking melatonin to help sleep. None of the strategies had any effect. In addition, Dolores appeared to lead a relatively healthy lifestyle: she liked her work and had a good relationship with her husband, she exercised moderately, ate a balanced diet, and had cut down on coffee, abstaining from drinking any coffee after 10 a.m.

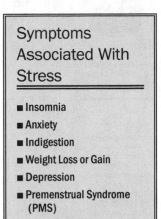

Symptoms Associated With Stress

■ Insomnia

■ Anxiety

■ Indigestion

■ Weight Loss or Gain

■ Depression

■ Premenstrual Syndrome (PMS)

■ Bad Breath or Body Odors

■ Muscle Spasms

Dr. Kruzel tested Dolores's adrenal gland cycle and DHEA levels using a salivary cortisol test. He found she had high cortisol levels late at night. Normally, the cortisol levels are high at 8 a.m., but Dolores' levels were high at midnight. Dolores had higher-than-normal levels of cortisol throughout the day as well. After taking Dolores' case history, he prescribed a single homeopathic remedy: *Carcinosin* 30C, once per day (two pellets). Although insomnia is one

For the **Adrenal Stress Index test**, contact: Diagnos-Tech, Inc., 6620 South 192nd Place, J-2204, Kent, WA 96032; tel: 800-878-3787 or 425-251-0596; fax: 425-251-0637.

of the indications for *Carcinosin*, the prescription was based not so much on Dolores' symptom profile, but on her family history of cancer, diabetes, and tuberculosis, Dr. Kruzel says. The name *Carsinocin* is derived from carcinoma, a type of cancer. According to the principles of homeopathy, *Carsinosin* is indicated when there are symptoms of various cancers in the family.[9]

Dr. Kruzel also prescribed phosphoserine, a combination of proteins, amino acids, and phosphorus, which is often successful in inducing sleep (500 mg twice a day), and pituitary glandular supplements (two tablets twice a day with meals).

Dolores was also placed on a vegetarian diet, based on her blood type. Dr. Kruzel says Dolores' diet wasn't so much an issue, but his clinic has almost all its patients follow the blood-type system. One concern was Dolores' high cortisol levels, which indicated a maladaptive stress syndrome. Even though Dolores appeared happy and calm, her body was signaling that she was under a great deal of stress. After

For **dietary recom-
mendations for sleep
disorders**, see Chapter
3: Improve Your Diet,
pp. 56-85.

For **glandular supple-
ments**, contact:
Standard Process
Laboratories, 1200
West Royal Lee Drive,
P.O. Box 904,
Palmyra, WI 53156;
tel: 800-232-8877 or
262-495-2122;
fax: 262-495-2512.

one month on the homeopathic remedy, Dolores was sleeping through the night about half the time, 6-8 hours per night. Her insomnia patterns persisted on the other nights, but Dolores began to feel much better because she was getting some rest, if not perfect sleep.

For the next year, Dolores saw Dr. Kruzel at six weeks, at eight weeks, at three months, and then at six months. After ten weeks, Dr. Kruzel increased the potency of the *Carcinosin* to 200C, which Dolores took in a liquid form, one dose that she drank in Dr. Kruzel's office, four or five drops in a little water. He did this to speed up Dolores' progress. Dolores stayed on the phosphoserine for three months, and continued with the diet. Dr. Kruzel stopped the pituitary supplements after one month. After about eight months, Dolores no longer needed any of the medicines and was sleeping through the night almost every night. "It took about eight or nine months for her to completely readjust her cycle, but by her last visit, she was doing fine. Her sleep pattern had returned to normal," Dr. Kruzel says.

Mind/Body Therapies for Better Sleep

According to Hans Selye, M.D., whether a person experiences stress as a positive motivational force or as a negative detrimental one depends on their perception of the stress.[10] People who perceive that they are in control of their lives and generally feel good about themselves (referred to as an "inner locus of control") will use life's stressors in a positive fashion. However, those who feel that their life circumstances are controlled by outside forces and other people ("outer locus of control") tend to react negatively to stress. The locus of control can be consciously shifted by deliberately "reprogramming" the mind, with positive instead of negative thoughts, through meditation and cognitive therapy. Relaxation therapies, such as biofeedback, hypnotherapy, guided imagery, flower remedies, and aromatherapy, among others, can help reduce your stress levels and relieve your sleep problems.

Meditation

Meditation is a safe and simple way to balance a person's physical, emotional, and mental states. It is easy to learn and can be useful for treating stress and sleep disorders. Meditation, in the broadest sense, is any activity that keeps the attention focused in the present. When the mind is calm and focused in the present, it is not reacting to past events or preoccupied with future plans, two major sources of chronic stress. The concept of "being here now" can be very important for reversing insomnia, because insomnia, by its nature, creates the opposite state—a person who is lost in the "mental movies" of the mind, out of touch with the body, and stressed. There are many forms of meditation, but they can be categorized into two main approaches, concentration meditation and mindfulness meditation.

Concentration meditation focuses the "lens of the mind" on one object, sound (mantra), the breath, an image, or thought, to still the mind and allow greater awareness or clarity to emerge. The breath is one of the most popular objects of focus in this type of meditation. As the person focuses on the ebb and flow of their breath, the mind is absorbed in the rhythm and becomes more placid, tranquil, and still. Mindfulness-based meditation entails bringing the mind to a still point, tuning out the world and bringing the mind to a halt as much as possible. Mindfulness meditation helps us practice non-judgment. The meditator sits quietly and simply witnesses whatever goes through the mind, not reacting or becoming involved with thoughts, memories, worries, or images. This helps the person gain a more calm, clear, and non-reactive state of mind.

Transcendental Meditation™ (TM), a popular form of concentration meditation, is the most well-documented regarding the physio-

A Simple Meditation Exercise

The first step to practicing meditation is learning to breathe in a manner that facilitates a state of calmness and awareness. Dr. Kabat-Zinn recommends the following exercise for achieving a sense of calmness—find a quiet place where you will not be disturbed and practice for several minutes each day:

■ Assume a comfortable posture lying on your back or sitting. If you are sitting, keep the spine straight and let your shoulders drop.

■ Close your eyes if it feels comfortable.

■ Bring your attention to your belly, feeling it rise or expand gently on the in-breath and fall or recede on the out-breath. Keep the focus on your breathing.

■ When your mind wanders off the breath, notice what it was that took you away and then gently bring your attention back to your belly and the feeling of the breath moving in and out. If your mind wanders away from the breath, your "job" is simply to bring it back to the breath every time, no matter what it has become preoccupied with.

Practice this exercise for 15 minutes every day, whether you feel like it or not, for one week and see how it feels to incorporate a disciplined meditation practice into your life.

logical effects of meditation, with over 500 clinical studies conducted to date.[11] Research shows that, during TM practice, the body gains a deeper state of relaxation than during ordinary rest or sleep.[12] Brain wave changes indicate a state of enhanced awareness and coherence and TM has been found to increase intelligence, creativity, and perceptual ability and reduce blood pressure and rates of illness by 50%.[13] TM also causes decreased blood levels of cortisol, a hormone responsible for many of the deleterious physiological changes seen with stress,[14] and increased EEG (electroencephalogram) alpha, a brain wave associated with relaxation.[15]

Mainstream institutions are starting to incorporate meditation. Several years ago, meditation teacher Jon Kabat-Zinn, Ph.D., author of *Wherever You Go, There You Are*, established the Stress Reduction Clinic at the University of Massachusetts Medical Center. The clinic's program teaches people how to meditate, reduce stress, and other techniques to heal themselves. In one experiment at the clinic, 22 patients suffering from panic attacks and anxiety went through an eight-week course in mindfulness meditation. When the course ended, 20 of them felt significantly less depressed and anxious. In other studies at the clinic, patients with chronic pain reported a 50% reduction in their suffering after learning how to meditate.[16]

"Through meditation, we can learn to access the relaxation response and to be aware of the mind and the way our attitudes produce stress," according to Joan Borysenko, Ph.D., a pioneer in the field of mind/body medicine and founder of the Mind-Body Clinic at Harvard Medical School's Deaconess Hospital. "By quieting the mind, meditation can also put one in touch with the inner physician, allowing the body's own wisdom to be heard." Instead of running to the doctor sleeping pills, for example, Dr. Borysenko advises us to pay attention to the body and ask ourselves, "What is going on in my mind or what's happening in my life that I need to attend to?"[17]

Biofeedback

Biofeedback training is a method of learning how to consciously regulate normally unconscious bodily functions (such as breathing, heart rate, and blood pressure) through the use of simple electronic devices. Biofeedback is particularly useful for learning to reduce stress, eliminate headaches, reduce muscle spasms, and relieve pain. Biofeedback can intercept a chronic fight-or-flight response and aid in revitalizing adrenal gland functions. By teaching patients relaxation techniques, biofeedback helps them reduce or eliminate sleep problems.

Biofeedback devices give immediate "feedback" or information about the biological system of the person being monitored, so that he or she can learn to consciously influence that system. For example, a person seeking to regulate their heart rate would train with a biofeedback device set up to transmit one blinking light or one audible beep per heartbeat. Electrodes are placed on the patient's skin (a simple, painless process). The patient is then instructed to use various techniques such as meditation, relaxation, and visualization to effect the desired response (muscle relaxation, lowered heart rate, or lowered temperature). The biofeedback device reports the patient's progress by a change in the speed of the beeps or flashes. By learning to alter the rate of the flashes or beeps, the person would be subtly programmed to control the heart rate.

The idea of biofeedback training is that the person will learn how to relax during the sessions with the machines, then use those relaxation techniques by themselves, in daily life, whenever stressful situations arise. For insomnia, biofeedback can be successful if the practitioner uses the biofeedback machine that corresponds to the patient's type of insomnia, according to Melvyn Werbach, M.D., director of the Biofeedback Medical Clinic in Tarzana, California. "Biofeedback is appropriate when insomnia is due to overactivation of the autonomic nervous system," Dr. Werbach says. "I use it particularly with people who have a problem with obsessive thinking when they try to go to sleep. This is when EEG biofeedback is most effective."

Similarly, Peter Hauri, Ph.D., says that people who have insomnia because of extreme muscle tension when they're trying to sleep can be helped using muscle-tension biofeedback. In two experiments, Dr. Hauri found that biofeedback had a lasting effect on insomnia. In the first study, at Dartmouth Medical School, 45 insomniacs kept written logs of their sleep habits and then spent three nights in the sleep laboratory. They were given biofeedback training and then continued with biofeedback at home. They returned to the lab for checkups after several weeks and again after nine months. The study showed that insomniacs who were tense and anxious were helped by biofeedback, but it didn't help people who were relaxed muscularly but still couldn't sleep. In a second study, 16 people with severe insomnia participated. All the subjects had suffered from chronic insomnia for at least two years. The subjects were evaluated during three nights at the Dartmouth Sleep Disorders Center and were given a series of questionnaires and interviews. Then they participated in biofeedback

For more information on **biofeedback**, contact: Association for Applied Biofeedback and Physiopsychology, 10200 W. 44th Avenue, Suite 304, Wheat Ridge, CO 80033; tel: 800-477-8892 or 303-422-8436; fax: 303-422-8894.

training. Sleep improved for the 16 subjects after the biofeedback training and continued through the nine-month checkup. But Dr. Hauri again emphasizes that this type of biofeedback works best for people who are muscularly tense.[18]

Hypnotherapy

Hypnotherapy has therapeutic applications for both psychological and physical disorders. A skilled hypnotherapist can facilitate profound changes in respiration and relaxation to create positive shifts in behavior and an enhanced sense of well-being. A physiological shift can be observed in a hypnotic state, as can greater control of autonomic nervous system functions normally considered beyond one's ability to control. Stress reduction is a common occurrence as is a lowering of blood pressure. Hypnotherapy can be a key to switching off insomnia because it provides a way to contact the deeper, unconscious self and to let go of old anxiety patterns and instead create healthy lifestyle changes.

Hypnosis works by accessing the unconscious mind and training it to react in a positive way, such as inducing an immediate sense of relaxation. Hypnotherapy can be a nurturing and highly relaxing experience. Certified hypnotherapists do not attempt to control your mind or take you into a state so deep that you do not have control over yourself. Most people are aware of everything that transpires during a hypnotherapy session, yet they are able to mobilize deeper levels of their mind to facilitate healing.

Hypnotherapy is currently taught in several allopathic medical programs and has been approved by the American Medical Association as a clinical adjunct in the management of chronic pain.[19] Some states certify the profession of hypnotherapy by requiring a certain level of training. Other types of practitioners, such as psychotherapists and body workers, may also use hypnosis as a tool to help their patients relax.

For **information and referrals for hypnotherapy**, contact: Bryan Knight, The International Registry of Professional Hypnotherapists, 7306 Sherbrooke Street West, Montreal, Quebec, Canada H4B 1R7; tel: 514-489-6733; fax: 514-485-3828; website: www.hypnosis.org.

See "Meditation," p. 339, and "Hypnotherapy," p. 306.

Visualization/Guided Imagery

Using the power of the mind to evoke a positive physical response, guided imagery and visualization can modulate the immune system and help with insomnia. It is similar to meditation, except that instead of focusing on the breath or a mantra, you allow your mind to dwell on a positive vision of what you would like to bring into your life. The patient uses the imagination to elicit positive physiological responses.

Self-Hypnosis for Relaxation and Sleep

Here are the basic steps that can induce a state of self-hypnosis:

1. Think of an affirmation and place it in the back of your mind. An affirmation is a simple statement of a goal about the future, made in the present tense as if that goal had already been achieved. Here are some examples of affirmations: "As I sleep soundly, I feel refreshed" or "Each breath enhances my relaxation" or "Every day, I feel calmer and calmer, stronger and stronger, healthier and healthier." The purpose of putting the goal in the present tense is so the subconscious knows it must make what is stated into a reality. The subconscious finds the best and fastest way to that goal.

2. Take three slow comfortable breaths. Close your eyes.

3. Signal to your body to relax from head to toe. You can suggest that each part feel relaxed, heavy, warm, or is letting go. Say to yourself: "My forehead is relaxed...the muscles around my eyes and mouth are relaxed...my jaw releases and drops open slightly, releasing all the tension in my face...my neck and shoulders are relaxed...my arms and hands are heavy and warm...my chest and belly are relaxed, as my breathing becomes smooth and calm...my hips and buttocks feel heavy and relaxed...my knees, calves, ankles, and feet feel heavy and warm...my toes are relaxed."

4. Count backward from 100 to 95. Visualize the numbers as you count, either on a large screen coming into focus and fading or seeing the numbers appear in changing colors.

5. Imagine a special place, where everything is exactly as you would like it to be. Is it a mountain forest with sunlight filtering through the trees? Is there a rippling stream or a sparkling lake or wildflowers in a field? Is it a tropical beach with crystal blue water? Fill in all the details (colors, sounds, textures, and smells) of this place. You may want to build a shelter of some kind there, as simple or as elaborate as you like—imagine the details of your shelter.

6. Repeat your affirmation three times.

7. Offer thanks to the universe for your creation or a positive occurrence.

8. When you feel ready, say good bye mentally to your special place and slowly open your eyes. The new thought, feeling, or goal is now part of your subconscious.

By directly accessing emotions, imagery can help an individual understand the needs that may be represented by an illness and can help develop ways to meet those needs. Imagery is also one of the quickest and most direct ways to become aware of emotions and their effects on health, both positive and negative.

Imagery is simply a flow of thoughts that one can see, hear, feel, smell, taste, or experience. According to Martin L. Rossman, M.D., of the Academy for Guided Imagery, in Mill Valley, California, while the sensory phenomenon that is being experienced in the mind may or may not represent external reality, it always depicts internal reality.

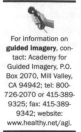

For information on **guided imagery**, contact: Academy for Guided Imagery, P.O. Box 2070, Mill Valley, CA 94942; tel: 800-726-2070 or 415-389-9325; fax: 415-389-9342; website: www.healthy.net/agi.

What Dr. Rossman means is that the sensations in the body that imagery creates are very real phenomena that can be measured via laboratory devices. Research using brain scans indicates that imagery activates parts of the cerebral cortex and centers of the primitive brain. During visualization, the visual (optic) cortex is active, and when sounds are imagined, the auditory cortex is active. It appears that the cortex can create imaginary realities and the lower centers (and perhaps every cell in the body) respond to this information. "If you are a good worrier," states Dr., Rossman, "and especially if you ever 'worry yourself sick', you may be an especially good candidate for learning how to positively affect your health with imagery, as the internal process involved in worrying yourself sick and 'imagining yourself well' are quite similar."

Here's an example of a visualization for someone with sleep problems: You are filling a tub with warm, aromatic, sudsy water. You get in and soak for 20 minutes. Then, you get out, dry off with a fluffy bath towel, yawn, and put on flannel pajamas. You pick up a cup of warm herb tea and sip it for a few minutes at your bedside. Then you climb into your warm, comfortable bed and fall easily asleep. You sleep soundly and deeply through the night, your body getting nourished by all the deep rest. Then, in the morning, the sun streams in the window and you wake up, feeling completely rested and refreshed, full of energy and vitality.

The whole visualization process could take up to 20 minutes. This is the same technique that some elite athletes successfully use to visualize winning tennis matches, being strong and poised at the finish line, or breaking world records. Try to repeat the visualization once or twice a day for a few days; as you're visualizing, feel free to elaborate and add more details. Then, see if you can reproduce the same script in real life.

Counseling

Each person with sleep problems has his or her own reasons—physical, emotional, or chemical—for disturbed sleep. In many cases, people need only counseling in what types of behavioral, dietary, or physical changes they need to make and some support in making those changes. Cognitive therapy is a form of counseling useful for those with sleep problems. It has been estimated the average human being has around 50,000 thoughts per day, according to Dr. Richard Carlson, author of *Don't Sweat The Small Stuff...And It's All Small Stuff*. Unfortunately, he reminds us, many of them are also going to be negative—angry, fearful, pessimistic, or worrisome. Up to 85% of the thinking we regularly engage in is negative and self-defeating.[20] The basis of cognitive therapy is to identify—through maintaining a journal and by introspection—the negative, self-defeating inner dialogue of thoughts (what cognitive therapists refer to as "automatic thoughts"). Positive, coping thoughts can then be used to counter the negative thoughts. The goal is to pull yourself out of reflexive self-destructive mental behavior that may be exacerbating your sleep problems and to bolster the positive, self-reliant aspect of your personality. Cognitive therapy does not focus on the root causes of psychological problems, rather it seeks to support health by interrupting the flow of negative thoughts. Countering each negative thought on paper with a list of positive responses to the same problem enables the mind to reframe the situation.

For more information on **cognitive therapy**, contact: University of Pennsylvania Center for Cognitive Therapy, 3600 Market Street, 8th Floor, Philadelphia, PA 19104, tel: 215-898-4100; fax: 215-898-1865. The American Institute for Cognitive Therapy, 136 E. 57th Street, Suite 1101, New York, NY 10022; tel: 212-308-2440.

In addition to counseling, there are specific coping strategies for typical disruptive habits that can disturb sleep.

1. For people who tend to have conditioned responses to certain stimuli, such as anxiety, when they go into the bedroom:

■ Go to bed only when sleepy.

■ Use the bed only for sleeping; do not read, watch TV, or eat in bed.

■ If unable to sleep, get up and move to another room. Stay up and do some relaxing activity until really sleepy, then return to bed. If sleep does not come easily, get out of bed again. The goal is to associate the bed not with frustration and sleeplessness, but with falling asleep easily and quickly. Repeat this step as needed. You may need to do it as many as ten times a night at first but that will lessen as your condition improves.

■ Set the alarm and get up at the same time every morning, regardless of how much or how little you sleep during the night. This helps the body to acquire a constant sleep/wake rhythm.

■ Do not nap during the day.

2. For people who feel they have no control over their lives, a frequent feeling of people who suffer from insomnia, and for people who feeling stressed in general:

■ Schedule 30 minutes or more of "worry time" at least three hours before bedtime. Write down what you are worrying about on index cards, then write the solution at the bottom of the card. The purpose is to get these thoughts out of your head and onto paper.

Sleep Check List

Each morning, check off the recommendations you followed the night before to prepare your mind and body for sleep:

Ate an early dinner _____
Filled out worry cards 3 hours before bedtime _____
Took a short walk after dinner _____
Avoided focused work after dinner _____
Avoided TV after dinner _____
Enjoyed light, relaxing activities _____
Drank herbal tea _____
Took a warm bath _____
Set alarm for 6-7 a.m. or earlier _____
In bed before 10 p.m. _____ If later, record time _____
Breathing exercises to relax in bed _____
Self-hypnosis to relax in bed _____
Woke up before 6-7 a.m. _____ If later, record time _____

Then put the cards into categories: financial, business, personal, children, mates, parents, etc. After you have written the cards, organized them, and given them some attention, deposit all the cards in a worry box before you go to bed. Take them out again, review them, add to them, or change them at the next scheduled worry time. If you find the worries creeping back into your mind as you're trying to sleep, say to yourself, "I've already worked that out."

Cranial Electrical Stimulation

Experimentation with low-level electrical stimulation of the brain was started in France in the early 1900s. It was originally called electrosleep as it was thought to be able to induce sleep. Newer names developed, such as transcranial electrotherapy and neuroelectric therapy. Research on the use of what is now called cranial electrical stimulation (CES) for treatment of anxiety began in the Soviet Union during the 1950s.[21]

For information on **cranial electrical stimulation**, contact: PATH Medical, 274 Madison Avenue, Suite 402, New York, NY 10016; tel: 212-213-6155; fax: 212-213-6188. For the **Alpha-Stim CES device**, contact: Electromedical Products International, 2201 Garrett Morris Parkway, Mineral Wells, TX 76067; tel: 800-FOR-PAIN or 940-328-0788.

According to Eric Braverman, M.D., CES devices work by stimulating brain tissue to produce more essential neurochemicals that may have been depleted due to stress or anxiety. These neurochemicals act to increase the beta endorphin levels in the brain—the substances that produce the "feel-good" or "runner's high" relaxed state.[22] The U.S. Food and Drug Administration has approved CES devices for treatment of insomnia, depression, and anxiety.

In 1996, Daniel Kirsch, Ph.D., a neurobiologist, reviewed 103 studies of CES involving 4,848 subjects. He found there were significant changes in relaxation levels in the subjects who received CES treatments, including slower electroencephalograms and reductions in blood pressure, respiration, and heart rate. In a survey of health-care practitioners who used CES on their patients, 71 of 74 patients who had insomnia reported 95% improvement after using the device.[23]

Some minor side effects reported with CES use are burning at the electrode site or some dizziness for a short time afterwards. For insomnia, Dr. Braverman recommends using the CES device before bed, but other physicians caution it can be too stimulating and should be used at least three hours before bedtime to induce sleep.

Herbal Therapy

There are specific herbs used for insomnia that have a sedative effect to ease stress and anxiety. Herbalist Terry Willard, director of the Wild Rose College of Natural Healing in Calgary, Alberta, recommends the following seven herbs for people with insomnia: valerian, hops, reishi mushrooms, skullcap, passionflower, kava-kava, and lemon balm.[24] Most of these herbs are available at health food stores or through your health-care practitioner.

■ Valerian (*Valeriana officinalis*): The odorous root of valerian has been used in European traditional medicine as a natural tranquillizer for centuries. In Germany, valerian root and its teas and extracts are approved as over-the-counter medicines for "states of excitation" and "difficulty in falling asleep owing to nervousness."[25] A scientific team representing the European community has reviewed the research on valerian and concluded that it is a safe nighttime sleep aid. These scientists also found that there are no major adverse reactions associated with the use of valerian and, unlike barbiturates and other conventional drugs for insomnia, valerian does not have a synergy with alcohol, meaning it is not dangerous to mix the two.[26] Possessing warming qualites, valerian is also effective in easing muscle pain when applied topically.[27] A randomized, double-blind study of 121 insomnia patients showed that those given 600 mg of valerian extract daily for four weeks slept better and were more rested than those in the control group. The valerian group reported a significant improvement in sleep quality by the end of the study; about 3% of the subjects in both groups reported side effects.

Willard recommends a dose of 300-400 mg of valerian

For more about **herbs or a referral to an herbalist**, contact: Herb Research Foundation, 1007 Pearl Street, Suite 200, Boulder, CO 80302; tel: 800-748-2617.

Acupuncture for Stress Reduction

To help patients cope with stress, as well as correct other imbalances that may be contributing to sleep disorders, practitioners of mind/body medicine often adjust a patient's energy fields. These fields, generally ignored by mainstream practitioners, link the emotions, consciousness, and physical body. "Other cultures recognize that there is a kind of energy that animates us," says Kristy Fassler, N.D., of Portsmouth, New Hampshire, a practitioner of both homeopathy and naturopathy. "It's called *qi* in China, *prana* in India."

In the Chinese model, *qi* is considered to be the life force that flows along specific pathways, called meridians, throughout the body. Points of heightened energy along the meridians are called acupoints. Sometimes the flow of *qi* in the body can become blocked, causing illnesses to develop. An acupuncturist uses the acupoints to stimulate the flow of *qi* and thus restore health to the body. In addition to its physical effects, acupuncture has a positive psychological effect as well. Acupuncture is equivalent to the effect of drug-based therapies in cases of depression, insomnia, and other nervous disorders, and its action is swift and lasting without the side effects of drugs.[28]

For information on **acupuncture** or a referral to an acupuncturist in your area, contact: American Association of Acupuncture and Oriental Medicine, 4101 Lake Boone Trail, Suite 201, Raleigh, NC 27607; tel: 919-787-5181.

extract (standardized to 0.5% of essential oil) taken about one hour before bedtime. It can be mildly habit-forming, with stronger doses required over time to get the same effect, so Willard recommends taking valerian for no more than a month at a time, or for occasional sleepless nights.[29] Rob McCaleb, president of the Herb Research Foundation in Boulder, Colorado, says valerian root extract is his top choice for treating insomnia, and he does not believe valerian is addictive. He says studies have shown that the extract reduces the time it takes to fall asleep and improves sleep quality. He recommends taking valerian 30-45 minutes before bed at one of the following doses: 1-2 g (about ½ oz) of the root in tea; 150-300 mg of the standardized herb extract; or one teaspoon of the tincture. He cautions that 10% of people are stimulated by valerian instead of sedated.[30]

■ Hops (*Humulus lupulus*): Hops has been used as a bittering and preservative agent in brewing for centuries. In Germany, hops is licensed for use in states of unrest and anxiety as well as sleep disorders, due to its calming and sleep-inducing properties. European medicinal plant researchers have approved the use of hops for such conditions as nervous tension, excitability, restlessness, and sleep disturbances, and as an aid to stimulate appetite. Unlike other types of sedatives, there are neither dependence nor withdrawal symptoms reported with the use of hops, nor are there any reports of adverse side effects. Hops tea is effective just before bedtime; use one heaping teaspoon of whole hops per cup of water for tea.[31] Dr. Hobbs recommends a valerian-hops preparation as a daytime sedative because it will not interfere with or slow reflexive responses[32]—again, unlike conventional pharmaceuticals.

■ Passionflower (*Passiflora incarnata*): Passionflower has enjoyed a long tradition of use for its mildly sedative properties. In Germany, passionflower is approved as an over-the-counter drug for states of "nervous unrest."[33] It is often added to other calming herbs, usually valerian and hawthorn. Pharmacological studies indicate antispasmodic, sedative, anxiety-allaying, and hypotensive (blood pressure-lowering) activity of passionflower extracts.[34] Passionflower is said to help in quieting worry and giving a feeling of well-being. For the anxiety and stress associated with sleep disorders, this can be an effective herb. For a tea, use boiling water over half a teaspoon of the dried herb; or use a tincture or extract.

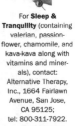

For **Sleep & Tranquility** (containing valerian, passionflower, chamomile, and kava-kava along with vitamins and minerals), contact: Alternative Therapy, Inc., 1664 Fairlawn Avenue, San Jose, CA 95125; tel: 800-311-7922.

■ Kava-Kava (*Piper methysticum*): An extract of the kava-kava plant (a slow-growing bushy perennial) acts as a natural tranquilizer. According to E. Lehmann, M.D., and colleagues, when 29 patients diagnosed with anxiety (including panic disorder and general tension) took kava-kava at the rate of 100 mg three times daily for four weeks, and were then evaluated using three standard psychological profiles of anxiety, all measures were significantly lower. No side effects or adverse reactions occurred, and benefits were noted as early as the first and second weeks.[35] In another study of 101 people, 100 mg of kava-kava extract taken three times daily produced significant improvement in anxiety and tension; the effects were noted from the eighth week of supplementation. Specifically, 20% of those taking kava-kava were rated "very much improved" according to a standard anxiety scale, while only 10.5% of the placebo group received a similar rating. After 24 weeks of taking the herbal extract, the percentages were 53.1% of the kava group and 30.2% of those taking a placebo.[36] Kava is useful when anxiety is a contributing factor in insomnia or other sleep problems. A typical recommended dose is 100 mg of kava extract (standardized to 70% kavalactones, the active ingredient) daily, divided into three equal doses.

■ Chamomile (German or wild, *Matricaria recutita*; Roman, *Anthemis nobilis*): The flower of the chamomile plant produces a calming effect, easing anxiety and reducing tension.[37] It can thus be helpful

Herbs Can Be Used in Many Forms

Whole Herbs: dried plants or plant parts that are cut or powdered. Depending on their source, whole herbs can have varying degrees of potency and contamination. Buy whole herbs from reputable manufacturers.

Teas: loose or teabag form; steeping in boiled water for a few minutes, releases the fragrance, aromatic flavor, and the herb's medicinal properties.

Capsules and Tablets: convenient and popular form of herbs; some herbs, such as goldenseal, have repulsive flavors which are hidden in a capsule or tablet.

Extracts and Tinctures: high concentrations of an herb that are more quickly assimilated by the body than tablets; Alcohol (or sometimes glycerin) is used as a solvent to extract non-water-soluble compounds from the herb and as a preservative. Tinctures usually contain more alcohol than extracts (sometimes 70% to 80% alcohol). Herbal tinctures and extracts should look and taste like the herb or plant it was derived from.

Essential Oils: distilled from various parts of medicinal and aromatic plants except oils of citrus fruits, which come directly from the fruit peel. Essential oils are highly concentrated and should be used sparingly for internal purposes. Dilute essential oils in water or in fatty oils if using topically except eucalyptus and tea tree oils, which can be applied directly to the skin without concern of irritation.

Salves, Balms, and Ointments: used for muscle aches, insect bites, or wounds; usually available in a vegetable oil base.

with overall anxiety, sleep disorders, and muscle tension. Its calming property has a beneficial effect on the gastrointestinal system as well. In Europe, chamomile is recognized as a digestive aid, a mild sedative, and an anti-inflammatory, notably in antibacterial oral hygiene and skin preparations.[38]

■ St. John's Wort (*Hypericum perforatum*): A remedy long used as an anti-inflammatory, wound-healer, mild sedative, and pain-reliever, St. John's wort has recently attracted medical attention. Traditionally used to treat neuralgia, anxiety, tension, and similar problems, it is now being increasingly recommended in the treatment of depression.[39] In Germany, St. John's wort is widely prescribed for depression (66 million doses in 1994 alone). In 23 separate clinical trials involving 1,757 patients who reported mild to moderately severe depression, taking 500-900 mg daily of St. John's wort extract (containing up to 2.7% hypericin, the active component of the herb) was three times more effective than a placebo and as effective as standard antidepressants such as Prozac and Zoloft. The researchers noted that it generally takes two to four weeks of steady use before the mood-elevating benefits of St. John's wort take effect.[40] Christopher Hobbs, L.Ac., founder of the American School

Chinese Herbal Formulas for Insomnia

Chinese medicine offers at least six premade herbal formulas (also known as "patent remedies") for restlessness and insomnia, according to acupuncturist/herbalist Lesley Tierra, L.Ac., Dip.Ac. These remedies are available at Chinese pharmacies or by mail order from Chinese herbal suppliers. Dr. Tierra offers the following list of insomnia symptoms matched with the appropriate formula:

For a mail-order source of **Chinese patent remedies**, contact: Mayway Corp., 1338 Mandela Parkway, Oakland, CA 94607; tel: 510-208-3113; fax: 510-208-3069.

Mental Agitation—This type of insomnia is accompanied by exhaustion, anxiety, mental agitation, excessive dreaming and thinking, red or irritated eyes, and poor memory. Remedy: An Mien Pien (four tablets, three times daily); do not eat hot greasy foods while using this remedy.

Night Sweats—Symptoms include restlessness, anxiety, palpitations, night sweats, vivid dreaming, and nocturnal emissions. Remedy: Emperor's Tea (Tian Wang Bu Xin Wan: eight pills, three times daily). This formula can also help students during times of prolonged study. Dr. Tierra cautions that this formula should not be used for more than two weeks at a time; discontinue for one week, then resume for two weeks, if needed. Do not eat hot greasy foods while using this remedy.

Nightmares—This type of insomnia is characterized by nightmares, restless sleep, night sweats, dizzyness, ear ringing, palpitations, and fatigue. Remedy: Shen Ching Shuai Jao Wan (20 pills, twice daily). Discontinue use after two weeks as overuse of this remedy can impair digestion; if necessary, resume again after a two-week hiatus, advises Dr. Tierra. Do not consume cold foods while using this formula.

Uneasiness—The accompanying symptoms include palpitations, poor memory, a sense of unease, excessive dreaming, restlessness, and dizziness. Remedy: An Sheung Bu Xin Wan (15 pills, three times daily)."

of Herbalism, has found St. John's wort useful in sleep disorders as well. He credits this to the same action behind the herb's antidepressant properties; that is, it maintains serotonin levels in the brain. Serotonin is a neurotransmitter (essential brain chemical) that influences mood and helps produce sleep.

■ Lemon Balm (*Melissa officinalis*): Lemon balm is an herb of the mint family that has long been used as a folk remedy for insomnia. It is a calming herb, used to relieve tension, anxiety, and other nervous disorders, and to reduce fevers and headaches. As a tea, Willard recommends steeping one to two teaspoons of the herb in a cup of hot, but not boiling, water.; lemon balm can also be mixed with other sedative herbs.

■ Reishi Mushroom (*Ganoderma lucidum*): Reishi has been used for thousands of years as a sedative and immune system tonic. It contains

For **referrals to homeopathic practitioners**, contact: International Foundation for Homeopathy, P.O. Box 7, Edmonds, WA 98020; tel: 206-776-4147. Homeopathic Academy of Naturopathic Physicians, 12132 S.E. Foster Place, Portland, OR 97266; tel: 503-761-3298. National Center for Homeopathy, 801 N. Fairfax, Suite 306, Alexandria, VA 22314.

a complex of phytochemicals that studies have shown to have anti-allergenic, anti-inflammatory, and antioxidant properties. It is used in traditional Chinese medicine for the treatment of high blood pressure, arthritis, insomnia and other nervous disorders, and to increase longevity. Reishi is Willard's herb of choice for insomnia—calming during the day, anxiety-reducing, and helpful in regulating sugar metabolism. He typically recommends three 1-gram tablets of reishi three times a day.[42]

■ Skullcap (*Scutellaria lateriflora*): Skullcap is also a member of the mint family, traditionally used as a nerve tonic and sedative. Skullcap's calming action comes mostly from the component scutellarin, which is antispasmodic.[43] Willard recommends using this herb in combination with reishi, hops, and valerian, or alone as a tincture of 15-40 drops, two to three times daily. As a tea, one to three teaspoons of the root per cup of water are recommended.

Homeopathic Remedies

Homeopathy was founded in the early 1800s by German physician Samuel Hahnemann. Today, an estimated 500 million people worldwide receive homeopathic treatment. Homeopathy is now practiced according to two differing concepts. In classical homeopathy, only one single-component remedy is prescribed at a time in a potency specifically adjusted to the patient; the physician waits to see the results before prescribing anything further. In complex homeopathy, a prescription involves multiple substances given at the same time, usually in low potencies.

Since there are more than 3,000 homeopathic remedies, derived from everything from plants to minerals to animals, choosing the right remedy can be a challenge. The key is uncovering the pattern of behavior or feelings that accompany the insomnia. In the short-term, for occasional insomnia, some basic remedies can be helpful. However, for chronic insomnia, you need what is called a constitutional formula, one that addresses not only the symptom but your underlying life pattern. For the constitutional formula, see a classical homeopath, who will normally thoroughly examine your lifestyle, habits, and medical history before prescribing a remedy.

Homeopathy is based on the principle of "like cures like." This means that the same substance that in large doses produces the symptoms of an illness in very minute doses cures it. The homeopathic remedies are "potentized" from tinctures, meaning they are diluted and then shaken, sometimes as much as 200 times or more. The result is that the final remedy is diluted to such a degree that it contains no molecules of the original substance, only its energetic vibration. According to homeopathic theory, the more times the remedy is potentized, the more powerful it is and the deeper effect it will have.

In classical homeopathy, the symptoms or disturbances clear up in the reverse order that they occurred, beginning with the presenting symptom, such as insomnia. As the more recent symptoms are resolved, new layers of underlying symptoms often present themselves for healing, and the practitioner will adjust the remedy accordingly. The underlying layers are often residues of fevers, trauma, or chronic disease that were unsuccessfully treated or supressed by conventional medicine.

Homeopathic Remedies for Sleep Vary with Symptoms—For occasional, acute, or short-term insomnia, here are some basic remedies. Take them in 30C dosage, one hour before going to bed for ten nights. Repeat the dose if you wake and cannot get to sleep again. For chronic insomnia, you will need to see a classical homeopathic practitioner (or one that is able to use that approach) to get a constitutional remedy.[44]

Aconite: Sleep problems worse after shock or panic; restlessness, nightmares, fear of dying.

Arsenicum album: Waking between midnight and 2 a.m., restless, worried, apprehensive, foreboding dreams of fire or danger.

Belladonna: Restlessness, irritability, overly sensitive to stimuli including light, noise, and touch; excited, angry, and trouble falling asleep.

Chamomilla: Feeling wide awake and irritable during first part of night; especially useful for children.

Coffea: Mind overactive as the result of good or bad news; inability to switch off.

Ignatia: Yawning but can't sleep; dread at not being able to sleep, especially after emotional upset; frequent nightmares; grief is also an indication.

Lycopodium: Mind very active at bedtime, going over and over work done during the day; frequent dreaming, talks and laughs in sleep, wakes around 1 a.m.

Natrum muriaticum: Anxiety, anxious dreams, becoming ill after emotional trauma; sensitive to sudden noise and heat.

Nux vomica: Sleeplessness due to great mental strain, overindulgence in food or alcohol, or withdrawal from alco-

For **homeopathic remedies**, contact: National College of Naturopathic Medicine, 11231 S.E. Market Street, Portland, OR 97216; tel: 503-255-7355.

hol or sleeping tablets; wakes around 3 a.m. or 4 a.m., then falls asleep just as it is time to get up; nightmares, irritable during the day.

Pulsatilla: Restless in early sleep; feels too hot, throws covers off, then feels too cold and lies with arms above head; not thirsty; insomnia worse after rich food.

Rhus toxicodendron: Irritable, restless, walks about, can't sleep, especially if there is pain or discomfort.

Coculus: Too tired to sleep, giddy.

Opium: Sharp senses, bed too hot.

In addition, Robert Milne, M.D., of Las Vegas, Nevada, traces many cases of insomnia to grief. For grieving individuals whose symptoms include irritability, sobbing, and muscle spasms, *Ignatia amara* is often used. Another remedy, *Muriaticum acidum*, is recommended for grief-stricken insomnia patients who are marked by extreme emotional sensitivity (another symptom may be an intolerance of sunlight).

Although there is some disagreement, many homeopaths believe remedies can be antidoted (rendered ineffective) if people consume or expose themselves to strong substances such as coffee, marijuana, mint, camphor, other strong tastes or scents, electric blankets, and dental procedures.

Aromatherapy

Essential oils from plants contain healing agents that are quite powerful. The word *aromatherapy* doesn't do them justice because it sounds as if the smell is the full treatment. "In actuality, the oils exert much of their therapeutic effect through their pharmacological properties and their small molecular size, making them one of the few therapeutic agents to easily penetrate bodily tissues," says Dr. Kurt Schnaubelt, director of the Pacific Institute of Aromatherapy. Dr. Schnaubelt says the chemical makeup of essential oils gives them a host of desirable pharmacological properties, including:

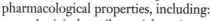

For information about **aromatherapy**, contact: American Alliance of Aromatherapy, P.O. Box 309, Depoe Bay, OR 97341; tel: 800-809-9850. For **aromatherapy oils**, contact: PhytoMedicine Company, 6701 Sunset Drive, Suite 100, Miami, FL 33143; tel: 305-662-6396; fax: 305-667-5619.

■ Antiviral, antibacterial, antispasmodic, diuretic (promoting production and excretion of urine), vasodilators (widening blood vessels), and vasoconstrictors (narrowing blood vessels).

■ Action on the adrenals, ovaries, and thyroid gland, and can energize or pacify, detoxify, and facilitate the digestive system.

■ Can treat infection, interact with the nervous system, affect immune response, and harmonize moods and emotions.

The essential oils are usually extracted from the plants by a special distillation method. Pure oils, without any extenders, are most desirable and have the highest therapeutic value, but are usually quite expensive. Many of the oils sold at health food stores have some type of synthetic or natural extenders added, says Marta Schreiner, a certified aromatherapist in Portland, Oregon. She says people may get some minor results from those oils, but if they want a true healing treatment, they need to buy the pure oils. "It takes a large amount of plant materials to make pure oils," says Schreiner. "But the pure essential oils are 75% more potent." She cautions that some manufacturers advertise "pure oils" but the products still may contain natural extenders. Since it is impossible to verify the purity without chemical analysis, she advises people buy from reputable sources and expect to pay more for a small bottle of oil.

For insomnia, lavender is the most frequently prescribed oil, either in a diffuser near the bed before sleep or in a bath to soak in before bed. Schreiner says her three favorite oils for insomnia are lavender, German chamomile, and marjoram. According to aromatherapist Peter Holmes, M.H., L.Ac., director of the Artemis Institute of Natural Therapies in Colorado, lavender is well-known for its action on the nervous system and particularly the brain. "It will act as a sedative or as a stimulant, depending on actual needs," Dr. Holmes says. "It will act as a sedative in conditions of emotional agitation and unrest, calming the mind, comforting and alleviating fears. With emotional depletion and depression, lavender has a distinctly stimulating effect, transforming depression and reviving the spirits as well as consciousness."[45] Along with lavender, oils of neroli (orange blossom), spikenard, Roman chamomile, and ylang ylang may be useful for insomnia treatments.

How to Use Aromatherapy

Drops of the oils can be placed on a heat diffuser, to disperse the essence and aroma into the air. Another option is to use aromatherapy rings, which are placed over a light bulb to heat the oils. Both are available at health food stores and through mail order.

Other options are to add drops of the essential oils to:

■ Massage oil, for an aromatherapy massage.

■ The bathtub, for a therapeutic soak.

■ Hot and cold compresses, to soothe minor aches and pains.

■ Floral waters, to spray into the air or spray on skin that is too sensitive to be touched.

■ Simple topical application of diluted oils. As a general rule, don't apply undiluted oils to the skin because they might elicit an allergic reaction or rash.

■ A pillow or eye shades, to waft the fragrance in while you sleep.

Flower remedies can help resolve repressed emotions and fears. They can also help deal with deep-seated fears that hinder the body's ability to relax.

Flower Remedies

Flower remedies directly address a person's emotional state in order to facilitate both psychological and physiological well-being. By balancing negative feelings and stress, flower remedies can effectively remove the emotional barriers to health and recovery. Flower remedies comprise subtle liquid preparations made from the fresh blossoms of flowers, plants, bushes, even trees, to address emotional, psychological, and spiritual issues underlying physical and medical problems. The approach was pioneered by British physician Edward Bach in the 1930s, when he introduced the 38 Bach Flower Remedies, based on English plants.

Today, an estimated 20 different brands of flower remedies, based on plants native to many landscapes, from Australia to India to Alaska, offer about 1,500 different blends for a diverse range of psychological conditions. The flower remedies each address a particular emotional issue: for example, Vine helps to increase feelings of self-worth, Impatiens is recommended for feelings of impatience with others and yourself, and Aspen is for feelings of fear. An individual formula can be made by combining four to six of the remedies and taking them orally or rubbing them into the skin. They can be taken for a short time to cope with a crisis or for a period of months.

Flower essences are initially made by floating fresh blossoms in spring water and letting them sit in the morning sun for three hours (or heat them by fire, as with some English essences). The blossoms are removed and what is left is the mother essence, which carries the vibratory energy—although no actual physical trace—of the flower. The essence is then diluted to the stock level, which is the form generally available commercially; the stock level can be diluted again to the dosage level. To use the essence directly from stock, place four drops under the tongue or in a little water; this dosage usually is taken four times a day. Another way to take the essences, especially if you are taking more than one, is to mix four drops of each into a large glass of water, stir, and sip it throughout the day. For baths, use about 20 drops of stock essence per tub. Stir the water to help potentize the remedies, then soak for about 20 minutes. For topical use, add 8-10 drops of stock essence per 1 oz of creme, oil, or lotion.

For more on **flower remedies**, contact: The Flower Essence Society, P.O. Box 459, Nevada City, CA 95959; tel: 800-548-0075 or 916-265-9163; fax: 916-265-6467. To order flower essences and books produced and used by society practitioners, contact: Flower Essence Services, P.O. Box 1769, Nevada City, CA 95959; tel: 800-548-0075 or 916-265-0258; fax: 916-265-6467.

Flower remedies are often selected according to their ability to work with a specific imbalanced emotional pattern, rather than a physical complaint such as insomnia. The imbalanced pattern is usually what is causing the physical symptoms. However, there are specific remedies recommended for insomnia or anxiety: Aspen, black-eyed Susan, chamomile, chaparral, dill, lavender, mugwort, red chestnut, St. John's wort, and white chestnut.[46] Flower essences can be useful for insomnia in the following ways:

■ They can help to ground and embody, bringing mental and spiritual components in alignment with a physical relaxation response.

■ They can open and clarify, to awaken consciousness. Sometimes when we awaken the consciousness, that allows the physical part of the body to go to sleep.

■ They can help resolve repressed emotions and fears. They can also help deal with deep-seated fears that hinder the body's ability to relax (traumas, such as physical injury or death of a loved one, as opposed to general fears and repressed emotions).

■ They can help hypersensitive people or highly allergic people who overreact to their environment.

■ They can help people who are reacting to geopathic stress by fostering the development of a healthier immune system.

7

Protection From a Toxic Environment

ELECTROMAGNETIC FIELDS ARE a type of low-level radiation generated by computer terminals, microwave ovens, and other electronic devices. The Earth itself produces some energy fields that are detrimental to human health as well, commonly referred to as geopathic stress. While the intensity of these fields is small, studies continue to show that they may be a factor in a number of chronic illnesses, including cancer, heart disease, and sleep disorders. In this chapter, we look at how electromagnetic fields affect the body, ways to detect them, and therapeutic options for protecting yourself from their harmful effects.

Success Story: Combating the Side Effects of Technology

Every night, Janice, 34, an executive secretary, had trouble staying asleep. She would wake up several times during the night, tense and stressed, unable to fall back to sleep for a half-hour or more. Tired all the time from such restless nights, Janice also suffered from headaches, red and irritated eyes, and frequent colds and flu. After months of trying different approaches on her own without success, Janice sought help for her sleeping problems.

Janice spent her workdays surrounded by electronic equipment such as computers, cellular phones, and fax machines. Those electronic devices produced waves of energy called electromagnetic fields (SEE QUICK DEFINITION). Her symptoms and a complete medical evaluation pointed to an extended overexposure to electromagnetic fields. We gave Janice two items to use in the office as protective devices. The first was a screen that Janice placed over her computer monitor; many companies now sell such screens, designed to shield the computer user from some of the electromagnetic fields generated by the monitor's electronic circuitry.

However, researchers disagree whether such screens are needed. Some say they are more essential for older video display terminals that can leak more EMFs, but not for the newer computers, which have been engineered to remove that problem. The need for the screen may depend on the person using the computer: some people are highly sensitive to the EMFs generated from video display terminals, while others report no adverse effects.

Enzyme specialist and researcher Lita Lee, Ph.D. says in her book *Radiation Protection Manual* that most screens block only the electric energy fields generated by terminals and do not block the magnetic energy fields. The dominant type of emission from video display terminals is extremely low frequency (ELF) magnetic fields. If so, then the screens are not offering complete protection from EMFs. If you purchase such a screen, check as to whether the screen blocks glare, electric fields, magnetic fields, or all three.[1]

Robert O. Becker, M.D., who has done more than 30 years of research in the area of electromagnetic energy, says the best advice is to put some distance between you and the monitor. He recommends using a detachable keyboard that can be placed at least 30 inches away from the computer and the monitor. He suggests people who do this

---

Alternative Medicine Plan for Reducing Toxic Exposure

- Avoidance Strategies
- Feng Shui
- The Energy-Friendly Bedroom
- Create a Comfortable Bedroom Environment
- Make Sure Your Mattress is Body-Friendly

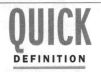

DEFINITION

Electromagnetic fields (EMFs) are a very low-level type of radiation that is generated when electric currents flow through wire coils. Every time you turn on an electric current, it produces these EMFs, even though you can't hear, see, or feel them. EMFs are measured in units called a gauss. They decrease with distance and will pass through wood, concrete, water, earth, and most metals. Common household and office appliances emit very low frequency (VLF) or extremely low frequency (ELF) electromagnetic fields. Those are measured in milligauss, or 1/1,000th of a gauss.

For **computer screens**, contact: Safe Technologies Corporation, 1950 NE 208 Terrace, Miami, FL 33179; tel: 800-638-9121 or 305-933-2026; fax: 1-305-933-8858. For the **Clearwave Professional**, contact: Clarus at 800-4-CLARUS. Pure Energies, P.O. Box 185, Goochland, VA 23063; tel: 800-700-5537 or 804-556-6844; fax: 804-556-6687; website: www.goqlink.com.

should have special corrective glasses made so they can see the monitor.[2] Dr. Becker says computers made after 1983 emit less electromagnetic radiation than the older models, but even the newer ones still pose a health risk for people using them for long periods of time.

In addition to adding the computer screen, Janice installed a Clarus Clearwave Professional device to her office. This is a digital clock that emits an invisible vibration to block electromagnetic fields in an area of about 2,500 square feet. The night after she installed the Clarus device, Janice began to sleep better. In three months, all her symptoms were gone, including the insomnia and restless sleep.

Electromagnetic Fields— The Dark Side of Technology

An electromagnetic field can be likened to an invisible energy web (shaped somewhat like the contour lines on a topographical map) produced by electricity that, in turn, creates a magnetic field. While EMFs are part of nature and in fact are radiated by the human body and its individual organs, the quality and intensity (called respectively frequency and gauss field strength) of the energy forming this contoured web can either support or destroy health. As a general rule, EMFs generated by technological devices tend to be much more harmful than naturally occurring EMFs.

Researchers once thought EMFs, especially very low frequency and extremely low frequency EMFs, were safe because they were of such low strength compared to other forms of radiation, such as those from a nuclear reactor or X rays. But now, as technology proliferates and people are using more electronic devices, some researchers suspect EMFs are contributing to a subtle assault on people's immune systems and overall health.

Electromagnetic changes in the environment can adversely affect the energy balance of the human organism and contribute to disease. We are surrounded by stress-producing, electromagnetic fields generated by the electrical wiring in homes and offices, televisions, computers and video terminals, microwave ovens, overhead lights, power lines, and the hundreds of motors that can generate higher than normal gauss strengths (magnetic energy measuring unit). EMFs interact with living systems, affecting enzymes related to growth regulation, pineal gland metabolism (regulation of the sleep hormone, melatonin), and cell division and multiplication.

In 1979, Nancy Wertheimer, Ph.D., and Ed Leeper, Ph.D., epidemiologists at the University of Colorado, found that children who had been exposed to high-voltage lines in their early childhood had a two to three times higher than normal risk of developing cancer, especially leukemia.[3] That was the first study to establish the direct link between EMFs and cancer. In 1987, a large-scale study conducted by the New York State Department of Health confirmed Dr. Wertheimer's findings and added that the EMFs from the high-voltage power lines also affected the neurohormones of the brain.[4] Since then, various studies have linked electromagnetic fields to increased incidence of heart disease, Alzheimer's disease, high blood pressure, headaches, sexual dysfunction, and blood disorders—the latter including a 50% increase in white blood count.[5]

At the same time, however, some researchers and medical professionals see promise in using very low currents of electromagnetic radiation to heal the body instead of harm it. Dr. Becker discovered that a small electrode implanted inside the body next to an unhealed bone fracture could speed healing.[6] Becker also has explored the possibilities for using electrical current to heal other conditions, including cancer, but cautions that more work needs to be done to establish solid scientific evidence.[7] Other medical professionals, such as physical therapists, acupuncturists, physicians, and chiropractors, use various kinds of devices, such as the TENS (transcutaneous electric nerve stimulation) unit or electro-acupuncture machine, that send a very small electromagnetic current into an injured part of the body, usually to reduce pain.

The EMFs, because they are on the weak end of the radiation scale, are categorized as non-ionizing radiation. That means the fields are not of sufficient energy to change atoms into charged particles called ions. Ionizing radiation, on the other hand, such as that generated by nuclear bombs or X rays, is strong enough to change the atoms into ions. No one who has seen the aftermath of a bomb explosion, or read reports about the health problems suffered by neighbors of Pennsylvania's Three Mile Island nuclear plant after its 1979 accident, needs to be convinced that ionizing radiation is harmful.

As to X rays, Dr. John W. Gofman, a noted physician and researcher in the field of radiation, has calculated that even relatively minor exposures increase the cancer risk.[8] Gofman has estimated that one million people could be spared death from cancer if medical and dental X-ray radiation doses were lowered. But as to the potential for harm from non-ionizing radiation, such as EMFs, emitted by your toaster or hair dryer, the rules and guidelines are still being established.

Electromagnetic Fields are Part of Nature

Electromagnetic energy is not only a phenomenon of technology. The life force itself, the Earth that we live on, and all living things are intricately connected to and by electromagnetic energy fields. Dr. Becker, twice nominated for the Nobel Prize, proved in a series of animal experiments that human and animal bodies carry their own electromagnetic currents, complete with positive and negative charges. In addition, he showed that trauma to the body creates an electromagnetic "current of injury" that stimulates the healing process and, in some animals such as salamanders, initiates regeneration. It was those experiments that led to his findings about how electric currents could be used to heal bone fractures.[9]

The Chinese long ago recognized our intimate link with energy fields by identifying energy pathways, which later came to be called acupuncture meridians, in the body. They use the word *qi* to describe the electromagnetic life force that flows through these meridians. The Chinese also honor the Earth's life force and electromagnetic energies through their science of feng shui (pronounced FUNG-shway), which studies ways of creating natural energy flows in a given environment that are beneficial to people and in harmony with nature. Much of traditional Chinese medicine consists of finding ways to keep the natural electromagnetic energies of the human body in alignment and in balance with each other.

But although electromagnetic energy is part of nature, there is serious concern about the health effects of the artificial, technology-generated electromagnetic fields. Some researchers think the artificial EMFs are upsetting the natural balance of our bodies as the number of EMF-generating devices increases.

Sources of EMFs

The greatest concern about EMFs is not from a one-time use of a hair dryer or an hour in front of a computer, but from cumulative exposures: hour after hour, day after day, continuous high levels of EMFs. For example, people who travel extensively in airplanes can have high exposure rates, up to 85 milligauss in the airplane cabin. The EMF exposure from hair dryers, heaters, electric shavers, and other appliances can be injurious to health over time. Food mixers, hair dryers, and vacuum cleaners emit EMFs that are 30 to 100 times greater than the suggested safe limit.[10] Ordinary household appliances tend to generate larger cumulative EMF exposures than power lines. The reason is proximity: most people do not live close enough to power lines to be greatly affected by their EMFs, but the situation is different with kitchen appliances, computers, cellular phones, televisions, even electrical outlets if they're located behind the head of a bed. Although the EMFs from appliances drop off at a distance of about 16 feet, people often stand or sit closer than this to the source of EMFs—typically 18 inches from computers, a few feet from televisions, and almost no distance from cellular phones.[11]

A unique type of EMF exposure is from electric blankets, which give you close-up exposure at high levels (50-100 milligauss) all night long. According to noted brain researcher Russel J. Reiter, Ph.D., electric blankets are dangerous because they expose the whole body to EMFs, they are close to the body, and they are thought to lower melatonin (SEE QUICK DEFINITION) levels. Because electric blankets are used at night, when the pineal gland is producing its highest amount of melatonin, they have the greatest chance of disrupting melatonin production and sleep.[12]

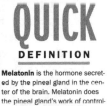

DEFINITION

Melatonin is the hormone secreted by the pineal gland in the center of the brain. Melatonin does the pineal gland's work of controlling sleeping and waking cycle and regulating the body's internal time clock, or circadian rhythm. The pineal gland adjusts its melatonin output based primarily on the body's exposure to light, although many other factors, including EMFs, can influence melatonin production.

Another concentrated source of EMFs is the fuse box where the electric power line branches off from the neighborhood utility pole to your house. That fuse box—which connects the outside line with the inside wiring—generates large amounts of EMFs on a continual basis. EMFs are able to penetrate through normal building walls, but they decrease in force dramatically as you move further away from the generating source. Another potential EMF source is the wiring in your home. Older wiring sometimes generates high amounts of EMFs at the electrical outlets where you plug in your appliances. Check the outlets with a gauss meter and, if necessary, either install new wiring or have a professional reconfigure the existing wiring pattern.

Outside the home, electric power lines can also be a major EMF source. Some scientists allege that exposure to electric and magnetic fields generated by electric power lines is reponsible for certain cancers, reproductive dysfunction, birth defects, neurological disorders, and Alzheimer's disease. Some activist groups believe the hazard to be so great that they are calling for closure of schools and other public facilities near power lines and restructuring of the entire electric power delivery system.[13] Dr. Becker says we are constantly exposed to a background level of EMFs generated by the electric power delivery system. In urban areas, this so-called ambient field level, which is inside and outside the home, could exceed three milligauss. In the suburbs, the ambient field ranges from 1-3 milligauss. Dr. Wertheimer and others said in their studies on power lines that constant surrounding levels of three milligauss or more were significantly related to increases in the risk of childhood cancer. Dr. Becker advocates one milligauss as a safe limit for continuous exposure to 60-hertz fields (the usual kind generated by electric power systems).[14]

Electromagnetic Fields and Sleep Disorders

Researchers suspect artificial EMFs cause sleep problems in a number of ways. First, the fields have a higher rate of oscillation (vibrate at a higher number of cycles) and strength than the natural electromagnetic energy fields of the body at rest. In addition, EMFs can disrupt the body's production of melatonin, a hormone that controls the body's sleep-wake cycle.

High Oscillation Rate and Strength Disrupts Sleep

The frequency at which an EMF is pulsed determines whether or not it is harmful. For example, the voltage of the electric current used in homes in the United States is 60 Hz (cycles per second). In contrast, the ideal frequencies of the human brain during waking hours range from 8 Hz to 20 Hz, while in sleep the frequencies may drop to as low as 2 Hz. The higher frequencies of EMFs generated by artificial electrical currents may disturb the brain's natural resonant frequencies and, in time, lead to cellular fatigue, according to John Zimmerman, Ph.D., president of the Bio-Electro Magnetics Institute in Utah.[15]

While common household electric currents oscillate at a rate of 50-60 Hz, this is slow compared to an FM radio station broadcast that comes to you on waves that oscillate at 100 million times per second, or 100 megahertz. Generally, the higher the frequency of the wave, the more energy it has and also the more potential it carries for damage.

But even 60-Hz EMFs are vibrating much faster than the human body's brain wave patterns at rest, says acupuncturist M.M. van Benschoten, O.M.D., based in Reseda, California. For example, if you have an electric clock radio on your bedside nightstand, it is generating 60-Hz EMFs probably not more than a foot or two from your head. This is a problem because your brain waves in deep sleep oscillate at 2-4 cycles per second (2-4 Hz), Dr. van Benschoten says. The EMFs from the clock radio could interfere with the rest pattern and prevent you from falling asleep or from staying in deep sleep. Dr. van Benschoten recommends removing all electric appliances from the bedroom or from close proximity to the bed.

Equally as important as the oscillation frequency of the EMFs are their strength. The strength of EMFs are measured in units called gauss. Most common appliances, which are very low frequency or extremely low frequency EMFs, are measured in units of milligauss, or one thousandth of a gauss. The milligauss level decreases as your distance increases from the appliance or device. For instance, an electric fan has an EMF at four inches of up to 900 milligauss; at three feet, it is only 5-20 milligauss. A computer monitor has an EMF measuring up to 600 milligauss at a four-inch distance; at one foot, it is only 3-30 milligauss. A microwave oven has an EMF of 40-90 milligauss at one foot; at three feet, it drops to 3-5 milligauss.[16]

EMFs Can Disrupt Melatonin Production

One of the main reasons why medical professionals and others are concerned about EMF exposure levels is a growing body of research showing EMFs have a negative impact on melatonin production in the body. EMFs from household sources are so small that the electrical currents they induce in the human body are actually weaker than those induced by electrical activity in nerve and muscle cells. Yet even these low-frequency EMFs can alter gene expression, the activity of enzymes involved in growth regulation, calcium balance in the cell, and the brain's metabolism of the hormone melatonin.[17]

Melatonin, a hormone produced by the pineal gland in the brain, was once thought to be unimportant. However, in recent years, researchers have found that it is present in every cell of the body and is essential in regulating the body's clock, or circadian rhythm, the mechanism that controls our sleep-wake cycles.

The pineal gland registers the amount of light in our surroundings, and if it finds no light, it increases the melatonin level, signalling it is time to go to sleep. If light is present, the melatonin production decreases and we feel more awake. Thus, restoring and maintaining adequate amounts of melatonin are crucial for people with sleep disorders.

For more on **melatonin and the body clock**, see Chapter 5: Resetting the Body Clock, pp. 120-145.

Other factors besides light decrease our melatonin supply, including aging, certain prescription drugs, stress, poor nutrition, and EMFs.

In addition to regulating sleep, researchers are discovering that adequate melatonin stores improve body immunity, have anti-cancer and anti-aging properties, can relieve depression, and may boost sexual function. Those types of health conditions are the same ones that researchers say can be hurt by EMF overexposure. The connection between melatonin and EMFs appears to be getting more solid evidence. A team of researchers in 1996, for example, found that blood melatonin levels in female rats decreased after exposure to 50-Hz magnetic fields, about the same frequency as most household appliances. Many similar studies on melatonin are now underway.[18]

At the same time, not being exposed to naturally occurring EMFs can have a negative impact on health, for they function as a kind of energy nutrient. Kyoichi Nakagawa, M.D., director of the Isuzu Hospital in Tokyo, Japan, observes that the amount of time people now spend in buildings and cars (tightly enclosed spaces) reduces their exposure to the geomagnetic field of the earth and may interfere with their health. Dr. Nakagawa calls this condition "magnetic field deficiency syndrome," noting it can cause headaches, dizziness, muscle stiffness, chest pain, insomnia, constipation, and general fatigue.

Geopathic Stress and Sleep Disturbances

The concept of geopathic stress has been well researched and substantiated in Germany since the 1920s. The theory is that the Earth (*geo*) in some locations generates energies that are detrimental (*pathic* as in pathological) to humans living or working in structures immediately above their source. These energies—electromagnetic or more subtle in nature—can put chronic stress on the body, eventually producing sickness.

Geopathic stress is an abnormal energy field, usually of an electromagnetic nature, generated deep underground by large mineral deposits, water streams, or geological faults. As British researcher Jane Thurnell-Read explains in *Geopathic Stress*, this abnormal energy occurs "when the Earth's magnetic field is disturbed, either naturally or artificially, and the background field we normally experience is changed." Artificial disturbances can be produced by mining, foundations for tall buildings, subways, and public utility piping, such as for sewers and public water, says Thurnell-Read.

If you work or, especially, sleep over an area of geopathic stress, European research confirms that you may get sick from continuous exposure to this abnormal energy. Sleep disorders are common, as are symptoms such as unaccountable irritation or depression, susceptibility to colds, waking up tired, and a slow deterioration in vitality, health, and mood.

While most of the emphasis on EMF exposure has to do with artificial, or technology-generated EMFs, natural patterns of electromagnetic energy can affect people. The Earth itself has an electromagnetic field of about 0.5 gauss, Dr. Becker says. Compared to the magnet that holds the refrigerator door closed, which has about a 200-gauss strength, the Earth's field is weak. However, living things are able to sense even minute fluctuations in the Earth's field—experiments with homing pigeons and even bacteria have shown this to be true. Scientists have identified magnet-like mechanisms in people and other creatures that act to align our energies with those of the Earth.[19]

Researchers around the world have documented cases where currents of energy coming from the ground were causing sleep disorders, headaches, depression, and other symptoms. The concept of geopathic, or pathogenic, influences from the earth, took root in Germany in 1929 when Baron Gustav Freiherr von Pohl made a systematic tour of the community of Vilsbiburg. It had 565 houses, 3,300 residents, and an unusually high rate of cancer. Von Pohl was acting on a hunch inspired from a survey of Stuttgart in the 1920s that showed a clear correlation between major geological faults in the city and those districts that had the highest cancer mortality rates. His tentative conclusion was that an unknown but noxious radiation emanating from the Earth faults might be an important and overlooked contributory cause of the cancers.

Baron von Pohl located all the major subterranean water veins (lying at a depth of 44-50 meters with a width of 3-4 meters) under Vilsbiburg, then mapped their courses onto the city street plan. Next, he cross-checked this with the residences of the 54 recent cancer fatalities and arrived at a startling conclusion: "The completed check of my map confirmed all the beds of the 54 cancer deaths were where I had drawn the radiation currents," von Pohl wrote in 1932 in his now classic *Earth Currents: Causative Factor of Cancer and Other Diseases*. Von Pohl himself presented dozens of cases in which rapid, perhaps miraculous, cures of numerous complaints, from insomnia to heart spasm, were achieved simply by moving the sleeper's bed out of the geopathic zone situated underneath the house.

"The effects of geopathic stress undermine and weaken a person's life force," says Thurnell-Read. "This does not mean that geopathic stress causes illness; rather, by weakening the body, it provides a fertile ground in which ill health can flourish." She says strong Earth energies can specifically influence brain rhythms, cellular renewal, functioning of specific body parts, the blood, and the electrical activity in the body.[20] These effects can have a detrimental influence on sleep.

In 1971, the theory of geopathic stress was supported by research showing that water flowing underground, especially subterranean streams that cross, produces measurable increases in magnetic anomalies; these conditions also increase electrical conductivity in the air and soil, and other physical changes. While the changes may be measurable though small (in the vicinity of ten inches square), they are still capable of contributing to the development of serious illness. One large-scale study published by the U.S. Department of Health, Education and Welfare reported that geopathic stress may be a factor in between 40%-50% of all human cancers, accounting for between 60%-90% of all cancers attributed to environmental radiation.[21]

"The magnetic field of the Earth is an important physiologic factor for living organisms," says Dr. Becker. "It appears that behavioral changes of an undesirable nature, either quite evident or subtle, may result from environments having lower or higher field strengths than normal."[22]

It is possible to measure Earth energies using a machine called a magnetometer, says Anthony Scott-Morley, M.D., Ph.D., of the Institute of Bioenergetic Medicine in Dorset, England. Dr. Scott-Morley says if people are particularly sensitive to geopathic stress, it can make it difficult for them to maintain their normal balance of health. Geopathic stress zones may be tiny, but shifting a bed a few feet in a geopathically troubled bedroom, says Dr. Scott-Morley, can make the difference between sleep and insomnia for the susceptible individual. The growing popularity of feng shui, the Chinese science of landscape interpretation and household exterior and interior design, is bringing the concept of geopathic stress to a larger audience in the West.

Success Story: Bedroom Feng Shui Helps a Child Sleep

David, an 8-year-old boy with brain damage from birth, was a restless and fitful sleeper. He had trouble falling asleep and, when he did sleep, would wake up every two hours and be unable to fall back asleep for at least a half-hour. David's parents, afraid he would hurt himself

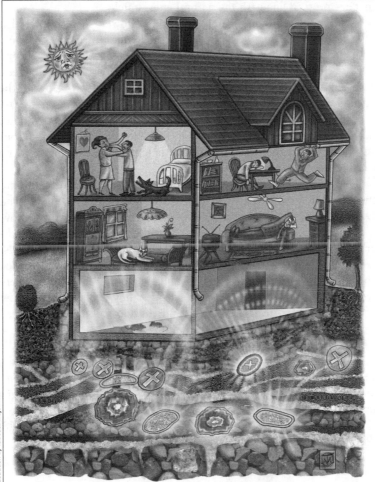

Illustration by Tadeusz Majewski.

Geopathic stress is an abnormal energy field generated underground by mineral deposits, water streams, or geological faults.

through tossing and turning or banging his head against the wall, were afraid to let him sleep alone and had to take turns sleeping with him.

David attended special physical therapy sessions during the day and took muscle relaxants, but his parents did not want to put him on sleeping pills. They took him to see Maureen Savereux Powers, a feng shui practitioner in Portland, Oregon. Feng shui is the Chinese art of placement. Its purpose is to create the most beneficial flow of *qi*, or life force energy, in an environment (home, office, or other setting) by arranging furniture, plants, decorations, buildings, or rooms in ways that are most in line with the natural energy field.

Using a feng shui formula, Savereux Powers determined that David was closely aligned with the Earth element, meaning he would be most comfortable around items related to nature, such as natural fabrics, earth-toned colors, plants, crystals, terra cotta pottery, trees, and stones. He would also be most comfortable sleeping close to the ground. David's bedroom, however, was not suited to this personality profile. It was decorated in all white, because David's parents did not believe he was able to perceive colors. His bed was high off the floor and there were no other decorations, the entire effect being one of a sterile hospital room.

The first thing Savereux Powers did was move David's bed onto the floor, to give him a feeling of being grounded. Then, she and David's parents painted the walls of the room a rich earthy yellow. They added items from nature on the walls and ceiling, such as feathers, Native American animal totems and symbols of peace, and crystals. They placed a hand-made Native American tapestry on the bed and terra cotta pots with plants around the room. The pillows were covered with colorful hand-made fabric. They replaced the carpet with a tile floor, to give a feeling of being outdoors. Finally, they added a window that opened out onto the family's garden, to give a feeling of freedom and connection with nature.

Within a week after the bedroom was redesigned, David was sleeping comfortably by himself. His periods of sleep began increasing in length until, by the end of the month, David was sleeping eight hours straight, without waking up in the middle of the night.

Alternative Medicine Plan for Reducing Toxic Exposure

A number of therapeutic options are available for dealing with EMFs and geopathic stress and returning to restful sleep. Reducing your daily exposure to electrical devices is the simplest way to help yourself. The Chinese art of placement, feng shui, can help you reallign your bedroom for better sleep. Finally, make sure that your bedroom environment and bedding materials are conducive to sound sleep.

"Prudent Avoidance" is a Good Policy
Given that the world around us is flooded by EMF-producing devices, what can be done to reduce our exposure? What is a "safe" level of

exposure, if there is one? Some agencies have made suggestions on exposure levels. In a 1995 report, the National Council on Radiation Protection (NCRP) Scientific Committee on Extremely Low Frequency Electric and Magnetic Fields recommended one milligauss as a target level for general exposure. The U.S. Environmental Protection Agency maintains that 2.5 milligauss is safe for the surrounding background EMF field.

For a **referral to a feng shui practitioner**, contact: Feng Shui Society of America, P.O. Box 488, Wabasso, FL 32970; tel: 407-589-9900.

For many people, it is not that easy to control the surrounding EMF field, unless they move to a home away from any power lines or transformer boxes. The most effective response to take is to reduce your personal EMF exposure—that is, EMFs from household appliances, tools, and office equipment. The U.S. Congress' Office of Technology Assessment recommends a policy of "prudent avoidance" of EMFs—becoming aware of potential EMF sources, measuring them, and acting to reduce exposures.

The first step is to find out what levels of EMFs you are currently exposed to in your home or office. You can check EMF levels with a gauss meter, an inexpensive hand-held device that can measure the milligauss of EMFs emitting from your appliances, computers, or office equipment. If you live in an apartment or condominium, be sure to check any shared walls around your bed for the presence of hidden junction boxes. (Your electric utility may also do this for you.) This will help you determine which sources pose the greatest danger and guide you on avoidance strategies.

There are some simple steps you can take immediately to reduce your EMF exposure at home:

■ In the bedroom, place all electric appliances at least three feet from the bed, including lamps, alarm clocks, televisions, and heaters. (You may even want to try pulling all circuit breakers before going to bed for three nights and see if there is any improvement in your sleep.) If you sleep on a water bed, turn off the heater before you get in and, in cold weather, preserve heat in the water with an insulating pad. Don't use an electric blanket except to heat the bed, then unplug it before you get in; don't leave it on through the night.

For information on **EMF exposure**, contact: National Institute of Environmental Health Sciences, P.O. Box 12233, Research Triangle Park, NC 27709; tel: 800-363-2383; website: www.niehs.nih.gov. For information about **gauss meters**, contact: Feng Shui Warehouse, P.O. Box 6689, San Diego, CA 92166; tel: 800-399-1599 or 619-523-2158; fax: 619-523-2165.

■ In the bathroom, avoid or reduce use of a hair dryer. Use a safety razor instead of an electric one.

■ In the kitchen, don't stand in front of the microwave oven or the dishwasher while they are in operation. Consider converting to a gas range if your stove is electric.

Protection From EMFs

A number of devices are available that may provide protection from harmful EMFs:

■ Computer shields can be mounted on monitors to reduce or block their emission of EMFs.

■ The Clarus Clearwave Professional is a digital clock that emits a vibration to block EMFs in an area of 2,500 square feet. Clarus also makes the Q-Link Pendant, a necklace that can neutralize the harmful effects of EMFs, according to Clarus.

■ The Sleepshield is a grounded, steel mesh screen that is mounted on the walls on two sides of the bed and on the floor beneath the bed to attract EMFs and then deflect them harmlessly away, says the manufacturer.

■ Electronic Smog Busters are units containing crushed crystals that you can stick on your computer or wear as a necklace to deflect electromagnetic fields, according to the manufacturer.

For **computer screens**, contact: Safe Technologies Corporation, 1950 NE 208 Terrace, Miami, FL 33179; tel: 800-638-9121 or 305-933-2026; fax: 1-305-933-8858. For **Clearwave Professional and the Q-Link Pendant**, contact: Clarus at 800-4-CLARUS. Pure Energies, P.O. Box 185, Goochland, VA 23063; tel: 800-700-5537 or 804-556-6844; fax: 804-556-6687; website: www.goqlink.com. For **Sleepshield**, contact: Bio Design, Inc., P.O. Box 1742, Easley, SC 29642; tel: 864-859-4900. For **Electronic Smog Busters**, contact: Feng Shui Warehouse, P.O. Box 6689, San Diego, CA 92166; tel: 800-399-1599 or 619-523-2158; fax: 619-523-2165.

Feng Shui for Fostering Sleep

Feng shui is a term from traditional Chinese culture to indicate the proper ways to arrange furniture, rooms, houses, offices, churches, and other human-made structures to maximize the favorable energies. The term, which literally means "wind and water" (although popularly it is known as the art of placement), is drawn from the ancient Chinese philosophy of Taoism, which linked energies of the solar system and Earth with human habitation and activities. Feng shui documents the flow or impedance of basic life force energy, or *qi*, through environments, building structures, homes, and rooms for the benefit or detriment of their inhabitants.

Qi is a Chinese word variously translated to mean "vital energy," "essence of life," and "living force." In Chinese medicine, the proper flow of *qi* along energy channels (meridians) within the body is crucial to a person's health and vitality. There are many types of *qi*, classified according to source, location, and function, such as activation, warming, defense, transformation, and containment. However, *qi* has two essential qualities: yang (active, fiery, moving, bright, energizing) and yin (passive, watery, stationary, dark, calming). According to this view, everything in the universe is subject to a constant interaction of yin and yang. Location, shape, size, color, weather, and other subtle influences all produce various levels of yin and yang energies. Feng shui seeks ways to harmonize and balance these energetic patterns.

These energies are categorized into five basic movements, commonly linked to the five elements of traditional Chinese astrology—south (fire), center (earth), west (metal), north (water), and east (wood). As you can see on the accompanying table (see "The Five Elements of Feng Shui," p. 190), these energy movements correspond with certain colors, shapes, and seasons of the year. Thus, in feng shui, objects, furniture, rooms, and buildings are not static but have particular energetic qualities that can affect our responses to them.

For example, most people have a favorite color, perhaps a particular shade of blue or green that you seem to naturally favor. One way of looking at your response is that the cool energy of blue corresponds to your attitude or personality type in some way. These subtle influences of color, shape, and space are the purview of feng shui. "Ordinarily our senses perceive the most obvious forms of motion—traffic passing by in the street or the cool rush of the wind against the skin," says Master Lam Kam Chuen, author of the *Feng Shui Handbook*. "We are less conscious of the subtle movements of energy as it passes invisibly through the space of an open room or the vibration of the patterns of energy in the walls and furnishings."[23]

The Nine Basic Cures—In feng shui, the cure or remedy for spaces that don't feel comfortable is to add items that help to stimulate, moderate, or move the *qi*. These cures can be very simple, such as adding a mirror, but on a subtle energy level they will create a difference that people will feel. In a bedroom, for example, it is advisable to add yin elements, such as water sounds, and avoid overly stimulating yang items, such as a television. The nine basic cures are:

1. Bright or light-refracting objects: mirror, crystal ball, lights; mirrors are considered the "aspirin" of feng shui because they cure many ills.

2. Sounds: wind chimes, bells.

3. Living objects: plants such as bonsai and flowers; aquarium or fishbowl.

4. Moving objects: mobile, miniature windmill, fountain.

5. Heavy objects: stones or statues.

6. Electrically powered objects: air conditioner, stereo, TV (not recommended for the bedroom because they are too stimulating).

The Five Elements of Feng Shui

	Fire	Earth	Metal	Water	Wood
DIRECTION	South	Center	West	North	East
SEASON	Summer	Indian summer	Fall	Winter	Spring
COLOR	Red	Yellow	White	Blue/Black	Green
SHAPE	Triangular	Square	Round	Horizontal and curving	Rectangular
REPRESENTATIONS	Candles, red objects	Terra cotta, ceramics, yellow objects	Wind chimes, metallic objects	Aquarium, fountain, black or blue objects	Plants, flowers, green objects

Sources— Richard Webster. *101 Feng-Shui Tips for the Home* (St. Paul, MN: Llewellyn, 1998). Master Lam Kam Chuen. *Feng Shui Handbook* (New York: Henry Holt, 1996).

7. Bamboo flutes.

8. Colors: most auspicious are red, green, blue, yellow.

9. Other items: for example, chalk under the bed to cure a back-ache.[24]

The Energy-Friendly Bedroom

Here are some ways to make your bedroom a health-enhancing, not health-draining, environment:

■ One factor to consider in bedroom placement is where it is located within the house. Since sleep is considered a yin activity according to traditional Chinese medicine, bedrooms should be on the yin, or non-solar, shady side, which is usually north or east. The solar side, usually west and south, gets more sun exposure and is better for yang activities, such as an office, living room, or kitchen. If it is not possible to put the bedroom on the non-solar side of the house, you may add some trees or water sounds, such as a fountain outside the window, to provide cooling, yin energy.

■ Where you put the bed is very important in feng shui. Ideally, it should be diagonally across from the room entrance, so that people in the bed have a full view of anyone coming in the door.[25] If you move your bed to straddle the corner, be sure to put a headboard or shelf behind it with plants, candles, stones, or other nurturing items. Corners are considered a place where *qi* can stagnate unless you add items that keep the *qi* flowing. If you can't place the bed catercorner

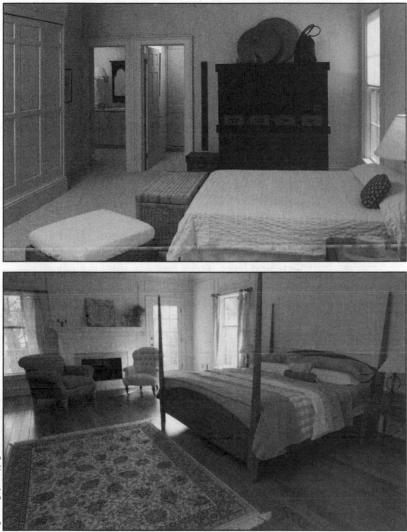

Feng shui documents the flow or impedance of basic life force energy, or *qi*, through environments, building structures, homes, and rooms for the benefit or detriment of their inhabitants. For sleep problems, it is important to create a soft, calm, and nurturing atmosphere in the bedroom. For example, the bed should be across the room from the entrance, so that people in bed have a full view of anyone entering. Other doorways (to the bathroom, for instance) should not be in direct line with the bed. Also, the bed should not be placed directly beneath a window as too much vital energy will be lost during the night. In general, avoid sharp angles and clutter, which can agitate the flow of energy in the room.

to the entrance for some reason, add a mirror to reflect the entrance way or place a wind chime between the entrance and the bed and keep the mirror opposite the entrance. Also, try to have the bed face the morning sunlight, if possible.

■ Avoid placing your bed next to a window because you will lose too much vital energy (*qi*) out the window during the night. Also, the energy coming in the windows at night could disrupt your body's yin energies and prevent sleep. But allow as much air and sunlight into the bedroom during the day as possible to accumulate *qi* to help replenish the body during sleep.

■ Besides the position of the bed, also pay attention to other details of *qi* flow. If you have a bathroom off the bedroom, for example, be sure to buffer the *qi* of the bathroom from the *qi* of the bedroom with a curtain, mirror, or other divider. If you have a desk in the bedroom, have it screened off or away from the main flow of *qi*.

■ Do not place your bed under an exposed beam. If it runs lengthwise down the bed, it may alienate the couple sleeping in the bed; if it crosses the bed at chest level, it may create health problems.

■ Do not place a mirror at the foot of the bed; waking up in the middle of the night, you may mistake your own visage for a ghost's.

■ Do not use your bedroom as a storage area, especially under the bed; negative or detrimental *qi* can accumulate.

■ Do place something "pleasant and attractive" or a beautiful scene (either a painting or a window view) beside your bed or in the line of vision from your bed so that, upon waking, you are greeted by this and start the day on a bright note.

■ Avoid harsh angles. Never place your bed under a low slanting ceiling or any other angular protrusion in your bedroom. These features can contribute to headaches, confused thinking, illness, and possibly financial or career problems.

■ Do not face sharp edges. The sharp edges from bookcases, dressers, and other furniture in the bedroom should not face where you lie in bed. The energy coming off the edges is sharp and can harm your health and create irritability.

■ Avoid "poison arrows." A bedroom with an irregular shape (in which edges such as a closet jut out) generates, geometrically speaking, "poison arrows." A sleeper regularly exposed to these influences is subject to minor health problems, mood swings, and loss of concentration. If you are stuck with a poison-arrowed corner or sharp-edged furniture, hang a crystal from the ceiling in front of the sharp edge or position a plant or folding screen to block them.

■ Remove electronic devices, such as televisions, from the bedroom—they are too stimulating. This applies especially to office equipment such as computers.

■ Try to use cooling colors, such as blues and greens, in darker shades, for your curtains and bedspreads. Bright colors such as reds or bright pinks are too stimulating. In general, try to create a soft, nurturing atmosphere.

■ Keep the *qi* fresh. Ultimately, feng shui is about managing the flow of *qi* for the best advantage of people within a given environment. *Qi,* say Li Pak Tin and Helen Yeap in *Feng Shui: Secrets That Change Your Life,* is "the animating life force that is everywhere; it permeates your home, physical surroundings, the rivers, roads, trees, and all people." The goal of feng shui is to constructively employ this *qi* and to "disperse, disrupt, or remove obstructions" in its free flow.[26]

For more on **feng shui**, contact: Feng Shui Guild, P.O. Box 766, Boulder, CO 80306; tel: 303-444-1548; website: www.feng-shuiguild.com. American Feng Shui Institute, 108 N. Ynez Avenue, Suite 202, Monterey Park, CA 91754; tel: 626-571-2757; fax: 626-571-2065; website: www.amfengshui.com. Feng Shui Association, 31 Woburn Place, Brighton BN1 9GA, England; tel/fax: 44-1-273-693-844; website: www.mistral.co.uk/fengshui. Feng Shui Society, 377 Edgware Road, London W2 1BT, England.

Steps to Relieve Geopathic Stress

How can you know if you suffer from geopathic stress? You could engage a skilled dowser, kinesiologist, or feng shui expert to assess your home; or, if you suspect the influence of geopathic stress, implement some of the following and see if you feel better. Certain of these recommendations will require the expert advice of a qualified dowser who can confirm and pinpoint the existence of problem areas underneath the house.

■ Move your bed: The average person spends 6-8 hours a day in the bedroom sleeping, making this part of the house the one most likely to transmit geopathic stress if it exists underground. As geopathic stress often occurs in thin bands, relocating the bed elsewhere in the room may take you out of the zone of influence.

■ Hang where the dog lies: Cats tend to sleep in places of geopathic stress, while dogs assiduously avoid them. If your dog has a favorite spot in the bedroom, relocate your bed there. If you suspect you have geopathic stress in your bedroom and your cat likes perching on your bed, move the bed. Feng shui experts also observe that ants, termites, bees, and wasps (as well as bacteria, viruses, and parasites) thrive in areas of geopathic stress, while chickens, ducks, and most birds do not.

■ Use cork tiles and plastic sheets: Lay untreated cork tiles under the bed or between the box spring and mattress for a few weeks; the cork apparently neutralizes the detrimental energies, at least temporarily. Plastic sheeting will also screen out geopathic energies for about a week, then must be replaced, says Karen Kingston in *Creating Sacred Space with Feng Shui*.[27]

■ Get a new bed: Kingston notes that if you have a metal bedframe or a mattress with metal springs and your bed sits over an area of geopathic stress, "the metal will conduct the harmful radiation throughout the bed." She recommends trading in your heavy metal springs for a wood-framed bed with a natural cotton mattress.

■ Pile crushed marble or quartz: Placing small piles (four to seven pounds each) of either crushed marble (such as garden centers sell) or quartz crystals at specific locations (identified by an expert, as cited above) within your bedroom and house may offset geopathic stress, says Thurnell-Read. It is believed that these stones somehow absorb the detrimental or negative energies. It is necessary to wash the crystals or marble regularly to remove any accumulations of such energy, she advises; soak the stones in a bucket into which cold water flows for 30 minutes.

■ Install copper coils: Thurnell-Read suggests placing several pairs of copper coils as high as possible in the house, even hung from the ceiling or placed in a loft; these will accumulate the detrimental energies. Each coil consists of ten revolutions of copper wire; in a pair, one is coiled clockwise, the other, counterclockwise. Like the marble and crystals, the coils need to be refreshed regularly, in the same manner.

■ Mirror it back down: Placing small mirrors in strategic locations in the bedroom can directly offset, neutralize, or reflect back to source the "rays" of unfavorable energies. In some cases, strips of aluminum foil (multiple layers work best) can also deflect detrimental energies, says Thurnell-Read. Often, both mirrors and foil work even when blocked by furniture or wallpaper, provided their size and positioning are correct.

■ Put magnets on the water pipes: It can be helpful to affix two to four magnets (800-1,200 gauss strength) on an incoming water pipe, with the magnets' south-seeking poles pointing inwards to the pipe, advises Thurnell-Read. Magnets may also be attached to walls, ceilings, or floors to work against geopathic stress.

■ Neutralize underground water streams: Australian engineer and architect George Birdsall cites the case of a bedroom in which three underground streams crossed under the bed of a child who was chronically sick. The presence of three "black streams," as feng shui experts call such streams, amplified the unhealthy energy. To correct this, Birdsall recommends inserting a $\frac{1}{2}$-inch thick copper pipe into the ground at the upstream end of the water flow, as determined by a skilled dowser. "After correction, the negative effects dissipate for some distance up and down stream," he says in *The Feng Shui Companion*.

■ Copper pipes yield sleep: Birdsall also advises using ½-inch copper pipe for removing the energy influences of a geological fault. He corrected a bedroom in which a seven-year-old boy had insomnia due to two geological faults passing through the room. Birdsall notes that the copper pipes, pounded into the ground at the upstream end (in terms of its energy flow) of the fault, should have a few twists at their tops.

Create a Comfortable Bedroom Environment

Once you have your bedroom arranged in a manner conducive to sleep, you can take care of the sensory elements such as light, sound, and temperature. First, the right room temperature during sleep can be crucial. The best sleeping temperature is between 60° F and 70° F. If the temperature is above 75° F, you may have nighttime awakening, increased movement in bed, and shallower sleep. Cold feet can also keep you awake. If your feet get cold, warm them in a foot bath or tub before going to sleep, then wear socks and use a heating pad to keep your feet warm.[28]

Be sure your bedroom is quiet and completely dark at night. Ear plugs and eye masks, available at most drug and department stores, are options for blocking noise and light. Eye masks can be useful if your window curtains or mini-blinds do not block enough light. For noise, another option is a "white noise" machine, which produces ocean sounds or other calming vibrations to mask the disruptive noise.

Snoring is another noise problem that not only ruins sleep, but relationships as well. If you have a snoring partner who is disturbing your sleep, your partner needs to get treatment, or at least be evaluated by a medical professional. Snoring, especially heavy snoring, may be a symptom of sleep apnea, in which a person temporarily stops breathing and has frequent awakenings during the night. Derek S. Lipman, M.D., author of *Snoring From A to ZZZZ*, says snoring used to be thought of as little more than a social handicap or nuisance, but is now considered a legitimate medical problem. As a first line of treatment, snorers who are overweight can try losing weight to see if that allows more breathing room around the throat and sinuses. If not, the snorer can try some of the antisnoring gadgets available, including a wrist bracelet that gives the sleeper a mild electric shock if he or she snores.

Make Sure Your Mattress is Body-Friendly

Part of making your bedroom a restful sleep haven is to have a bed that

Treatment Guidelines for Sleep Apnea

■ Use a CPAP—the continuous positive airway pressure (CPAP) device is a mask that forces air through the nose to keep the throat open.

■ Lose weight—reduces fat in the throat and can open up the airway.

■ Sew a tennis ball into the back of the person's pajama top—to prevent sleeping on the back.

■ Stop smoking—cigarettes can cause nasal and throat swelling.

■ Avoid alcohol, tranquilizers, sleeping pills, and antihistamines in the evening—these can relax throat muscles to the point of collapse.

■ Use nasal tape—available over-the-counter, nasal strips pull the sides of the nose outward, holding the nasal passages open.

■ Eliminate allergens in the home—dust, mold, or other allergens may cause nasal congestion.

■ Raise the head of the bed or add pillows—sleeping with your head raised helps drain congestion and open your airways.

■ Develop a consistent sleep schedule—regular sleeping may help keep breathing stable and decrease snoring.

■ Wash out your sinuses—a process called pulsatile nasal irrigation uses a WaterPik with a special attachment to clear out thick secretions. Ask your health-care practitioner.

■ Get a custom dental splint—good for people with large tongues, the dental splint holds the jaw forward so that the tongue can't fall back toward the throat and obstruct breathing.

is firm enough to support your body weight but cushioned enough to let you sleep through the night. Mattresses generally start to deteriorate after about eight years. If yours is relatively new, you may only need to add a top layer of extra cushioning. Try spreading a sleeping bag on top of your mattress and see if you sleep better and are more comfortable. If so, you can buy an inexpensive foam pad or mattress pad that will cover your mattress and give you the extra cushioning you need.

Besides cushioning, you also want to test your mattress for sag. Try putting a sheet of plywood under the mattress and sleep on it for a few nights. If you feel better, you need either a firmer mattress or you can leave the plywood in place. Once you decide that you need a new mattress, you have many options: you can buy a ready-made mattress and box-spring off the shelf or have one custom made; a water bed can feel soft and warm, but it doesn't breathe and tends to sag under your body's heaviest parts; air beds are more adjustable, but can be expensive and sometimes the vinyl core is hot; a high-density foam mattress is firm, but some people may also find it too hot. Because of these reservations, most people choose innerspring mattresses because they have different choices in firmness, are cooler and drier because air can circulate around the coils, and they are widely available.

Innerspring mattresses consist of rows of tempered steel coils sandwiched between insulation and cushioning. Firmness and durability are based on thickness of the wire and number of turns per coil. The thicker the wire and the more turns per coil, the stronger and firmer the mattress. Also, the higher the coil count, the firmer the mattress. A standard 500-coil mattress is considered somewhat soft; look for 720 coils if you want a firmer mattress.

The top layers of cushioning in a mattress are important, not only for their firmness, but for their ability to cool. At night, even though our metabolism slows down while we sleep, our bodies still produce up to 80 watts of heat. Often the top layers of mattresses are polyester and cotton on top of polyurethane foam—these materials do not have very good absorption and breathability. The optimum material for these layers is wool, which wisks moisture away from the body.[29]

When you're in the store buying your mattress, lie down in the position you usually sleep in, and have a friend check your alignment for sags and a scrunched posture. Most people do well with a medium-firm mattress with a medium-soft top layer of padding to cushion hips and shoulders. However, if you sleep on your side or stomach, you might need a medium-firm top. If you sleep on your back, and have a lot of curve in your low back, you might need a softer mattress to support and cushion your spine.

Avoid Bedding Materials That Make You Sick—People who are sensitive to chemicals and synthetic fabrics can get severe allergic reactions to toxic materials in certain types of sheets, pillows, and mattresses. For some people, the reaction can develop into a syndrome called multiple chemical sensitivity (MCS). Symptoms could include headaches, nausea, breathing problems, and joint pain, according to Lynn Marie Bower, author of *The Healthy Household: A Complete Guide for Creating a Healthy Indoor Environment*.

For **natural bedding products**, contact: Garnet Hill at 800-622-2216; website: www.garnethill.com. Seventh Generation, One Mill Street, Box A-26, Burlington, VT 05401-1530; tel: 800-456-1191 or 802-658-3773; fax: 802-658-1771. The Natural Bedroom, 11134 Rush Street, South El Monte, CA 91733; tel: 800-365-6563.

Buy your bedding and carpets from companies that use natural fabrics, such as wool and cotton. Make sure the companies don't coat their fabrics with chemicals to keep them from wrinkling. For example, avoid polyester and polyester-blend percale sheets, which are coated with formaldehyde to resist wrinkling—the formaldehyde gives off gases for the life of the sheets. In people with formaldehyde sensitivity, the gases can cause insomnia, coughing, throat and eye irritation, headaches, nausea, and nosebleeds. Look instead for high-density, combed-cotton percale sheets, without a "no-iron" or "easy-care" designation. Similar problems can come from mattresses and pillows stuffed with polyurethane foam; try natural cotton mattresses, futons, and cotton or buckwheat pillows.[30]

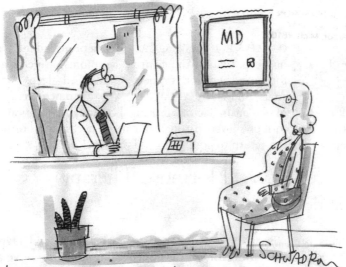

"I'M TAKING YOU OFF VALIUM AND PUTTING YOU ON SOMETHING THAT HASN'T BEEN DEBUNKED."

CHAPTER

8 Balancing Your Hormones

ORMONE LEVELS CAN have a profound influence on sleep. One of the primary symptoms of menopause for both men and women is disturbed sleep. Aging, stress, and an increasingly toxic environment are some of the main factors causing hormonal disruption. By rebalancing hormone levels through nutrition, herbs, and hormone therapy, you can return to getting a good night's sleep.

Success Story: Hormone Therapy for Better Sleep

Phyllis Bronson, a Ph.D. candidate in biochemistry, and Harold Whitcomb, M.D., directors of the Aspen Clinic for Preventive and Environmental Medicine in Aspen, Colorado, report that almost all of the perimenopausal women they see are suffering from either depression, anxiety, or other emotional disturbances caused by hormonal imbalance. Bronson and Dr. Whitcomb relate the following case which illustrates the powerful influence hormones have on mood and how insomnia can be reversed with the proper balance of supplements and natural hormone therapy:

Margaret was 50 when she came to see us. At that age, Margaret was nearing menopause and had irregular periods. She had sleeping difficulties and a lack of clar-

---

In This Chapter

- Success Story: Hormone Therapy for Better Sleep
- Hormonal Imbalance and Sleep Disorders
- Causes of Hormone Problems
- Are Your Hormones Imbalanced?
- Alternative Medicine Plan for Balancing Hormones

ity in her thinking, a condition referred to as brain fog. She also suffered from chronic depression, for which she had been prescribed numerous antidepressants over the last ten years. She experienced persistent sadness, cried frequently, continually gained weight, and retained water. Other symptoms included hot flashes, sex drive loss, and mood swings.

Margaret's insomnia and emotional disturbances were consistent with low levels of estradiol, which is how we measure estrogen status. Her estrogen level was 54.3 whereas a woman her age should have a level between 90 and 130. Margaret's progesterone level was 0.2 whereas a normal reading for her would have been 25. Her testosterone was around 14; the acceptable reference range for women is 14 to 76, but for menopausal women we like to see it around 40 to 60. With a low level of 14, Margaret had no sex drive.

We also checked her DHEA level, which was 90. For a woman of this age to be optimally healthy with a low risk of degenerative disease, the DHEA count should be above 400 and preferably 500 to 600. Low DHEA levels such as Margaret's are often correlated with extreme exhaustion and flu-like symptoms without apparent medical basis.

Estrogen-deficient women often are low in pregnenolone, an essential hormone which is a precursor to progesterone. Pregnenolone appears to have a great calming effect because it activates receptor sites in brain cells for GABA (itself a calming agent), enabling more GABA to be absorbed by the cells.

Using a procedure called electrodermal screening (SEE QUICK DEFINITION), we discovered that Margaret had many food sensitivities, specifically to grains such as wheat, rice, rye, kamut, and spelt. A blood test showed that Margaret was deficient in histidine, an amino acid (SEE QUICK DEFINITION) associated with allergies; histidine deficiencies are often correlated with a hormonal imbalance. To address the food allergies and depression, we prescribed histidine (200 mg, once daily) and another amino acid, tyrosine (500 mg, before meals), vitamin B5 (pantothenic acid; 500 mg, with meals), and a supplement called Doctor's Brand 007, containing amino acids needed to produce serotonin, a key brain chemical involved in sleep.

Alternative Medicine Plan for Balancing Hormones

- Dietary Recommendations
- Natural Hormone Therapy
- Herbal Therapy
- Homeopathy

EDITOR'S NOTE
Phyllis Bronson is a nutritional biochemist and a Ph.D. candidate in biochemistry with 20 years of clinical experience in the nutrient effects of depression and anxiety.

Harold Whitcomb, M.D., is a board-certified internist with an emphasis in environmental and preventive medicine. They may be contacted at: Aspen Clinic for Preventive and Environmental Medicine at Internal Medicine Associates, 100 East Main Street, Aspen, CO 81611; tel: 970-920-2523 or 970-925-5440; fax: 970-920-2282.

QUICK
DEFINITION

Electrodermal screening is a form of computerized information gathering, based on physics, not chemistry. A blunt, noninvasive electric probe is placed at specific points on the patient's hands, face, or feet, corresponding to acupuncture points at the beginning or end of energy meridians. Minute electrical discharges from these points serve as information signals about the condition of the body's organs and systems, useful for the physician in evaluation and developing a treatment plan.

Amino acids are the basic building blocks of the 40,000 different proteins in the body, including enzymes, hormones, and the key brain chemical messenger molecules called neurotransmitters. Eight amino acids cannot be made by the body and must be obtained through the diet; others are produced in the body but not always in sufficient amounts. The body's main "amino acid pool" consists of: alanine, arginine, aspargine, aspartic acid, carnitine, citrulline, cysteine, cystine, GABA, glutamic acid, glutamine, glycine, histidine, isoleucine, leucine, lysine, methionine, ornithine, phenylalanine, proline, serine, taurine, threonine, tryptophan, tyrosine and valine.

We also gave Margaret a natural estrogen called E1,E2,E3 Tri-estrogen (E123), which contains 100 mg of progesterone in cream form, and a transdermal DHEA gel. Margaret applied the E123 cream twice daily and the DHEA gel once daily, rubbing them into the skin at soft tissue sites such as the stomach and thighs; applying each in a different place and spacing the applications at least an hour apart.

To resolve her sleeping problems, we started Margaret on melatonin, a brain hormone, but she felt agitated after each dose, a reaction we sometimes observe in women with preexisting hormonal imbalances. As a substitute, we gave her inositol, a nutrient considered part of the vitamin B complex (650 mg, at bedtime). This quickly ended her sleeping difficulties.

After the first six weeks, Margaret's energy picked up, she started sleeping deeply and woke feeling refreshed. She reported a marked clarity in her thinking as one of her most significant symptoms, brain fog, had lifted. Her libido returned and, with it, the interest for a romantic relationship. Four months into the program, Margaret's progesterone level had climbed to 5.6. Her estrogen levels came up more slowly, which is often the case with natural estrogens. Now, more than a year after beginning with us, Margaret's estrogen is at 95, progesterone at 8, DHEA at 350, and testosterone at 42. Margaret says she "feels great" and has plenty of energy. Her insomnia and emotional disturbances have been resolved by rebalancing her hormones naturally.

Hormonal Imbalance and Sleep Disorders

The word *hormone* comes from the Greek *hormao*, meaning "to stir up." They are released by the various endocrine glands in the body in order to regulate energy production, growth, sexual development, stress responses, and many other functions. Because minute quantities of hormones can "stir up" so many activities in the body, when they are thrown out of balance the result can be system-wide. One of the symptoms of a hormone problem is insomnia and other sleep problems.

Women's Hormones and Sleep Disorders

For women at midlife, the natural interplay between the two primary female hormones, estrogen and progesterone (see "A Hormone Glossary," p. 206), takes on a new significance. As a woman approaches menopause, even as long as 10-15 years from menopause onset, hormone levels begin to shift. Many women don't realize that they may start having some symptoms of menopause long before what is still referred to as "The Change" is due; this early onset of symptoms is called perimenopause. These symptoms, including insomnia, night sweats, fluctuating moods, little interest in sex, and memory loss, among others, are indications that the levels of the basic female hormones are shifting or out of balance. Perimenopause has been likened to "PMS from hell," an apt comparison because both are brought on by rising estrogen levels and declining progesterone levels. This transition period of hormonal imbalances has been associated with a significant increase in sleep disturbances.[1]

When progesterone is in short supply women become "estrogen dominant," a condition that women's health expert John R. Lee, M.D., describes as "toxic to the body."[2] Estrogen dominance

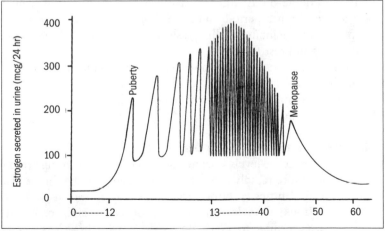

Peaks and Troughs of Estrogen Secretion Throughout a Woman's Life.

can damage the pituitary gland and put stress on liver function. The liver is required to detoxify estrogen and to convert thyroid hormone to its active form. If the liver is not working properly, it will perpetuate the cycle by allowing estrogen to build up. Estrogen-dominant women also tend to retain fluids and salt and to crave carbohydrates, which can lead to blood sugar problems and insulin imbalances, both factors in disturbed sleeping patterns. Excess estrogen can interfere with the function of the thyroid and the action of thyroid hormones, causing hypothyroidism, which can contribute to sleep problems.[3]

The cycle of estrogen release is closely linked with the activities of the adrenal glands. Estrogens are necessary for the smooth functioning of the sleep cycle, so when women enter menopause and their estrogens start to fluctuate and diminish, they are likely to experience disturbances in their sleep. Levels of estrogen can directly alter the circadian pattern of neurotransmitters affecting sleep, particularly serotonin and norepinephrine (adrenaline). In one study, 25 menopausal women classified as "bad sleepers" (based on questionnaires about their sleep patterns) were placed on a program of hormone replacement therapy with an estradiol transdermal gel. After three months, 18 of the women now rated as "good sleepers," a 72% response rate.[4] A randomized, double-blind study involving 63 postmenopausal women over a seven-month period found that hormone therapy "improved sleep quality, facilitated falling asleep, and decreased nocturnal awakenings and restlessness."[5]

Hormone fluctuations can also cause insomnia indirectly because of the increased frequency of hot flushes and night sweats during menopause. It has been shown that hormonal variations influence body temperature and disrupt sleep.[6]

Men's Hormones and Sleep Disorders

A man's testosterone levels start to slowly decrease beginning around age 30, then more rapidly around age 60. Usually by the time a man reaches his mid-fifties (although symptoms may appear in one's forties), indications of "male menopause," also called andropause, are noticeable, according to Gary Ross, M.D., who practices in San Francisco, California. According to Dr. Ross, the andropause complex of symptoms includes fatigue, lack of energy, obesity, a loss of sexual interest and possibly some sexual dysfunction, depression or emotional malaise, panic attacks, decrease in short-term memory, and insomnia, among others.

These are signs that a man's hormones—their levels and ratios one to another—are in flux, shifting into a new configuration at midlife. "Men experience a 'lite' version of menopause, physically," says Theresa L. Crenshaw, M.D., author of *The Alchemy of Love and Lust*. "Their hormones and neuropeptides diminish, albeit less abruptly. Their bodies sag and change shape. Sexual functioning is often compromised by hormonal imbalance, disease, medications, mind, or mood. Their stamina and temperament alter as well. Yet often they are less well-equipped to deal with these extremes than women."[7]

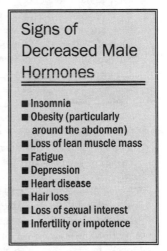

Signs of Decreased Male Hormones

- Insomnia
- Obesity (particularly around the abdomen)
- Loss of lean muscle mass
- Fatigue
- Depression
- Heart disease
- Hair loss
- Loss of sexual interest
- Infertility or impotence

This hormonal shift can lead to sleep problems in a number of ways. Testosterone is involved in blood sugar control. Decreased levels of the hormone are associated with increased insulin output, a factor for the development of sugar imbalances and insomnia. Decreased testosterone levels can lead to an increase in blood levels of the stress hormones adrenaline and cortisol. If this state occurs for an extended period of time, sleep disturbances can result. "Testosterone has been shown to be an antagonist of the stress hormones," says Eugene Shippen, M.D., author of *The Testosterone Syndrome*. "More testosterone, less stress hormone production."[8]

There also appears to be a direct relationship between testosterone levels and REM sleep, according to a clinical study. Testosterone levels in four male subjects were measured at 10-20 minute intervals throughout the night. Researchers found a pattern of increases in testosterone concentrations just prior to the onset of periods of REM sleep.[9] Researchers on another study confirmed this finding, stating that there were "positive associations between sleep efficiency, decreased latency to onset of REM, and number of REM episodes, and circulating testosterone."[10] Thus, fluctuations in testosterone during male menopause could have a profound effect on sleep.

A Hormone Glossary

Estrogen, a female sex hormone produced mainly in the ovaries, regulates the menstrual cycle. Estrogen is important for adolescent sexual development, prepares the uterus for receiving the fertilized egg, and affects all the body's cells; its levels decline after menopause. Estrogen slows down bone loss, helps reverse the incidence of heart attacks, and acts as an antiaging factor.

Progesterone is a female sex hormone (produced in the ovaries) which prepares the uterus for a fertilized egg and then stops the cell proliferation in the uterus if pregnancy does not occur. When estrogen is high (days 7-14 of a woman's cycle), the level of progesterone is at its lowest. Its levels climb to a peak around days 14 to 24 and then drops off again just before the start of menstruation. Around age 35, a woman usually starts producing less progesterone.

Pregnenolone is the parent hormone for DHEA and other key hormones. As a brain power hormone, pregnenolone enhances memory, improves concentration, reduces mental fatigue, and generally keeps the brain functioning at peak capacity.

DHEA (dehydroepiandrosterone) is naturally produced by the human adrenal glands and gonads with optimal levels occurring around age 20 for women and age 25 for men. As an antioxidant, hormone regulator, and the building block from which estrogen and testosterone are produced, DHEA is vital to health. Low DHEA levels have been associated with diabetes, hypertension, obesity, heart disease, Alzheimer's, and immune dysfunction illnesses. Test subjects using supplemental DHEA reported improved sleeping patterns, better memory, an improved ability to cope with stress, and decreases in body fat.

Testosterone is the primary male sex hormone, important for the development of male sexual characteristics. Testosterone can help reverse male impotency, heighten virility, and increase muscle mass. After "male menopause" at midlife, testosterone levels decline.

Cortisol is a hormone secreted by the adrenal glands, which are located atop the kidneys. Cortisol secretion (as well as the adrenal gland's other hormones, DHEA, adrenaline, and aldosterone) occurs in daily cycles, peaking in the morning and having the lowest values at night. Cortisol promotes protein building, regulates insulin and glycogen synthesis, and helps produce prostaglandins. Under conditions of stress, high amounts of cortisol are released; chronic excess secretion is associated with obesity and suppressed thyroid function.

Causes of Hormone Problems

A number of factors can cause hormone imbalances in women and men. Hormone levels generally decline as a result of aging, but they can also be affected by dietary choices, mineral deficiencies, environmental toxins and synthetic chemicals, medications, smoking, and stress.

Causes of Hormone Imbalances in Women

Estrogen dominance (the excess of estrogen in relation to progesterone) can be created by numerous factors. Eating a diet high in estrogenic foods is often double exposure, because many of the foods that naturally contain estrogen are from animals which have also been pumped full of synthetic hormones to increase their weight or egg or milk production. Estrogen-mimicking chemicals, known as environmental estrogens or xenoestrogens, are found in our food, air, and water. Herbicides, pesticides, by-products of plastics manufacture, and many other poisons mimic estrogen once they enter the body. The body responds as if it is real estrogen and the result is estrogen dominance and all the problems that imbalance carries with it.

Environmental estrogens are increasingly prevalent in Western societies; once in the body, they accumulate and persist for decades. There is no doubt that something is seriously interfering with normal human hormonal and endocrinal functioning, states Theo Colborn, Ph.D., a senior scientist with the World Wildlife Fund and an environmental author. Since 1945, synthetic chemicals (such as DDT, DES, PCBs, dioxins, among many others) have been released into our air, water, soil, food, and body. At least 51 of these have been conclusively shown to disrupt the human endocrine system. Each year, an estimated 1,000 new synthetic chemicals enter the world market, swelling the planetary total to well over 100,000. All of these are completely foreign and potentially harmful to endocrine function; almost none have been thoroughly tested for long-term, trans-generational health effects. Evidence is accumulating that these chemicals, even at very low concentrations and exposures, can, by disrupting the endocrine system, cause "hormone havoc."[11]

Progesterone normally exerts a balancing effect on estrogen that neutralizes it, but stressful situations can disrupt the estrogen-progesterone balance. Betty Kamen, Ph.D., a psychologist and nutritionist based in Novato, California, and author of *Hormone Replacement Therapy: Yes or No?*, says that under prolonged stress, the body uses progesterone to make cortisol, one of the adrenal hormones.[12] As progesterone is used up in cortisol production, there is nothing left to balance or offset the effects of estrogen.

If a woman has chronic constipation or toxic buildup in her intestines, the excess estrogen is reabsorbed by the body instead of being eliminating, further adding to the imbalance of the hormonal ratio. Another contributing factor to estrogen dominance is perimenopause (the ten to 15 years before the actual cessation of menses),

Ten Reasons Why Women's Hormones are Imbalanced

Estrogen dominance (too much estrogen in relation to progesterone) can be created by both an excess of estrogen and a deficiency of progesterone. Here is how it happens.

Too much estrogen may be caused by:

1) foods that have hormones added to them, such as commercially produced meat, milk, eggs, and dairy products

2) herbs that have an estrogenic effect in the body, such as licorice, black cohosh, and damiana

3) birth control pills that have high levels of estrogen

4) environmental toxins that mimic the actions of estrogen (known as xenoestrogens); the largest source of xenoestrogens is pesticides

5) exposure to radiation, which increases estrogen levels in the blood

6) chronic constipation, which interferes with the body's ability to eliminate estrogen properly; estrogen then builds up in the colon and can be reabsorbed by the body

7) synthetic estrogen supplements as part of a hormone replacement therapy for menopausal symptoms

Too little progesterone may be caused by:

8) an underactive thyroid gland (hypothyroidism)

9) chronic stress

10) frequent anovulatory cycles (menstruation without ovulation)

which depletes progesterone supplies and skews the estrogen-progesterone ratio.

Chronic stress can exhaust the adrenal glands, two small glands nestled atop the kidneys. The adrenal glands respond to stress by producing the hormones adrenaline and noradrenaline. Progesterone is the primary raw material the glands use for producing the adrenal hormones; the more adrenaline, the more progesterone needed. This is how chronic stress can lead to a state of progesterone deficiency (or estrogen dominance) as supplies of progesterone become depleted. When hormonal levels become imbalanced, emotional disorders can occur, potentially leading to sleep disturbances.

Causes of Hormone Imbalances in Men

The concept that men go through major physiological changes in their fifties—the "male menopause"—of potentially equal impact as women's menopause is beginning to gain acceptance. But most men still remain unaware that they experience a predictable decline in hormone production at midlife, notes Julian Whitaker, M.D., a nationally recognized alternative medicine educator and editor of *Health and Healing*. As noted above, a man's testosterone levels naturally start to decrease around age 30, with a more rapid decline around age 60.

Dietary factors can influence a man's hormone levels as well. The typical Western diet with its high levels of dietary fat and low levels of fiber may have a direct influence on testosterone production, according to clinical studies.[13] Other foods that have been found detrimental to hormone balance include saturated fats (commonly found in fast foods, processed foods, and red meats), hydrogenated oils, preservatives, and products containing refined sugar.

The minerals zinc, copper, and selenium are necessary for normal hormone production in men. In one study, a group of patients was given 1.4 mg of zinc daily while a second group received 10.4 mg per day. While blood levels of zinc did not vary between groups, the low-zinc group had significantly lower levels of testosterone.[14] Selenium, in addition to being required for testosterone production, helps protect the male sex glands against free radicals and heavy metals.[15] If these minerals are lacking in the diet, hormone imbalances may occur.

As with women, men's hormones may be thrown out of balance by environmental estrogens, foreign compounds and/or chemical toxins that mimic the effects of estrogen. Environmental estrogens, also called xenoestrogens, are present primarily in pesticides (such as DDT, PCBs, and dioxin) and industrial by-products. According to some researchers, environmental estrogens may contribute to testicular cancer, urinary tract disorders, and low sperm count. In men, a high level of estrogen slows down the production of testosterone.[16] Exposure to lead, mercury, cadmium, and other heavy metals also inhibits testosterone production.[17]

Men's hormone levels can be adversely affected by certain lifestyle choices. Smoking, in particular, may be a factor in reduced production of testosterone. Animal studies have shown that nicotine and related substances in cigarettes increase the activity of enzymes that deactivate male hormones such as testosterone.[18] Excessive consumption of alcohol decreases levels of testosterone and increases estrogen levels in men. However, modest alcohol intake has not been shown to affect hormone levels.[19] In addition, physical or mental/emotional stress can inhibit hormone production, particularly the adrenal hormone DHEA. Under conditions of chronic stress, the adrenal glands switch from producing DHEA to producing cortisol. Since DHEA is a precursor of the male hormones, less DHEA can severely limit testosterone production. A high level of cortisol also leads to blood sugar imbalances, depressed immune function, and sleep disturbances.[20]

Aging: Sleep Problems Are Not Inevitable

It is commonly believed that as we get older, we should expect to sleep poorly, but we disagree with that conclusion. How well you will sleep as you age depends to a large extent on your lifestyle. If you are a senior citizen who has spent most of your life drinking alcohol and caffeinated beverages, not exercising, and eating poorly, your body will then pay you back with sleep problems. Many people in their seventies and eighties sleep wonderfully well because they have had healthy lifestyles. Some lifestyle changes that you can make to improve your sleep include:

- Get plenty of exercise each day.
- Go to bed at a regular time each night and get up at the same time every morning.
- Eliminate distractions—turn off lights and the television.
- Avoid all caffeine prior to bedtime.
- Don't smoke—nicotine is a stimulant.
- Avoid sleeping pills (if you do use them, never use for more than three nights in a row).
- Avoid alcohol.
- Don't use your bed for eating or watching television.[21]

"The most consistent change with aging is in sleep quality, not in sleep duration," says Charles M. Morin, Ph.D., author of *Relief from Insomnia: Getting the Sleep of Your Dreams*. The proportion of time spent in deep sleep (Stages 3-4) decreases from about 20%-25% of the night during young adulthood to 5%-10% during your sixties. "This deep slumber virtually disappears," Dr. Morin says.[22] He adds that,

as the deep sleep disappears, the lightest sleep (Stage 1) increases, meaning people are more easily awakened by noise, movements of a bed partner, or by a full bladder. He says it is not unusual for a 65-year-old to be awakened two to five times a night, for only a few minutes or as much as 30 minutes.

Not only is sleep not as deep, but it is not as efficient with aging. Older people spend more time in bed, but a lesser percentage of that time is spent in sleep. "For example, a 20-year-old without insomnia sleeps on average about 95% of the time spent in bed; in contrast, a 70-year-old without insomnia sleeps just over 80% of that time," Dr. Morin says.[23] He says those are normal changes with aging: true insomnia does not have to happen as we age.

Another common problem with aging is advanced sleep phase syndrome, or falling asleep too early and then awakening before dawn. About one-third of adults over 65 tend to fall into that pattern, says James Perl, Ph.D., author of *Sleep Right in Five Nights*. This problem can be corrected with bright light therapy, melatonin supplements, or napping. Dr. Perl says that if you're going to nap, don't nap after 3 p.m. and don't nap for more than an hour. Also, try to stay up until 10-11 p.m.; if you get sleepy earlier, take a walk or do indoor exercise.[24]

Older adults also tend to have less dramatic ups and downs in their body clock, or circadian rhythms. "The polarity between nighttime sleep and daytime wakefulness decreases as night and day blend together," says Dr. Perl. The core body temperature of a young adult is about 2° F lower during the night, while a 75-year-old may have a temperature difference of only 0.5° F or less. This lessening of daytime/nighttime temperature variation is a factor in sleep disturbances.

For more on **melatonin**, see Chapter 5: Resetting the Body Clock, pp. 120-145.

As we age, melatonin levels decline; since melatonin is the hormone that puts the body to sleep, it makes sense that older adults would have more sleep problems.[25] In a study of elderly insomniacs, researchers found a connection between deficient levels of melatonin and an increased prevalence of sleep disorders with advancing age. The study involved 95 elderly patients with insomnia, 25 elderly patients without sleep disorders, and 12 young men without sleep disorders. The melatonin levels in the elderly insomniacs were only half those of either the young men or the elderly people without insomnia. "Melatonin deficiency seems to be a key component in the incidence of sleep disorders in elderly subjects and melatonin replacement therapy may be of benefit," the researchers concluded.[26]

Are Your Hormones Imbalanced?

The first step in treating a hormonal imbalance is to get an accurate measurement of your hormone levels. Blood or 24-hour urine tests, which can be ordered by your physician, are the standard conventional method of determining hormone levels. However, saliva tests provide a noninvasive and simple alternative to a blood test that can also be used during the therapeutic process to determine your progress.

Aeron LifeCycles Saliva Test

If you want information about your hormone levels, you can test your saliva at home to find out where you stand. The test, called the Aeron LifeCycles Saliva Assay Report, can be ordered by both consumers and physicians and provides graphs of individual hormone levels. It can measure up to eight different hormones. Changing levels can be plotted over time on the same graph if supplementation or subsequent testing is done. Although hormones are present in saliva only in fractional amounts compared to the blood, "clinically relevant and highly accurate levels of hormones can be determined in saliva," says John Kells, president of Aeron LifeCycles in San Leandro, California. "Saliva testing provides a means to establish whether or not your hormone levels are within the expected normal range for your age."

The saliva assay has several advantages over traditional blood testing for hormones. It is painless and noninvasive, and tests can be performed simply at any time or place. As DHEA, cortisol, estrogen, progesterone, and testosterone levels are highest in the morning, it is far more convenient to be able to test them at home (and then immediately ship the saliva sample to Aeron's laboratory). As the test is less expensive than blood testing, you can do frequent testing to monitor changes (brought on by interventions such as diet, exercise, herbs, stress reduction, or acupuncture) and to adjust dosages of over-the-counter hormones, says Kells. In general, Kells explains that it is best to establish a baseline level of saliva hormones first, then after intervention (which can include hormone supplementation), test a second time to measure the changes.

For information on the **hormone saliva test**, contact Aeron LifeCycles, 1933 Davis St., Suite 310, San Leandro, CA 94577; tel: 510-729-0375 or 800-631-7900; fax: 510-729-0383. For the **Adrenal Stress Index test**, contact: Diagnos-Tech, Inc., 6620 South 192nd Place, J-2204, Kent, WA 96032; tel: 800-878-3787 or 425-251-0596; fax: 425-251-0637.

Are Your Adrenal Glands Stressed?

The Adrenal Stress Index (ASI) can pinpoint whether an imbalance in the adrenal glands might be contributing to hormonal imbalance and weight gain. This test evaluates how well one's adrenal glands are functioning by tracking hormone levels over a 24-hour cycle (circadian rhythm). Four saliva samples taken at intervals throughout the day are used to reconstruct the adrenal rhythm in the laboratory. These samples are used to determine whether the three main stress hormones are being secreted in proper proportion to each other, and at the right times. Based on the results, a physician can prescribe the appropriate treatment to restore the balance of hormones and correct the circadian rhythm.

Alternative Medicine Plan for Balancing Hormones

If your hormones are imbalanced, one of your priorities should be to detoxify your body systems of accumulated toxins. Both the liver and gastrointestinal system are involved in the normal processing of excess levels of hormones. When these organs are not functioning properly, your hormones may become imbalanced, contributing to a number of health problems, including sleep disorders. Holistic practitioners generally recommend tending to these systems first in order to normalize the body's functions. Alternative medicine also offers a number of therapies to balance your hormones, including dietary and nutritional support, hormone replacement, herbal medicine, and homeopathy.

For more on **detoxification**, see Chapter 4: Detoxify Your Body, pp. 86-119.

Therapies for Women

Rather than artificially manipulating your estrogen levels with synthetic hormones and ignoring the reasons behind the imbalance, it is more valuable to determine why you have the estrogen buildup or progesterone deficiency in the first place. Depending on the source of the relative excess estrogen, restoring hormonal balance can be more effectively achieved with dietary changes and nutritional supplements, natural progesterone cream, and herbal therapy.

Dietary Support—Eating soybeans and soybean-derived products, particularly fermented soybean foods such as tempeh and miso, can help counteract the negative effects of excess estrogen. These foods contain high levels of genistein, a substance that has a chemical structure similar to estrogen and can be used by the body as a mild estrogen surrogate. Substances like genistein are known as phytoestrogens, which are plant compounds that block estrogens from attaching to cell receptor sites—the places where estrogens exert their effect on the body. Phytoestrogens tend to balance estrogen in the body.[27] Other than soy, foods that are high in phytoestrogens include flaxseeds, apples, whole grains, nuts, celery, and alfalfa.[28] Ellen Brown and Lynn Walker, Pharm.D., M.Ac., D.H.M., authors of *Menopause and Estrogen*, suggest the following foods to help balance estrogens: raw fruits, fresh fruit and vegetable juices (especially green juices), leafy green vegetables, garlic, figs, dates, cabbage, avocados, grapes, apples, beets, spirulina, chlorella, seaweed, wheat germ, and wheat germ oil.[29]

Supplementing with essential fatty acids (EFAs—SEE QUICK DEFINITION) can be important for balancing your hormones. "Many women actually eat themselves into hormonal dysfunction," says nutritionist Ann Louise Gittleman, M.S., C.N.S., of Bozeman, Montana. "They overindulge in carbohydrates and they don't get enough protein, which is needed to support the adrenal glands. They deprive themselves of needed fats and end up lacking the building blocks of the essential sex-related hormones, which derive from fats." In the effort to cut down on fats, many women have stopped consuming the ones their bodies need.[31] Only one or two tablespoons per day of EFAs is often all it takes to restore balance to the hormones. EFAs, both omega-3s and omega-6s, can be a prime source of relief. Flaxseed oil (one tablespoon) and evening primrose oil (500 mg, twice daily) are excellent sources of EFAs.

Dr. Lee recommends taking the following antioxidant (SEE QUICK DEFINITION) vitamins to help cleanse the body of harmful pollutants and toxins that can lead to excessive estrogen: 1,000-2,000 mg of vitamin C daily; 400 IU of vitamin E daily; 500 mg of quercetin (a bioflavonoid) twice daily; 50 mg of B-complex vitamins daily, and 500-1,000 mg of magnesium (in the gluconate or citrate form).[32]

Natural Progesterone Therapy—To restore progesterone levels in the body, Dr. Lee recommends taking a progesterone supplement, which can help turn fat into energy and reduce water retention.[33] While progesterone supplements are available in sublingual (under-the-tongue) drops and capsules, using a progesterone skin cream or oil is best. Applying progesterone to the skin allows it to be absorbed into fat layers under the skin, where it can be taken up by the blood as needed. If taken in a capsule form, it is more difficult for the body to regulate the amount of progesterone entering the blood.

Natural progesterone can be manufactured in the laboratory from a substance called diosgenin, which is found in wild yam or soybeans. However, the body cannot manufacture progesterone from the raw diosgenin found in these foods. Dr. Lee therefore recommends using products that have been preconverted in the laboratory into progesterone, rather than try to obtain it from dietary sources. He advises consumers to check labels to make sure that a product lists the actual concentration of progesterone.

The recommended application of progesterone cream is between $1/8$ and $1/2$ teaspoon per day, or three to ten drops of the oil. Premenopausal women with average menstrual cycles (28 days) should apply the cream during days 12 to 26 of their cycle. Those with longer cycles should apply it from days 10 to 28. For menopausal women, Dr. Lee indicates that there can be more flexibility in applying the cream. He recommends using it over a 14-21 day period, and then discontinuing use until the following month. The cream can be applied to the palms of the hands, the face and neck, the upper chest and breasts, the insides of the arms, and behind the knees. Alternating applications among these sites will increase absorption.[34]

Various creams are available in health food stores and by mail order. When you purchase a product, there are two points to keep in mind. First, make sure it contains natural progesterone, not just wild yam (*Dioscorea villosa*). Don't be misled by claims that wild yam creams are the same as progesterone creams. As an herbal supplement, wild yam can have a mild hormone-balancing effect, but it does not provide natural progesterone. Second, make sure you use a brand of cream that has enough natural progesterone in it to make a difference. Dr. Lee advises using only creams that have at least 400 mg of progesterone per ounce.

Herbal Therapy—Herbs that are helpful for hormone balancing include unicorn root (*Aletris farinosa*), an herb used in folk remedies for premenopausal women, and black cohosh (*Cimicifuga racemosa*). These herbs promote the normal production and conversion of the healthier forms of estrogen and contribute to the proper balance of estrogen and progesterone. Other herbs that may be helpful include dong quai (*Angelica sinensis*), licorice (*Glycyrrhiza glabra*), and Siberian ginseng (*Eleutherococcus senticosus*), which contribute to proper hormone regulation.[35]

Linda Ojeda, C.N.C., Ph.D., author of *Menopause Without Medicine*, generally suggests using certain herbs for their hormone-stimulating properties. Unlike synthetic hormone replacement therapy, the action

Dietary Guidelines for Balancing Your Hormones

Women's health expert John R. Lee, M.D., of Sebastopol, California, who coined the term *estrogen dominance*, offers the following general dietary recommendations for maintaining balanced hormone levels:

- Avoid refined sugars and processed foods; instead, eat whole organic foods, emphasizing fresh vegetables and fruit, whole grains, legumes, and nuts.
- Consume modest amounts of meat (chicken, beef, or pork) two or three times per week at most; preferable sources of protein are eggs, yogurt, and coldwater ocean fish (4-5 servings per week).
- Avoid hydrogenated oils (in margarine and processed foods); use primarily olive oil instead. Limit total dietary intake of fat to 20%-25%.
- Eliminate colas and other sodas and reduce alcohol consumption; drink plenty of clean water daily.[30]

of herbs is safe and gentle. Dr. Ojeda cites the following herbs as estrogen-stimulating: black cohosh, alfalfa, hops, sweetbriar, horsetail, buckwheat, sage, rose, and shepherd's purse. Among the herbs she recommends to support progesterone are: wild yam, chastetree berry (*Vitex agnus-castus*), sarsaparilla, and yarrow. The herbs can be taken as supplements or teas.[36]

In addition to a healthy lifestyle, Chinese herbal supplements can be very helpful in strengthening the kidney essence, says Harriet Beinfield, L.Ac., of San Francisco, California. Dr. Beinfield recommends the herbs ginseng, lotus seeds, and longan fruit for a woman with a kidney essence weakness that results in a heart yin deficiency. Symptoms of this condition are insomnia, hot flashes, anxiety, palpitations, emotional instability, unusual thirst or perspiration, premenstrual build-up, with scanty bright flow. For women with a kidney essence deficiency that results in a liver weakness, Dr. Beinfield recommends white peony root and lycii berries. Symptoms of this imbalance are dry eyes, skin, hair, nails, or vaginal mucosa, irritability or hypersensitivity, headaches, muscle tension or cramping, dizziness or vertigo, and uneven or intermittent menstrual flow.[37]

Chinese Medicine, Menopause, and Insomnia

In traditional Chinese medicine, insomnia is seen as an imbalance between the yin and yang energies of the body. Yin is the calming, slow, quiet, wet, dense, feminine life energy, while yang is the fast, bright, strong, loud, expansive, masculine life energy. In menopause, a decrease in a woman's kidney essence, or reproductive force, can trigger a yin/yang imbalance in the associated organ systems, such as kidney, liver, or heart. If a woman does not maintain a lifestyle that keeps her kidney energy strong—good nutrition, exercise, plenty of rest, low stress, positive outlook—she could develop menopausal symptoms including insomnia.

Success Story: Acupuncture and Herbs Outperform Drugs—Lynn, a 28-year-old woman, was three months pregnant when she developed insomnia that kept her awake all night. Lynn first tried conventional sedatives to try to get some sleep, but she was concerned about potential side effects, ranging from memory loss to headaches to poor muscle coordination. She was also worried about potential harm to the baby and the medications were not even working for Lynn. After two more months of insomnia, Lynn came to acupuncturist Edythe Vickers, N.D., L.Ac., in Portland, Oregon.

As soon as Dr. Vickers inserted the hair-thin acupuncture needles into Lynn's body, Lynn fell asleep on the table, which Dr. Vickers indicated was a favorable sign because it showed Lynn's body responded well to acupuncture. Dr. Vickers used 21 needles: ten on Lynn's back and 11 on the front side of her body at her feet, hands, knees, neck and forehead. The needles were placed at specific points along energy pathways in Lynn's body called meridians. At those specific points, the needles serve to unblock the *qi*, or life force energy, that circulates in the meridians, according to traditional Chinese medicine (TCM). The *qi* becomes blocked from various traumas or stresses such as poor diet, overwork, emotional tension, viruses, or, as in Lynn's case, from changes due to the pregnancy.

After the treatment, Dr. Vickers gave Lynn a Chinese herbal formula, focused on the herbs ginseng and longan, to strengthen Lynn's kidney and heart energies so that the two systems could work together. In Lynn's case, the kidney energy, a water element in TCM, was being diverted to care for the baby, which left the heart energy, a fire element, blazing out of control, causing anxiety, restlessness, and insomnia. In addition, Dr. Vickers gave Lynn zizyphus, a Chinese herb used for insomnia because it strengthens the yin, or the cooling, feminine energy of the body. Yin is the energy that governs sleep and rest, while yang refers to the active, masculine, bright qualities of energy. In general, TCM practitioners say that most types of insomnia are either from too much yang energy or not enough yin. Lynn took one teaspoon of the herbs before bed and another teaspoon every time she woke up.

Dr. Vickers often recommends that pregnant women with insomnia take the naturally calming minerals calcium and magnesium supplements in liquid form before bed. The liquid form is more readily absorbed, she says. A quick-acting and safe anti-insomnia method such as minerals is best for pregnancy, when women cannot take any drugs and must also be careful with herbal supplements.

That night, without any medications, Lynn fell asleep within 20 minutes, which was an unusually short time for her, and slept for four hours straight. Thereafter, Lynn slept through the night, aided by acupuncture treatments three times a week for several weeks and continued herbal therapy. After the first few weeks, Lynn continued once-a-week acupuncture treatments throughout the rest of her

For **liquid calcium and magnesium supplements** (available to health-care providers), contact: NF Formulas Inc., 9775 S.W. Commerce Circle, C5, Wilsonville, OR 97070; tel: 800-547-4891.

pregnancy, as well as continuing the herbs. Her insomnia did not return until she became pregnant again two years later, when she again sought treatment from Dr. Vickers.

Therapies for Men

Once you've determined that your hormones are imbalanced, a number of alternative therapies are available to normalize them. Dietary adjustments can have a significant impact on your hormone levels, along with other therapeutic support such as nutritional supplements, hormone therapy, homeopathy, and herbs.

Dietary Recommendations—To help rebalance the hormones, the consumption of refined sugar products, saturated fats, and food preservatives must be reduced, according to Dr. Ross. He advises men to eat more fresh fruit and vegetables with a high nutrient content. Increase your intake of legumes (especially soy), dark-green leafy vegetables (for their protective antioxidant content), essential fatty acids (flaxseed, evening primrose, and borage oils), and nuts and seeds (a good source of zinc).

During male menopause, low levels of testosterone may lead to a relative excess in estrogen; this female hormone can reduce the effects of testosterone in the body. Dr. Shippen also emphasizes eating more soy, which contains phytoestrogens that can block the action of estrogen in the body. He recommends eating plenty of cruciferous vegetables, such as cauliflower and broccoli, as these vegetables help rid the body of excess estrogen.[38] Maintaining an adequate level of dietary fiber is also important for clearing estrogen from the body.

Since environmental estrogens and other toxins are a factor in male hormonal imbalances, you should reduce or eliminate your exposure to these substances. One way is to select meats produced without the use of hormones or antibiotics, eat free-range chicken, and choose organic sources for your dairy products, fruits, and vegetables.

Dr. Whitaker emphasizes that men who supplement with testosterone should closely monitor their prostate-specific antigen (PSA) levels, as excess testosterone has been linked to prostate cancer.

Testosterone Replacement Therapy—According to Dr. Whitaker, easing male menopause requires its own hormone therapy, testosterone replacement. Studies have shown that testosterone replacement can heighten sex drive, increase bone density, and improve mood and sleep patterns, among other effects. If you are considering testosterone replacement, the first step is a blood or saliva test to assess your levels of the hormone, says Dr. Whitaker. If your levels are low or even average for your age, testosterone therapy can help alleviate andropause symptoms and improve overall health, he explains.

The goal of supplementation is to restore blood testosterone levels to those of a healthy 25- to 30-year-old man. For this, Dr. Whitaker recommends weekly injections of testosterone cypionate (100 mg) or biweekly injections of testosterone enanthate (200 mg). These long-acting versions of the hormone are considered the safest and most effective preparations for use in testosterone replacement, says Dr. Whitaker. As injection guarantees consistent absorption, he considers this to be the preferred method of testosterone supplementation. Skin patches and oral lozenges can also be effective, he reports. However, Dr. Whitaker advises against oral testosterone in pill form. "With oral testosterone, there is a potential for liver dysfunction and a decrease in protective HDL [high-density lipoprotein] or 'good' cholesterol levels," he cautions. In addition to the benefits of testosterone replacement cited above, according to Dr. Whitaker, further positive effects include increased lean muscle mass and protection for the heart, as certain forms of testosterone can improve the ratio between "good" and "bad" cholesterol and lower cholesterol levels overall.[40]

Another option is a gel called Libidex Creme, which can be applied to the skin to stimulate testosterone production and support the endocrine system. Developed by Michael Borkin, D.C., N.M.D., of Santa Monica, California, Libidex contains DHEA, androstenedione (a testosterone precursor), alpha-lipoic acid, oat extract (*Avena sativa*),

Supplements for Male Hormone Support

Sandra Cabot, M.D., author of *Smart Medicine for Menopause*, offers a nutritional strategy that men can apply to start improving the functioning of their endocrine system (the source of all hormones). Here are Dr. Cabot's daily male menopause recommendations:

- Vitamin E: 500 IU
- Magnesium: 500 mg
- Zinc: 50 mg
- Selenium: 50 mcg
- Manganese: 5 mg
- Ginseng: 2,000-4,000 mg
- Royal Jelly: 2,000-4,000 mg
- Vitamin B complex: 1 tablet
- Evening primrose oil: 3,000 mg

These supplements, taken daily, are designed to help the male body cope with the natural decline of testosterone. Ginseng, for example, acts as a glandular tonic, helping to improve the function of the testicles. Royal Jelly, rich in choline, indirectly helps improve sexual performance and response. Evening primrose oil supplies fatty acids that aid the production and release of hormones. Zinc can boost male virility and reduce prostate problems such as swelling. Vitamin E and magnesium strengthen the heart and circulation, including blood supply to the pelvic region.[39]

Success Story:
Raising Hormone Levels for Better Sleep

Cyril, 55, turned out to be "dreadfully low" in the key male hormones when he came to see Gary Ross, M.D. A professional writer, Cyril wasn't sleeping well and complained of a slump in his mental abilities; he wanted his mind to feel sharper.

Based on a male hormone profile developed from urine collected over 24 hours, Dr. Ross found that Cyril's DHEA (a key adrenal gland hormone) was very low at 0.11 (normal is 0.2 to 2.0); his testosterone was also in the basement at 4.95. A blood test also showed plasma levels of testosterone were low, at 319. In addition, Cyril's level of human growth hormone (made in the brain, with levels declining with age) was low. As it was only 138, compared to 250 and higher, considered the norm for optimal functioning, this was worrying. "In general, Cyril's male hormone levels were at the bottom of the barrel," Dr. Ross notes.

His treatment plan for Cyril called for the following supplements and substances: the amino acid tryptophan to help regulate his sleeping; Sexativa, a green oat extract (two tablets, twice daily), to release and elevate the level of free testosterone; Libidex Creme (a transdermal gel containing nutrients, herbs, hormones, and flower essences); and homeopathic growth hormone stimulator called Vital, given in liquid form (ten drops in water, three times daily) to encourage the body to produce its own hormone.

After only a short time on this therapy regimen, Cyril starting sleeping better and his other symptoms improved as well. Dr. Ross reports that "clinically, he's definitely feeling better."

Gary S. Ross, M.D., 500 Sutter Street, Suite 300, San Francisco, CA 94102; tel: 415-398-0555; fax: 415-398-6228. For **Sexativa:** GeroVital Intl., 520 Washington Blvd., Suite 240, Marina Del Rey, CA 90292; tel: 800-406-1314 or 800-929-9726; fax: 800-559-3535. For **Vital:** Liddell Homeopathic Formulae, 1036 Country Club Drive, Moraga, CA 94556; tel: 800-460-7733 or 925-631-0257; fax: 925-631-7948.

Michael Borkin, D.C., N.M.D.: 310 26th Street, Santa Monica, CA 90402; tel: 310-451-8599; fax: 818-248-5434. For **Libidex Creme** (available to health-care practiioners only), contact: Market Resource International, 310 26th Street, Santa Monica, CA 90402; tel: 888-674-9556. For **ginseng supplements**, contact: Nature's Herbs, 600 East Quality Drive, American Fork, UT 84003; tel: 800-437-2257 or 801-763-0700. Futurebiotics, 145 Ricefield Lane, Hauppauge, NY 11788; tel: 800-FOR-LIFE or 516-273-6300.

saw palmetto, colloidal silver, vitamins A, B12, and E, plus homeopathic support and ten flower remedies. The typical daily dosage is $^1/_8$ to $^1/_2$ teaspoon, depending on age, applied to areas of soft skin, preferably upon rising in the morning.

Herbal Medicine—As an accompaniment to andropause treatment, Dr. Whitaker generally suggests taking the herb saw palmetto (120-360 mg daily). This medicinal plant has been shown to reduce the conversion of testosterone into dihydrotestosterone, a stronger version of the hormone. Too much testosterone has been linked to various health problems, including prostate cancer.

Thyroid Problems Can Ruin Sleep

Low thyroid hormone levels are a key cause in insomnia, says Lita Lee, Ph.D., an enzyme specialist in Eugene, Oregon. The thyroid gland, one of the body's seven endocrine glands, is located just below the larynx in the throat. The thyroid is the body's metabolic thermostat, controlling body temperature, energy use, the rate at which organs function, and the speed with which the body uses food; it affects the operation of all body processes and organs. Of the hormones the thyroid synthesizes and releases, T3 (tri-iodothyronine) represents 7% and T4 (thyroxine) accounts for almost 93%. The secretion of both these hormones is regulated by thyroid-stimulating hormone, or TSH, secreted by the pituitary gland in the brain.

The thyroid plays a key role in the interaction between REM and non-REM sleep cycles and patterns of hormone secretion from the endocrine system during the night. Both TSH and T4 show a definite circadian pattern and levels of TSH directly affect the onset of REM sleep periods.[43] Dr. Lee says people with low thyroid generally also have low blood sugar. When the blood sugar is low, the body produces adrenaline to compensate, and the adrenaline induces the "fight-or-flight" stress response that wakes people up and makes them tense. The low blood sugar often happens at night and the person develops sleep-maintenance insomnia.

Common symptoms of hypothyroidism are chronic fatigue, aches and pains, depression, weight gain, cold limbs, poor hair and skin quality, and insomnia. Dr. Lee will often prescribe whole-food thyroid glandular extract, such as Armour Thyroid, if needed (a glandular extract is a purified nutritional and therapeutic product derived from animal glands). When people with insomnia improve their thyroid function, they usually start sleeping better in a short time, says Dr. Lee.

Lita Lee, Ph.D.:
P.O. Box 516, Lowell, OR 97452;
tel: 541-937-1123;
fax: 541-937-1132.

The herb ginseng has an ancient history and has accumulated much folklore about its actions and uses. One variety, Oriental ginseng (*Panax ginseng*), has received a great deal of attention as a potential aid to virility and animal studies have shown that *Panax ginseng* does increase testosterone levels.[41] Ginseng should not be abused, however, as serious side effects can occur, including headaches, skin problems, and other reactions. For this reason, the proper dosage for the individual should be determined and respected.

Studies indicate that Chinese wolfberry (*Lycium chinense*) may be able to boost testosterone levels.[42] Oats (*Avena sativa*) have traditionally been used as an energy and nerve tonic and may be useful for stimulating male hormone levels.

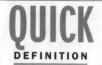

Homeopathy—"The first step in andropause treatment is to balance and correct the hormone deficiencies," says Dr. Ross. Here he finds certain complex homeopathic (SEE QUICK DEFINITION) remedies helpful, either alone or in conjunction with prescribed hormones. Among these are *Testis compositum*® (stimulates male sexual, brain, and adrenal function and reduces fatigue); *Coenzyme compositum*® (a multiple vitamin in homeopathic form, containing vitamin C and several B vitamins needed for metabolism); *Cerebrum compositum*® (enhances brain and nervous system function and memory, reduces anxiety and depression); and Galium-Heel® (for body detoxification and reduction of inflammation). Depending upon each individual's case, any or all of these homeopathic preparations can be used in the treatment plan, says Dr. Ross. Response time can vary from quickly to several months, he adds.[44]

For information on **complex homeopathic remedies**, contact: Heel/BHI, 11600 Cochiti Road SE, Albuquerque, NM 87123; tel: 800-621-7644; website: www.heelbhi.com.

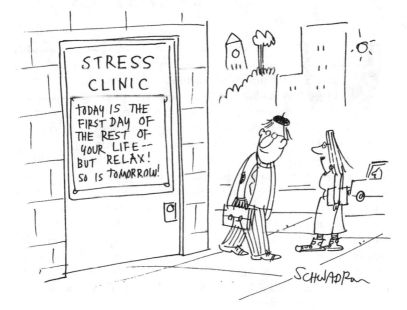

Correcting Structural Imbalances

WE'VE SEEN HOW STRESS and emotional tension can disturb sleep. Similarly, physical stress and muscular tension may be keeping you awake at night. While exercise and physical activity are important components of any healthy lifestyle, they are an absolute necessity for people who suffer from sleep disorders. The exercise program should target flexibility, circulation of blood and lymph fluid, and relaxation. And you don't need to become a marathon runner in order to benefit from regular exercise. Exercises from the East, such as *qigong* and yoga, increase flexibility as well as relaxing an anxious mind. Daily exercise should be further augmented by chiropractic, massage, acupressure, or other physical therapies that promote relaxation and improve the circulation of nerve impulses, blood, and lymphatic fluid. In this chapter, we discuss some of the most widely available physical therapies so that you and your health-care professional can determine which one would be most beneficial.

Structural Imbalances and Sleep Disturbances

Hans Selye, M.D., a pioneering researcher on stress, determined that any neurological pressure, at any point, affects the function of the entire spinal cord. So the whole function of the human body is affected by any kind of neurological blockage or impingement. That means that almost any symptom can be fully or partially caused by spinal dysfunction.

The spinal column, or backbone, is made up of twenty-four bones called vertebrae that surround and protect the spinal cord. Between each vertebra, pairs of spinal nerves exit and extend to every part of the body, including muscles, bones, organs, and glands. The nervous system itself is comprised of three overlapping systems: the central nervous system, which includes the brain and spinal cord; the autonomic nervous system, which controls involuntary functions such as heart rate, digestion, and glandular function; and the peripheral nervous system, which connects the central nervous system to all the body tissues and voluntary muscles.

Health relies upon the balance and equilibrium of these three interrelated nerve systems, which can be easily disrupted by spinal injury, misalignment, stress, or illness. When vertebrae get out of alignment (subluxations), pressure is placed on the nerves in that area. As a result, the nerves cannot carry out their proper function and this can lead to dysfunction, disharmony, and eventually disease.

Chiropractic, like traditional Chinese medicine (TCM), espouses the notion that disease is the lack of homeostasis due to an excess or deficiency of energy (*qi* in TCM and nerve energy in chiropractic). Chiropractors speak of the parasympathetic and sympathetic "tone" of the autonomic nervous system. The sympathetic nervous system controls the "fight-or-flight" stress response and activates the body; the parasympathetic calms the body and conserves energy. Subluxations can throw this system out of balance. "Subluxations restricting the parasympathetic or exciting the sympathetic nerve flow would

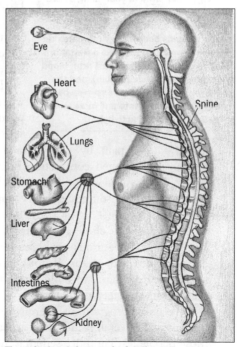

The spinal vertebrae and related organ systems.

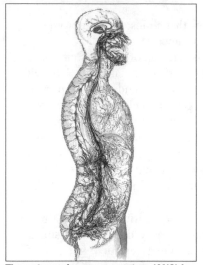

The autonomic nervous system (ANS) is like your body's automatic pilot. It keeps you alive through breathing, heart rate, and digestion, without your being aware of it or participating in its activities. The ANS has two divisions: the sympathetic, which expends body energy (prepares us physically when we perceive a threat or challenge by increasing heart rate, blood pressure, and muscle tension), and the parasympathetic, which conserves body energy (slows heart rate and increases intestinal and gland activity).

Tim Leasenby, D.C.:
4260 Westbrook Drive,
Suite 106, Aurora,
IL 60504;
tel: 630-851-9222.

result in sympathetic dominance," explains Tim Leasenby, D.C., of Aurora, Illinois. "Sympathetic dominance leads to too much energy in the legs in restless legs syndrome and too much energy in the mind/brain in insomnia."

Subluxations of the spinal vertebrae can also affect the body in less obvious ways. A subluxation can have a direct effect on an organ's function when it impedes the proper nerve flow to that organ. When the vertebrae are properly aligned, the spine remains mobile, allowing the electrical impulses from the brain to travel freely along the spinal cord to the organs, thus maintaining healthy function. However, when subluxations occur, they interrupt the normal flow in the nerve structures which, in turn, affects the normal functioning of the organ.

In addition, muscle tension, whether from normal activity, awkward movement, lack of exercise, or stress, contributes to muscle fatigue and pain by compressing nerve fibers in the muscle. Prolonged contraction interferes with the elimination of chemical wastes in the muscles and surrounding tissues, and can cause frequent nerve and muscle pain. The lymphatic system (SEE QUICK DEFINITION) relies on physical activity and movement to eliminate wastes from the body. However, if the lymph stagnates, serious problems can result as the body becomes overburdened with toxins. If not properly addressed these body tensions have a tendency to build into chronic patterns of stress, potentially leading to sleep disturbances.

A regular program of exercise can help you sleep better and improve your overall health. Researchers have consistently found that those people leading more sedentary lives have a higher incidence of insomnia. One of the reasons for the increasing incidence of sleep disorders in older people may be their decreasing level of physical activity. In addition, chiropractic, massage, and other forms of bodywork can help relieve physical tension and structural imbalances contributing to disrupted sleep.

Exercise

Most health-care professionals endorse exercise as a sleep-promoter—if it is done at the right level, at the right time of day. "I don't think there's a single thing in life that's as therapeutic as the right kind of exercise program applied over time," says John Hibbs, N.D., of Bastyr University in Seattle, Washington, "but misapplied, it can be just another stressor." As early as 1978, researchers were crediting exercise with producing more restful sleep.[1] In a more recent study, 50 men and women over the age of 67 were split into two groups—half did 45 minutes of aerobic exercise three times a week and the other half did stretching exercises with the same frequency. After six months, they all came to a sleep lab for testing. Those in aerobics group were getting 33% more deep sleep than before the study began. Also, some of the exercisers picked at random were found to be secreting 30% more human growth hormone (HGH—SEE QUICK DEFINITION). Not one person in the stretching group showed any changes in levels of either deep sleep or HGH.[2] The release of HGH is closely tied to the circadian rhythm of sleep. The reason for the increased HGH production with exercise is that muscle tissue requires more HGH for maintenance than fat does: in other words, a fitter body demands more deep sleep before it will produce the hormone.

Other researchers speculate that exercise later in the day raises the body temperature very slightly until bedtime, and the extra heat seems to drop the body deeper into sleep. That's one of the reasons that a hot bath (researchers call it "passive heating") before bedtime can induce deep-

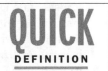

DEFINITION

The **lymphatic system** consists of lymph fluid and the structures (vessels, ducts, and nodes) involved in transporting it from tissues to the bloodstream. Lymph fluid occupies the space between the body's cells and contains plasma proteins, foreign particles, and cellular waste. Lymph nodes are clusters of immune tissue that work as filters or "inspection stations" for detecting and removing foreign and potentially harmful substances in the lymph fluid. While the body has hundreds of lymph nodes (more than 500), they are mostly clustered in the neck, armpits, chest, groin, and abdomen. The lymphatic system is the body's master drain, collecting and filtering the lymph fluid and conveying it to the bloodstream, thereby clearing waste products and cellular debris from the tissues.

Human growth hormone (HGH), naturally secreted by the pituitary gland in the brain, is a small, protein-like hormone similar to insulin. HGH is secreted in very brief pulses during the early hours of sleep and remains in circulation for only a few minutes. During adolescence, when growth is most rapid, production of HGH is high. After age 20, HGH production declines progressively at an average rate of about 14% per decade; by age 60, it is not uncommon to measure a growth hormone loss of 75% or more. In the early 1980s, growth hormone extracts were used to correct disturbances in normal growth; later it was synthesized for adult use. Benefits from HGH include increased muscle mass; improved physical strength; reduced fatigue; decreased fat; increased bone strength; revitalization of liver, kidney, spleen, and brain functions; strong kidney blood flow and efficiency; improved cardiac function; and a general enhancement in the sense of well-being.

er sleep. Karla A. Kubitz, M.D., of the Department of Kinesiology at Kansas State University in Manhattan, Kansas, says that the beneficial effect is dependent on the time of day that you exercise as well as the intensity and duration of the exercise. "I find that many more patients have normalization of sleep patterns with regular exercise than disruption of their patterns," says Dr. Kubitz. "When there is a disruption, it is usually related to timing, such as exercising just before bedtime." Dr. Kubitz has found exercise can increase slow wave (deep) sleep and total sleep time. Exercise may also decrease the time it takes to fall asleep and reduce REM (dream) sleep time.[3]

Experiments in South Africa have found exercise significantly improves sleep quality. In one study, nine young women entered a 12-week aerobic training program. The program involved cycling three times a week on a bicycle at a heart-rate intensity of 155-165 beats per minute, 15 minutes per session initially, increasing to 60 minutes for the last four weeks. Also, the women participated in sprints of 100, 200, 400, and 800 meters, and a four-kilometer road run once a week (increasing to 8K in weeks 11 and 12). The exercise, which was done between 4 p.m. and 7 p.m., shortened the time it took for the women to fall asleep. However, the study found that the women had decreased levels of deep sleep as the result of exercising before bedtime. The women exercised at about 70% of their maximum energy output, or what is called a "submaximal" level.[4]

The timing of exercise seemed to be a factor in sleep quality improvement in a study in Finland, involving a random sample of 1,600 people, aged 36 to 50. Light to moderate exercise early in the evening was found to promote sleep and improve its quality. However, exercise late in the evening was found to be somewhat less beneficial. In the study, 65% of the respondents said they felt better in the morning when they had exercised the previous evening. When asked their feelings on sleep-promoting activities, 33% of the respondents said evening exercise promoted sleep and improved its quality.[5]

How to Start Exercising

The most important thing is to get moving. This may mean developing a workout schedule or simply returning to regular participation in your favorite physical activity or sport. Before beginning any exercise program, consult your physician and have a thorough exam to rule out any health conditions that may need attention. If you have heart disease, diabetes, or are at high risk for these or other serious illnesses, begin an exercise program only with your physician's approval. Inactive men over the age of 40 and women over 50 should also con-

Exercises for specific parts of the body

These exercises target the head, neck, shoulders, and back. For many people, stress and tension tend to build up in these areas, causing muscle contractions and pain. Do these exercises two to three times per day to stretch contracted muscles. When doing these stretches, concentrate on breathing to provide a deeper, more relaxed stretch.[6]

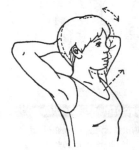

Base of head and neck

A. With chest up, tuck chin down and in, as if rocking head on neck. Do not bend neck or bob head. Do not hold breath while nodding.

B. Turn head to left and repeat A, then turn head to right and repeat A.

Neck, shoulders, and upper back

This is the starting/ending position. Can be done sitting or standing.

While exhaling, turn head slightly and pull head/neck down in a diagonal direction. Release pressure from hand on head.

When head reaches the end point in B, maintain pressure and rotate head away from arm about 40°. Repeat this rotation motion several times before returning to position A, then repeat. Do to both sides.

Exercises for specific parts of the body

Upper Back Stretch

With chin in, arms straight, raise upper back toward ceiling, inhale. Relax, exhale, and lower spine letting shoulder blades come close to each other.

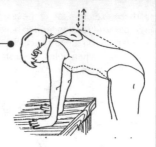

Upper Chest, Shoulders

With hands at prescribed level, lean in toward corner keeping chest up and exhaling.

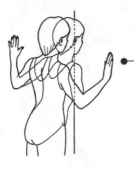

Shoulder & Middle Back

Interlock fingers and raise arms as high as possible while exhaling. Keep chest up, chin in.

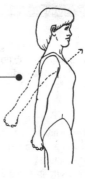

Shoulder Rotation

Holding rubber tubing move hands apart while exhaling and pinching shoulder blades together slightly. Keep elbows bent to 90° and at sides, chest up.

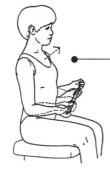

sult their physician. If you have been physically inactive for some time, consult with your physician to determine if you may need to undergo a detoxification program before you begin exercising.

According to the President's Council on Physical Fitness and Sports, a balanced physical fitness program incorporates the following elements:[7]

■ Warming Up—Begin gradually. Start with some basic warm up exercises, which can include gentle stretching or a short, slow walk for five to ten minutes.

■ Cardiorespiratory Fitness—Endurance athletes, such as long-distance runners or swimmers, have the stamina for their physically demanding sports because they have good cardiorespiratory fitness. The heart and lungs are able to deliver oxygen and nutrients to the tissues and remove wastes over sustained periods of activity. After you have warmed up your muscles and you are breathing more deeply, begin your activity and gradually pick up the pace. This may mean moving from a slow walk to a brisker pace or increasing the speed on a treadmill. If it has been a long time since you have exercised regularly, begin slowly. Your first session may consist of five minutes of warming up and another five to ten minutes of walking. Always be sure to cool down afterward. Avoid stopping your exercise abruptly without giving your body a chance to slow down and cool off. To see improvement, it is recommended that you exercise for 20 minutes at least three times a week.

■ Muscular Strength—A muscle's capacity to exert force for a brief period of time can be developed by participating in sports or by specific weight-training exercises. By regularly working individual muscle groups, they increase in strength. Begin a weight resistance program. Join your local gym and learn how to use the free weights or perform activities that require regular lifting, such as chopping wood and gardening. Be certain you are observing proper lifting stances to protect your back and joints from injury. Strive for at least two sessions of 20 minutes of free weights a week.

■ Muscular Endurance—The muscle's ability to undergo repeated contractions or to continue applying force against a fixed object; performing 100 pushups requires this kind of endurance. Groups of muscles are recruited to perform a certain activity over a sustained period of time. Try to incorporate at least three 30-minute sessions of exercises such as pushups, sit-ups, and similar calisthenics for overall training of all the major muscle groups. Public parks often have an "obstacle course" that includes many of these exercises at designated stations. Again, other activities involving vigorous work around the house, such as washing the car, can provide similar benefits.

For more **fitness tips**, contact: The President's Council on Physical Fitness and Sports, 200 Independence Avenue SW, Room 738-H, Washington, DC 20201; tel: 202-690-9000; fax: 202-690-5211; website: www.surgeongeneral.gov/ophs/pcpfs.htm.

■ Flexibility—Flexibility is the ability to move your muscles freely through a full range of movement. Dancers rely on their excellent flexibility, but everyone can benefit from increased flexibility as it can prevent injury. Try to incorporate about 10-15 minutes of gentle, non-bouncing stretching exercises into your workouts. This can be done before you set off on a walk or bike and also at the end of the session. If you are familiar with yoga or tai chi, both are excellent for increasing flexibility.

Calories Burned by Moderate Activities

In the table below, the calories burned are indicated for a 150- to 160-pound person; a lighter person would burn fewer calories and a heavier person more.[8]

Activity	Calories Burned
Cooking and preparing food for 30 minutes	25
Walking the dog for 30 minutes	125
Raking leaves for 30 minutes	150
Washing and waxing the car for 60 minutes	300
Going up a flight of stairs three times a day	15
Walking 10 minutes to public transit, riding 30 minutes, walking 5 minutes to work	60
Walking at the mall for 60 minutes	240

Moderate Activity Can Help You Sleep—For many people it is more realistic to include activities of moderate exertion, such as walking the dog or taking stairs instead of the elevator, to get their daily exercise. Including more physical activity throughout your day can help you maintain a basic level of fitness. Park your car a block away from your destination and walk. If you can perform certain errands, such as going to the post office or the grocery store, by walking or biking, do so. Walking more frequently and using less timesaving devices can burn additional calories and help keep you active.

For many years, the prescription for health maintenance included three to five 30-minute sessions of exercise per week. Current recommendations from the American College of Sports Medicine and the U.S. Centers for Disease Control and Prevention state that nearly everyone should strive for 30 minutes daily or alternately divide that amount into three eight- to 10-minute bouts per day.[9] Research has shown that people exercising in more frequent, shorter intervals reap the same health benefits as those participating in longer sessions of exertion. Even if you are seriously short of time, set a minimum goal of three daily walking sessions of ten minutes each.

Qigong: Good for Overall Health as Well as Insomnia

Qigong (also referred to as chi-kung) is like acupuncture without doctors, says Roger Jahnke, O.M.D., of Santa Barbara, California, because you can manipulate and enhance your own energy. *Qigong* has three aspects: the regulation of posture and movement, the regulation of the breath, and the regulation of the mind through meditation and relaxation. *Qigong* means working with a person's *qi* or subtle life energy. "The presence of healthy *qi* is obvious," says Dr. Jahnke. "It is what produces radiance and vitality. Its absence is also obvious: fatigue, pain, and disease."

Qigong practice can range from simple calisthenic-type movements with breath coordination, to complex exercises where brain-wave frequency, heart rate, and other organ functions are altered intentionally by the practitioner. When practiced regularly, *qigong's* combination of movement, deep relaxation, and breathing can improve strength and flexibility, reverse damage caused by prior injuries and disease, and promote relaxation, awareness, and healing. Traditional Chinese medicine holds that *qigong* stimulates and nourishes the body's internal organs by circulating *qi*. *Qigong* can break down energy blocks and facilitate the free flow of energy throughout the body, promoting blood and lymph flow and the even flow of nerve impulses necessary for proper health maintenance. "The overall benefit of *qigong* is to mobilize and harmonize the body's naturally occuring healing resource (*qi*)," according to Dr. Jahnke.

Like acupuncture, *qigong* activates the electrical currents that flow along the meridian pathways of the body. This affects the entire body and it is responsible for maintaining the function of the organs and tissues. For example, one *qigong* exercise involves breathing regulation and deep relaxation while lifting the arms and rising upward on the toes. According to Dr. Jahnke, this exercise

See "Qigong,"
pp. 426-430.

For more about
qigong, contact:
American Foundation
of Traditional Chinese
Medicine, 505 Beach
Street, San Francisco,
CA 94133;
tel: 415-776-0502.

can help prevent tension headaches, constipation, insomnia, and other disorders by improving circulation of the cardiovascular and lymphatic systems, as well as modulating brain chemistry.

Dr. Jahnke recommends a daily practice of *qigong* for 30 minutes to an hour. Regular practice, in addition to helping irradicate insomnia, can reduce stress, improve circulation and provide increased resistance to disease. Dr. Jahnke says that *qigong* produces the following health-promoting effects:

■ Initiates the "relaxation response," which decreases the sympathetic function of the autonomic nervous system. This decreases heart rate and blood pressure, dilates the blood capillaries, and optimizes the delivery of oxygen to the tissues.

■ Alters the neurochemistry profile (neurotransmitters bond with receptor sites on cells to excite or inhibit their function), moderating pain, depression, and addictive cravings, as well as optimizing immune capability.

■ Improves resistance to disease and infection by accelerating the elimination of toxic metabolic by-products from the tissues, organs, and glands through the lymphatic system.

■ Coordinates right/left brain hemisphere communication, promoting deeper sleep, reduced anxiety, and mental clarity.

■ Induces alpha and theta brain waves, which reduce heart rate and blood pressure, facilitating relaxation.

■ Moderates the function of the hypothalamus, pituitary, and pineal glands, as well as the cerebrospinal fluid system of the brain and spinal cord, which mediates pain and mood, facilitates immune function, and regulates sleep.

Yoga

Yoga is one of the most ancient systems of self-healing practiced today. Yoga teaches a basic principle of mind/body unity: if the mind is chronically restless and agitated, the health of the body will be compromised. Similarly, if the body is in poor health, mental clarity will be adversely affected. The practice of yoga can help integrate mind, body, and spirit.

Classical *Ashtanga* (meaning eight limbs) yoga is divided into eight branches or "limbs" that give guidance as to the proper diet, hygiene, detoxification regimes, and physical practices to help the individual integrate their personal, psychological, and spiritual awareness. The most well-known type of yoga is Hatha yoga, which teaches certain *asanas* (postures) and breathing techniques to create profound changes in the body and mind. One important aspect of yoga is to harness and increase the flow of *prana*, or life energy (similar to the Chinese *qi*). The blockage of *prana*, through improper diet, lifestyle stressors, or imbalance in one's physical, emotional, or spiritual health, can lead to illness. Breathing techniques and duration of holding certain postures remove blockages to the flow of *prana*.

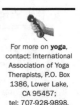

For more on **yoga**, contact: International Association of Yoga Therapists, P.O. Box 1386, Lower Lake, CA 95457; tel: 707-928-9898.

The main reason yoga can help people with sleep disorders, in addition to its ability to relax tight muscles, is that regular yoga practice restores the connection between mind and body, says yoga teacher Beryl Bender Birch. As this happens, your brain waves begin to slow down, fostering more relaxation. "Yoga is about learning to pay attention," she says. "Yoga means to unite, and it's about joining the mind and body." When people are connected, they are relaxed and their stress is reduced, she says. Regular yoga practice can have a therapeutic, balancing, and purifying effect on the body's metabolism and hormone system. This can help sleep disorders that are caused by hormone imbalances, poor digestion, or malnutrition, says Bender Birch.

The safest and most reliable way to use yoga therapeutically is to follow a balanced program of postures to achieve an overall normalizing and health-inducing effect. It is best for the beginner to start with a simple program of basic postures. A structured course can teach the fundamental breathing techniques and postures for exercises later practiced on one's own.

Success Story: Yoga Transforms Sleep by Transforming Life—Brad, a 51-year-old successful, high-profile attorney, was unable to turn off his mind when he went home at night. The details of his cases, the intensity, drama, and stress of mediating battles in other people's lives

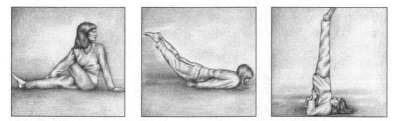

Yoga postures or *asanas*: half spinal twist, locust, and shoulder stand.

Breathing Awareness with Yoga

Well-known yoga teacher Beryl Bender Birch, author of *Power Yoga*, says one of the gifts of yoga is that it trains you to pay attention to your breath. "As long as you can stay focused on your breath, you're in the present moment," says Bender Birch. "You can't be with your breath and also be worried about a fight you had this morning, and you can learn to use yoga breathing techniques to loosen that stranglehold, that stress." For people with stress and anxiety, she recommends a yoga breathing technique called *ujjayi* breathing. *Ujjayi* breathing is deepchest breathing that lengthens the breath through glottal control, a slight conscious constriction of the throat that creates a unique hissing sound.

Here are step-by-step instructions for *ujjayi* breathing:[10]

1. Begin by whispering an "ahh" or " urr" sound with the mouth open on an exhalation. Completely empty the lungs as you make the sound.

2. Inhale by making the same "ahh" or "urr" sound. Completely fill the lungs.

3. Repeat this process with the mouth closed. You will notice a soft aspirant sound on the inhale, and a throaty sibilant sound on the exhale—much like a closed-mouth whisper. Continue to breathe with the mouth closed and inhaling and exhaling through the nose only. You should feel your diaphragm rising and falling and notice an increasing sensation of relaxation as you continue to breathe this way.

churned over and over in his mind, and he could not relax. Despite a heavy exercise routine that included marathon running and weight-training, it was a rare night that Brad could fall asleep easily or sleep through the night. He also suffered from hypertension and poor circulation.

Brad's osteopath was treating him for numerous running injuries, such as inflammation and tightness in the leg muscles and knee joint problems. The osteopath suggested to Brad that he start doing yoga as a preventative measure to keep his muscles and joints flexible and so avoid more injuries. Brad signed up for classes at Holiday's Health and Fitness Yoga Center in Portland, Oregon.

"There's the energetics, the hook of the negativity of that profession [lawyer]," says Holiday Johnson, the center director and one of the yoga teachers. "I think that is a reason why he couldn't sleep. His profession is not harmonious, it's so full of discord." Whatever the reason for the insomnia, it's the imbalance in his life that's the main problem, she adds. "That's why yoga works so well, because it brings people back to noticing how much their lives are out of balance. Sleep isn't the problem—the lack of sleep is trying to tell them to pay attention."

At first, Brad was not able to let go during yoga class, nor during the relaxation session at the end of class. He would be unable to lie down, and instead would pace around the room. After several weeks, though, Brad began to unwind. Friends who knew him as an attorney told Johnson they couldn't believe he was the same person when they saw him in yoga class.

See "Yoga," pp. 475-480.

Brad began attending three to five classes a week. Over the course of a year, he gradually began making changes in his lifestyle and relationships, adding more balance and finding a new partner who supported him in learning to relax. He noticed that he slept better when he was out of town and away from the telephones, so Brad began sched-

Beryl Bender Birch: Hard & Soft Astanga Yoga Institute, 325 East 41st Street #203, New York, NY 10017; tel: 212-661-2895.

uling more vacations and treating himself better. He continues to attend yoga classes and is sleeping through the night on a regular basis.

Chiropractic

Osseous manipulation is the repositioning of bones, including the joints of the spinal column, cranium, and other moveable joints. Chiropractors as well as naturopathic or qualified osteopathic physicians are trained and licensed to practice this type of therapy. Chiropractic is concerned with the relationship of the spinal column and the musculoskeletal structures of the body to the nervous system. The nervous system holds the key to the body's incredible potential to heal itself because it controls the functions of all other systems of the body. The spinal column acts as a "switchboard" for the nervous system. When there is interference, caused by slight misalignments of the spine (subluxations), the transmissions of the nervous system can be altered, like an electrical wire that has been impinged. This can not only cause localized pain in the spine, but can interfere with neurological information being transmitted to the major organs and cause dysfunction or disease. By adjusting the spinal joints to remove subluxations, normal nerve function can be restored.

Types of Chiropractic Treatment

The primary feature of chiropractic treatment is the chiropractic adjustment. During an examination, if localized areas of dysfunction are apparent, treatment is begun specifically to increase spinal motion. The chiropractic physician may use a combination of touch (palpation), active motion (having the patient bend or stretch in different ways), and passive movement (in which the doctor assists the patient) to initiate a specific adjustment.

One type of adjustment is a maneuver in which the joint is gently and precisely stretched to just beyond its normal range of motion. An audible, painless click is often heard, which is caused by the release of gases from the joint fluid. The patient will usually notice an increased range of movement and any soreness should rapidly disappear.

Some chiropractors prefer to use "non-force" techniques, applying gentle touch along the spine, skull, and pelvis. No forceful adjustment is used and no "popping" sounds are heard when the vertebral subluxations are corrected. Another option is the use of a hand-held instrument called an Activator™, a small instrument with a rubber tip used to gently and painlessly move the vertebrae.

Applied kinesiology deals not only with the placement of bones, but with the muscles that hold them in position. Chiropractors employing applied kinesiology use special techniques to help balance opposing muscles attached to a misaligned bone. Their approach restores normal muscle function in order to allow the adjustments to be more effective.

Network chiropractic was developed by Donald M. Epstein, D.C., of Boulder, Colorado, who observed from clinical experience that not all subluxations of the spine are the same. Network chiropractic combines a variety of chiropractic techniques to enable the practitioner to adjust subluxations with the precise amount and type of force suggested by clinical findings. "This is different from attempting to match the vertebra being adjusted to a specific technique," Dr. Epstein explains. "The difference lies in the sequence of the adjustments and the 'networking' of the various methods."

Just as there are several types of adjustments, there are also several types of chiropractic physicians. Though they are usually split into two groups, those who combine chiropractic with other modalities (mixers) and those who deal only with locating and removing subluxations (straight chiropractors), there are many variations within the two groups.

Success Story:
Chiropractic Brings Relief From Insomnia

Jerry, a 35-year-old writer, had been self-treating his insomnia with all types of natural products—herbs, vitamins, minerals, and homeopathic remedies—for years, with no success. Jerry had difficulty falling and staying asleep; in fact, there were long periods of time when he got no sleep at all. The episodes of insomnia had recurred regularly for the previous 15 years. "Sometimes days went by when he had little to no sleep," says chiropractor David Waldman, author of *What You Don't Know Can Heal You*, who practices in Portland and Mt. Angel, Oregon. "At times he would fall asleep and then wake up and not be able to get back to sleep. Other times, he just couldn't fall asleep." Jerry came to Dr. Waldman for help with his chronic upper and middle back pain.

For information about **chiropractic**, contact: American Chiropractic Association, 1701 Clarendon Blvd., Arlington, VA 22209; tel: 703-276-8800. International Chiropractic Association, 1110 N. Glebe Road, Suite 1000, Arlington, VA 22201; tel: 800-423-4690. Association for Network Chiropractic, 444 N. Main Street, Longmont, CO 80501; tel: 303-678-8101.

During the exam, Jerry told Dr. Waldman about his unsuccessful experiments with natural products to cure his sleep problems. He said he was taking what Dr. Waldman says were toxic levels of the sedative herbs valerian and St. John's wort, various B-vitamins, L-tryptophan, and other substances. Because the natural treatments had not helped him, Jerry had resigned himself to living with the insomnia. Also, Jerry had problems with his digestion, including frequent indigestion after meals, gas and bloating, and a queasy stomach.

Dr. Waldman evaluated Jerry's spinal function through an exam and other tests and found that Jerry had inflammation and joint dysfunction in the middle and upper (thoracic) spine. Dr. Waldman then began a series of spinal manipulations, or adjustments, in that area. Dr. Waldman also used therapeutic touch in the middle part of the spine, using his hands to unblock energy in Jerry's back.

Jerry saw Dr. Waldman six times over the next three weeks. At the end of the three weeks, Jerry's pain was reduced and all of his sleep and digestive problems were gone. Jerry discontinued the array of herbal remedies that he was taking for sleep. Since that time, Jerry has had some isolated episodes of insomnia, two or three times a year. As soon as those arise, however, he comes back for treatment and his sleep is restored.

"There were two factors involved in Jerry's inability to sleep," Dr. Waldman says. "One was that he couldn't get into a comfortable position so he was feeling physical discomfort, which created an inability to relax and fall asleep; that's the obvious piece. The other piece is that whenever there is any kind of neurological compression, studies have shown that it affects the functioning of the entire nervous system, which can manifest in innumerable ways." One of them can be neurological irritation and irritability; there is a natural relaxation response when this stimulus is removed.

Craniosacral Therapy

Craniosacral therapy refers to correcting imbalances in the relationship among breathing, the sacrum (the base of the backbone, attached to the pelvis), and the bones of the skull (cranium), especially the occiput. The sacrum acts as a pump to propel cerebrospinal fluid up the spine to the brain; the cranial bones contract and pump it back down. Health depends on a smoothly functioning sacro-occipital pump. Restrictions that result from injury, inflexibility of the joints of the spine and cranium, or from dysfunctions in other parts of the body, can all cause abnormal motion in the craniosacral system. The abnormal motion leads to stresses in the cranial mechanism, which can contribute to dysfunction and poor health, especially in the brain and spinal cord.

For information on **craniosacral therapy,** contact: The Upledger Institute, 11211 Prosperity Farms Road, Suite D-325, Palm Beach Gardens, Florida 33410-3487; tel: 800-233-5880 or 561-622-4334; fax: 561-622-4771; website: www.upledger.com.

The purpose of craniosacral therapy is to enhance the functioning of this important system. Craniosacral therapy, as delivered by a chiropractor or other trained practitioner, is a light-touch adjustment that restores the sacrum to full motion and balance with respect to the cranial bones. The proper functioning of the craniosacral system implies health for the central nervous system. The proper alignment of the craniosacral system allows the nervous system to rest at a more stress-free level.

Individuals who experience craniosacral treatment describe profound states of relaxation, of feeling lighter and more integrated. "When there is synchronous movement in the craniosacral system, the physiology of the central nervous system functions more efficiently and the nerve tissue is, in general, healthier," says Robert Norett, D.C., of the Stillpoint Health Center in Venice, California.

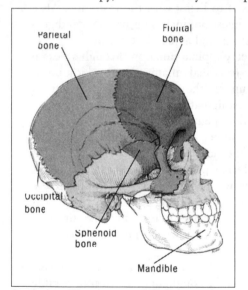

Parietal bone

Frontal bone

Occipital bone

Sphenoid bone

Mandible

Craniosacral therapy corrects imbalances in the relationship among breathing, the sacrum (the base of the backbone), and the bones of the skull (cranium), especially the occiput.

Neuro-Emotional Technique (NET)

NET is a process developed by from Scott Walker, D.C., a chiropractor in Encinitas, California, using principles from chiropractic and acupuncture. In NET theory, physical problems are almost always caused by a Neuro-Emotional Complex (NEC), a combination of: a spinal vertebra out of alignment; an acupuncture meridian out of balance; a specific emotion being activated; a memory picture of an event in the past; and various other muscle and body system conditioned responses. The NET practitioners, who are mostly chiropractors, use applied kinesiology (SEE QUICK DEFINITION), case history, and examination to identify the NEC, and then perform a spinal adjustment plus reflex point manipulation, thereby releasing the NEC and the emotional pattern that goes with it. Once the NEC is released, the physical problem usually clears up.

Dr. Walker says he has an estimated 90% success rate treating people with insomnia. Sleep disorders seem to respond well to NET, perhaps because there is frequently an emotional component—such as anxiety, fear, worry, sadness, or depression—to the sleep disorder pattern. In diagnosing some types of insomnia, Dr. Walker uses the Chinese clock, which states that the life force (*qi*) energies run through the 12 major acupuncture meridians on a daily cycle. By asking people what time they usually wake up at night, he can determine what meridian is affected. Often it is during liver time (1-3 a.m.) or gallbladder time (11 p.m. to 1 a.m.).

The Chinese clock can be a useful starting place for checking reflex points, Dr. Walker says. For example, if a person says he always

Treatment Options for Restless Legs and Periodic Limb Movements

- Exercise regularly, such as walking or cycling.
- Soak in a hot bath; then do ten deep knee bends.
- Stretch the legs, particularly the calves.
- Regularly massage your legs or use a heating pad on your legs.
- Eliminate coffee, tea, and chocolate from your diet.
- Supplement with vitamins C and E, folic acid, and the minerals iron, calcium, and magnesium.
- Participate in a local support group; more than 150 are established throughout the country.

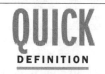

QUICK DEFINITION

Applied kinesiology, first developed by George Goodheart, D.C., of Detroit, Michigan, is the study of the relationship between muscle dysfunction (weak muscles) and related organ or gland dysfunction. Applied kinesiology employs a simple strength resistance test on a specific indicator muscle that is related to the organ or part of the body that is being tested. If the muscle tests strong (maintaining its resistance), it indicates health. If it tests weak, it can mean infection or dysfunction.

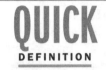

For **a referral to an NET-trained practitioner**, contact: One Foundation, 1991 Village Park Way #201A, Encinitas, CA 92024; tel: 800-638-1411; website: www.onefoundation.org.

QUICK DEFINITION

Neuropeptides are chains of amino acids formed in the DNA of neurons and released into the extracellular fluid. To date, approximately 609 neuropeptides have been discovered. These substances are part of a large group of messenger molecules called informational substances, and are the carriers and mediators of emotions. Neuropeptides are also manufactured by other tissues in the body and can be transported to the brain. When manufactured and released from the endocrine system cells, they are called hormones, and when released from the immune system, they are called immunotransmitters.

wakes up at midnight, the practitioner knows to check the gallbladder reflex points. If muscle testing finds a weakness in the gallbladder reflex points, the practitioner knows the gallbladder meridian is disrupted. Next, the practitioner will hold a reflex point for emotional issues on the person's forehead to see if the imbalance has an emotional component. If the muscle again tests weak, then the practitioner knows emotions are involved and that NET can be useful.

The person is encouraged to relax and let any memories surface as he answers questions from the practitioner, a process Dr. Walker calls "semantic testing." The semantic testing involves stirring up concepts in the patient's memory in an effort to stimulate memories. When a clear picture of a painful memory emerges, the patient describes it to the practitioner. Then, the patient holds the memory picture in his mind, touches the relevant reflex points, and the practitioner gives the patient a spinal adjustment, simultaneously releasing both the body memory and the emotional picture. Sometimes only one memory release cures the insomnia, but there can be layers of memories to be released. Dr. Walker estimates the typical insomnia patient gets significant relief in three to seven visits.[11]

Dr. Walker explains that NET is based on a "triad of health"—like an equilateral triangle—with one side being structure or spinal alignment, the second side being biochemistry, and the third side being emotions. A person's health is dependent on each side of the triangle being in harmony. The biochemistry side refers mainly to information substances that circulate in the body fluids such as hormones and neuropeptides (SEE QUICK DEFINITION).

What this means, Dr. Walker says, is that emotions aren't necessarily generated in the mind and that they can be accessed in various parts of the body via the neuropeptides. When a specific emotional trauma takes place, the body chemistry itself takes a "picture" of that trauma and memorizes the physiological responses—in other words, the body preserves the biochemical response to the emotional trauma through the neuropeptides. Over time, that traumatized body response pattern will weaken the acupuncture meridians and other body structures associated with the event, ultimately causing symptoms or a disease until the traumatic response pattern is released. "NET is really about the physiological aspects of emotions," Dr. Walker says.

Bodywork

The term *bodywork* refers to therapies such as massage, reflexology, and acupressure, which are employed to improve the structure and functioning of the human body. Bodywork in all its forms helps to reduce pain, soothe injured muscles, stimulate blood and lymphatic circulation, and promote deep relaxation—all helpful for sleep disorders.

Massage

Massage is used for general well-being, stress reduction, resolution of embedded emotions or psychological problems, recovery from sports injuries or muscle soreness, or as an adjunct therapy for medical conditions. Within the past decade, an overwhelming accumulation of scientific evidence has supported the claim that massage therapy is beneficial.[12] According to John Yates, Ph.D., author of *A Physician's Guide to Therapeutic Massage*, massage can benefit such conditions as muscle spasm and pain, spinal curvatures, soreness related to injury and stress, headaches, whiplash, temporomandibular joint

For information on **massage**, contact: American Massage Therapy Association, 820 Davis Street, Suite 100, Evanston, IL 60201; tel: 312-761-2682.

(TMJ) syndrome, and tension-related respiratory disorders such as bronchial asthma or emphysema. Massage can also help reduce swelling, help correct posture, improve body motion, and facilitate the elim-

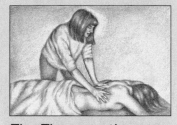

The Therapeutic Effects of Massage

Gertrude Beard, R.N., R.P.T., former associate professor of Physical Therapy at Northwestern University Medical School, summarizes the findings of numerous research studies on the therapeutic effects of massage. Studies indicate that massage helps to:

■ Sedate the nervous system and promote voluntary muscle relaxation

■ Relieve certain types of pain

■ Provide effective treatment of chronic inflammatory conditions by increasing lymphatic circulation

■ Improve circulation through the capillaries, veins, and arteries, and increase blood flow through the muscles

■ Trigger reflex actions in the body to stimulate organs

■ Promote recovery from fatigue

Beard adds that these uses of massage should be applied only under the direction of a knowledgeable practitioner or physical therapist.

Reflexology Massage to Promote Sleep

For a better night's rest, you can learn a simple self-massage to do before bed. For best effect, take a relaxing soak in a hot tub with a few drops of calming essential oils before you do the self-massage. You can also rub diluted essential oils directly on your skin as a further relaxer. Here's a simple reflexology foot massage technique:[16]

1. Sit comfortably with your left leg crossed over the right so you can easily reach your left foot.

2. Use the knuckles of your right hand to massage the sole of the foot. Press firmly, moving slowly in small circles. Pay particular attention to areas of tenderness.

3. After massaging the sole, massage the top of the foot to the ankle, using only the tips of your fingers, not the fleshy pads; press gently but firmly. Massage firmly with your thumb between the long tendons that run from your ankle to each toe.

4. Massage the bottom of the heel with your thumb and forefinger.

5. Grasp your foot with both hands, and press hard top and bottom, sliding out to the edge of the foot.

6. Grasp your big toe with your thumb and forefinger, pull gently, then shake the toe; repeat with the other toes.

7. Repeat the entire procedure on your right foot.

ination of toxins from the body.[13] Lymphatic massage, for example, can move metabolic waste through the body to promote a rapid recovery from illness or disease. Other studies show that massage can be used as an adjunct in the treatment of cardiovascular disorders and neurological and gynecological problems, and can often be used in place of pharmacological drugs.[14]

Tim Silva, a licensed massage therapist in Portland, Oregon, says massage is a natural way to treat sleep disorders because it already has the goal of relaxing and releasing muscle tension. The benefits of massage are also improvements that would ease sleep disorders, including the following: improved blood circulation, increased lymphatic fluid circulation, release of toxins, release of tension, mind/body integration, and reduction of stress.[15]

Reflexology

Reflexology is based on the idea that there are reflex areas in the hands and feet that correspond to every part of the body, including the organs and glands. Eunice Ingham, a physiotherapist, pioneered the discipline in this country in the late 1930s. He mapped out reflexes on the feet and developed techniques for inducing healing effects in those areas. Practitioners often focus on breaking up lactic acid and calcium crystals accumulated around any of the 7,200 nerve endings in each foot. By applying gentle but precise pressure to these reflex points, reflexologists can release blockages that

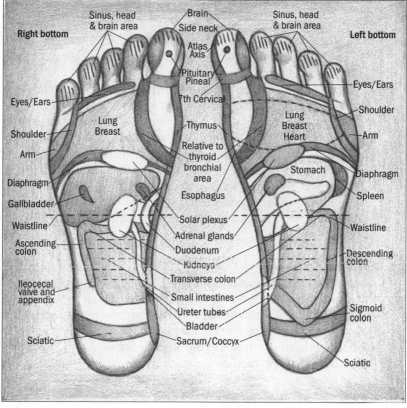

Right bottom

Sinus, head & brain area

Brain

Side neck

Atlas Axis

Sinus, head & brain area

Left bottom

Pituitary Pineal

7th Cervical

Eyes/Ears

Eyes/Ears

Shoulder

Shoulder

Lung Breast

Thymus

Lung Breast Heart

Arm

Arm

Relative to thyroid bronchial area

Diaphragm

Stomach

Diaphragm

Esophagus

Spleen

Gallbladder

Solar plexus

Waistline

Adrenal glands

Waistline

Ascending colon

Duodenum

Descending colon

Kidneys

Transverse colon

Ileocecal valve and appendix

Small intestines

Ureter tubes

Sigmoid colon

Bladder

Sciatic

Sacrum/Coccyx

Sciatic

Foot reflexology chart.

inhibit energy flow and cause pain and disease. This pressure is believed to affect internal organs and glands by stimulating reflex points of the body. Typically, practitioners use their thumbs to press on the various zones, or areas of the feet, that correspond to organs or other structural components of the body. For sleep disorders, reflexology can help to detoxify organs such as the kidneys and liver, as well as stimulate sluggish glands like the thyroid and adrenals.

For information on **reflexology**, contact: International Institute of Reflexology, P.O. Box 12462, St. Petersburg, FL 33733; tel: 813-343-4811.

Barbara, 44, was diagnosed with multiple sclerosis. Around the same time, as part of that crippling disease, she developed constant foot pain that was so severe she had trouble walking and had to use a cane. The foot pain prevented her from sleeping, even though Barbara bought a metal "lift" to put under her bed covers to keep the sheets and blankets off her feet. She also tried chiropractic treatments, special shoes, heel lifts, and podiatrist visits, all to no avail. "They took X-rays of my feet to see if there was something wrong, but they couldn't find anything," says Barbara. Barbara also suffered from constipation and leg cramps as part of the multiple sclerosis. She went to see Jim Hughes, a licensed massage therapist and foot reflexologist in Vancouver, Washington.

During the first visit, a half-hour where Hughes kneaded, massaged, and pressed on the many knots of muscle tension on the bottom of her feet, Barbara felt a great deal of discomfort. But after three treatments, Barbara's foot pain was substantially reduced. She saw Hughes two or three times a week for the next six months and massaged her feet at home as well. By the end of that time, Barbara's foot pain was gone and she was able to sleep again. She also began having more regular bowel movements, and her leg cramps disappeared. The relief has lasted, with occasional tune-ups, for the past five years.

Oriental Bodywork

The oriental body therapies, such as acupuncture or acupressure, work to balance the flow of *qi* (vital life energy) throughout energy meridians. These meridians run throughout the body and are associated with different organs—if there is a block in the energy meridian, it will be expressed as health problems in the organs associated with the blocked meridian. Blocked *qi* can be released by applying pressure to specific points along the energy meridians. Acupuncture uses needles, while acupressure (such as shiatsu and *Jin Shin Do*) uses rubbing, kneading, or other types of pressure from the fingers and hands.

Shiatsu means "finger pressure" in Japanese and was originally developed from the ancient Chinese acupressure techniques. Shiatsu uses a sequence of firm rhythmic pressure applied to specific points for 3-10 seconds and, like acupuncture, is designed to awaken, calm, and harmonize the meridians. Shiatsu affects not only the acupressure point, but the entire mind and body, making it one of the most effective forms of bodywork for sleep disorders. *Jin Shin Do* is another Japanese bodywork technique based on the original *Jin Shin Jyutsu* founded by Jiro Murai. Master Murai based his system on moving *qi* through the meridians by using certain combinations of acupressure points in a special sequence. Pressure is held for a minute or more until the practitioner can feel the flow of blood and *qi* through the point. Opening and releasing sequences are important to move the *qi* in the proper direction.

See "Bodywork," pp. 97-118.

For more about **acupressure techniques and a practitioner referral**, contact: American Oriental Bodywork Association, 6801 Jericho Turnpike, Syosset, NY 11791; tel: 516-364-5533.

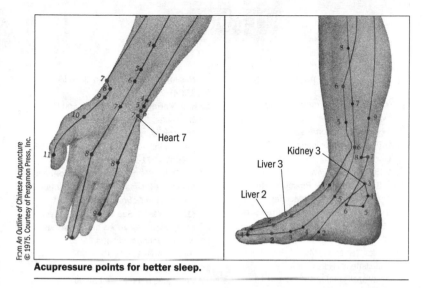

Acupressure points for better sleep.

Acupressure Self-Help for Insomnia—The simplest approach to self-massage is to work what the Chinese call the microsystems, says Dr. Jahnke. There are three microsystems in the body: the ears, the feet, and the hands. The whole body is represented by and can be affected at specific points in the microsystems. You start the massage by rubbing the whole microsystem (each ear, for example) vigorously for a few minutes. Then, you begin the massage again, this time going more slowly and looking for areas of particular soreness. When you find sore spots, spend a few minutes focusing on them, using firm and steady pressure. Dr. Jahnke says you can do a good whole-body workout using the three microsystems in about 15 minutes. He recommends that people with insomnia try to do at least one 15-minute session a day.

Here are some specific acupuncture points to massage if you can't sleep:

Liver 2 or 3: Find the fleshy space on the top of your foot between your big toe and second toe. Feel for the sorest spot and massage or press firmly for a minute or two.

Heart 7: Find the bony prominence on the inside of your wrist, opposite the thumb. Massage or press firmly just inside the prominence.

Kidney 3: Find the fleshy part on the inside of your ankle just behind the bony prominence and massage or press firmly.

Endnotes

Chapter I: The Basics of Sleep

1 "Brain Basics: Understanding Sleep." Available from: National Institute of Neurological Disorders and Stroke, Office of Communications and Public Liaison, P.O. Box 5801, Bethesda, MD 20824; website: www.NINDS.nih.gov.

2 R.J. Reiter. "Oxidative Processes and Antioxidative Defense Mechanism in the Aging Brain." *FASEB Journal* 9:7 (1995), 526-533.

3 Ibid.

4 Dun-Xian Tan et al. "Melatonin: A Potent Endogenous Hydroxyl Radical Scavenger." *Endocrine Journal* 1 (1993), 57-60.

5 R.J. Reiter. "The Indoleamine Melationin as a Free Radical Scavenger, Electron Donor, and Antioxidant: In Vitro and In Vivo Studies." *Advances in Experimental Medicine and Biology* 398 (1996), 307-313.

6 R.J. Reiter et al. "Melatonin in Relation to Cellular Antioxidative Defense Mechanisms." *Hormonal and Metabolic Research* 29 (1997), 363-372.

7 Ibid.

8 Russel J. Reiter. "Novel Intracellular Actions of Melatonin: Its Relation to Reactive Oxygen Species." *Frontiers of Hormone Research* 21 (1996), 160-166.

9 E. Reimund. "The Free Radical Flux Theory of Sleep." *Medical Hypotheses* 43 (1994), 231-233.

10 G.J. Maestroni. "T-Helper-2 Lymphocytes as Peripheral Target of Melatonin Signaling." *Journal of Pineal Research* 18 (1995), 84-89.

11 R.J. Reiter et al. "The Role of Melatonin in the Pathophysiology of Oxygen Radical Damage." In: M. Müller and P. Pévet, eds. *Advances in Pineal Research*, Vol. 8 (London: John Libbey, 1994), 278.

12 K.M. Morrey, J.A. McLachlan, and O. Bakouche. "Activation of Human Monocytes by the Pineal Hormone Melatonin." *Journal of Immunology* 153 (1994), 2671-2680.

13 L.A. Toth. "Sleep, Sleep Deprivation, and Infectious Disease: Studies in Animals." *Advances in Neuroimmunology* 5:1 (1995), 79-92. See also: J.M. Krueger et al. "Sleep, Microbes and Cytokines." *Neuroimmunomodulation* 1:2 (March/April 1994), 100-109.

14 A. Rechtschaffen et al. "Physiological Correlates of Prolonged Sleep Deprivation in Rats." *Science* 221:4606 (July 8, 1983), 182-184.

15 D. Mueller-Wieland, B. Behnke, and W. Krone. "Melatonin Inhibits LDL Receptor Activity and Cholesterol Synthesis in Freshly Isolated Human Mononuclear Leukocytes." *Biochemical and Biophysical Research Communications* 203:1 (1994), 416-421.

16 N. Birau, U. Peterssen, and J. Gottschalk. "Hypertensive Effect of Melatonin in Essentoal Hypertension." *IRCS Medical Science* 9 (1981), 906.

17 S.H. Kennedy, S. Tighe, and G.M. Brown. "Melatonin and Cortisol 'Switches' During Mania, Depression, and Euthymia in a Drug-Free Bipolar Patient." *Journal of Nervous and Mental Disease* 177:5 (1989), 300-303. P. Monteleone et al. "Depressed Nocturnal Plasma Melatonin Levels in Drug-Free Paranoid Schizophrenics." *Schizophrenia Research* 7 (1992), 77-84.

18 Arthur C. Guyton, M.D., and John E. Hall, Ph.D. *Textbook of Medical Physiology* 9th Edition (Philadelphia: W.B.

Saunders, 1996), 761.

19 Ibid.

20 S. Gabel. "Information Processing in Rapid Eye Movement Sleep: Possible Neurophysiological, Neuropsychological, and Clinical Correlates." *Journal of Nervous and Mental Disorders* 175 (April 1987), 193-200.

21 P. Maquet et al. "Functional Neuroanatomy of Human Rapid-Eye-Movement Sleep and Dreaming." *Nature* 383 (September 12, 1996), 163-166.

22 U.D. McCann et al. "Sleep Deprivation and Impaired Cognition: Possible Role of Brain Catecholamines." *Biological Psychiatry* 31:11 (June 1, 1992), 1082-1097. See also: C.P. Maurizi. "The Function of Dreams (REM Sleep): Roles for the Hippocampus, Melatonin, Monoamines, and Vasotocin." *Medical Hypotheses* 23:4 (August 1987), 433-440.

23 A. Karni et al. "Dependence on REM Sleep on Overnight Improvement of Perceptual Skill." *Science* 265 (July 29, 1994), 679-682.

24 J. De Koninck et al. "Language Learning Efficiency, Dreams, and REM Sleep." *Psychiatric Journal of the University of Ottawa* 15.2 (June 1990), 91-92.

25 M. Nesca and D. Koulack. "Recognition Memory, Sleep, and Circadian Rhythms." *Canadian Journal of Experimental Psychology* 48:3 (September 1994), 359-379.

26 S. Gabel. "Information Processing in Rapid Eye Movement Sleep: Possible Neurophysiological, Neuropsychological, and Clinical Correlates." *Journal of Nervous and Mental Disorders* 175 (April 1987), 193-200.

27 Roger Fritz, Ph.D. *Sleep Disorders: America's Hidden Nightmare* (Naperville, IL: National Sleep Alert, 1993), 30.

28 C.P. Maurizi. "The Function of Dreams (REM Sleep): Roles for the Hippocampus, Melatonin, Monoamines, and Vasotocin." *Medical Hypotheses* 23:4 (August 1987), 433-440.

29 William Dement, M.D., Ph.D., with Christopher Vaughan. *The Promise of Sleep* (New York: Delacorte Press, 1999), 271.

30 "Brain Basics: Understanding Sleep." Available from: National Institute of Neurological Disorders and Stroke, Office of Communications and Public Liaison, P.O. Box 5801, Bethesda, MD 20824; website: www.NINDS.nih.gov.

31 Ibid.

32 N. Ishida, M. Kaneko, and R. Allada. "Biological Clocks." *Proceedings of the National Academy of Sciences of the United States of America* 96:16 (August 3, 1996), 8819-8820.

33 Ibid.

34 Russel J. Reiter, Ph.D., and Jo Robinson. *Melatonin: Your Body's Natural Wonder Drug* (New York: Bantam Books, 1995), 17.

35 J.Z. Nowak and J.B. Zawilska. "Melatonin and Its Physiological and Therapeutic Properties." *Pharmacy World and Science* 20:1 (1998), 18-27.

36 Ray Sahelian, M.D. 5-HTP: *Nature's Serotonin Solution* (Garden City Park, NY: Avery Publishing, 1998), 29.

37 A.J. Lewy, T.A. Wehr, and F.K. Goodwin. "Light Suppresses Melatonin Secretion in Humans." *Science* (December 1980), 210.

38 Russel J. Reiter, Ph.D., and Jo Robinson. *Melatonin: Your Body's Natural Wonder Drug* (New York: Bantam Books, 1995), 161.

39 M.L. Rao, B. Muller-Oerlinghause, and H.P. Volz. "Blood Serotonin, Serum Melatonin and Light Therapy in Healthy Subjects and in Patients with Nonseasonal Depression." *Acta Psychiatrica Scandinavica* 86 (1992), 127-132.

Chapter 2: Sleep Disorders and Their Causes

1 National Sleep Foundation. "2000

Omnibus Sleep in America Poll." Available from: National Sleep Foundation, 1522 K Street NW, Suite 500, Washington, DC 20005; fax: 202-347-3472; website: www.sleepfoundation.org.

2 Ibid.

3 National Commission on Sleep Disorders Research. *Wake Up America: A National Sleep Alert*, Volume 1 (Bethesda, MD: National Institutes of Health, 1993).

4 William C. Dement, M.D., Ph.D. with Christopher Vaughan. *The Promise of Sleep* (New York: Delacorte Press, 1999), 308.

5 National Sleep Foundation. "2000 Omnibus Sleep in America Poll." Available from: National Sleep Foundation, 1522 K Street NW, Suite 500, Washington, DC 20005; fax: 202-347-3472; website: www.sleepfoundation.org.

6 National Institutes of Health and National Heart, Lung, and Blood Institute. "Insomnia." *NIH Publication* No. 95-380 (Washington, DC: U.S. Department of Health and Human Services, October 1995).

7 National Sleep Foundation. "2000 Omnibus Sleep in America Poll." Available from: National Sleep Foundation, 1522 K Street NW, Suite 500, Washington, DC 20005; fax: 202-347-3472; website: www.sleepfoundation.org.

8 Ibid.

9 Ibid.

10 National Institutes of Health and National Heart, Lung, and Blood Institute. "Sleep Apnea." *NIH Publication* No. 95-379. (Washington, DC: U.S. Department of Health and Human Services, September 1995).

11 Christensen Damaris. "Allergies May Be Linked to Obstructive Sleep Apnea." *Medical Tribune* (February 1997), 3.

12 Derek S. Lipman, M.D. *Snoring From A to Zzzz* (Portland, OR: Spencer Press, 1996), 71-72.

13 Victor Hoffstein. "Is Snoring Dangerous to Your Health?" *Sleep* 19:6 (1995), 506. See also: Paul L. Enright et al. "Prevalence and Correlates of Snoring and Observed Apneas in 5,201 Older Adults." *Sleep* 19:7 (1997), 529.

14 U. Koehler and H. Shäfer. "Is Obstructive Sleep Apnea (OSA) a Risk Factor for Myocardia Infacrtion and Cardiac Arrhythmias in Patients with Coronary Heart Disease?" *Sleep* 19:4 (1995), 283.

15 National Institutes of Health and National Heart, Lung, and Blood Institute. *Sleep Apnea NIH Publication* No. 95-379 (Washington, DC: U.S. Department of Health and Human Services, 1995).

16 American Sleep Apnea Association. "Sleep Apnea Fact Sheet." Available from: American Sleep Apnea Association, 1424 K Street NW, Suite 302, Washington, DC 20005; tel: 202-293-3650; fax: 202-293-3656; website: www.sleepapnea.org.

17 National Institutes of Health and National Heart, Lung, and Blood Institute. *Sleep Apnea NIH Publication* No. 95-379. (Washington, DC: U.S. Department of Health and Human Services, 1995).

18 Jacques Montplaisir et al. "Persistence of Repetitive EEG Arousals (K-Alpha Complexes) in Patients Treated with L-DOPA." *Sleep* 19:3 (1995), 200.

19 National Institutes of Health and National Heart, Lung, and Blood Institute. "Narcolepsy." *NIH Publication* No. 96-3649. (Washington, DC: U.S. Department of Health and Human Services, 1996).

20 Ibid.

21 Ibid.

22 Martin Moore-Ede, M.D., Ph.D., and Suzanne LeVert. *Complete Idiot's Guide to Getting a Good Night's Sleep* (New York: Alpha Books, 1998), 184.

23 James Perl, Ph.D. *Sleep Right in Five Nights* (New York: William Morrow, 1993).

24 James B. Maas, Ph.D. *Power Sleep* (New

York: HarperPerennial, 1999), 194.

25 Jane Brody. Personal Health." *The New York Times* (January 17, 1996), B8.

26 Roger Fritz, Ph.D. *Sleep Disorders: America's Hidden Nightmare* (Naperville, IL: National Sleep Alert, 1993), 106.

27 Martin Moore-Ede, M.D., Ph.D., and Suzanne LeVert. *Complete Idiot's Guide to Getting a Good Night's Sleep* (New York: Alpha Books, 1998), 175.

28 Michael S. Aldrich. *Sleep Medicine* (New York: Oxford University Press, 1999).

29 John F. Simonds and Humberto Parrago. "Prevalence of Sleep Disorders and Sleep Behaviors in Children and Adolescents." *Journal of the American Academy of Child Psychiatry* 21 (1982), 383-388.

30 Michael S. Aldrich. *Sleep Medicine* (New York: Oxford University Press, 1999).

31 Martin Moore-Ede, M.D., Ph.D., and Suzanne LeVert. *Complete Idiot's Guide to Getting a Good Night's Sleep* (New York: Alpha Books, 1998), 176.

32 Diagnostic Classification Steering Committee. Michael J. Thorpy, ed. *The International Classification of Sleep Disorders: Diagnostic and Coding Manual* (Rochester, MN: American Sleep Disorders Association, 1990).

33 Terry Chisholm and Rachel L. Morehouse. "Adult Headbanging: Sleep Studies and Treatment." *Sleep* 19:4 (1995), 343.

34 Ibid.

35 Martin Moore-Ede, M.D., Ph.D., and Suzanne LeVert. *Complete Idiot's Guide to Getting a Good Night's Sleep* (New York: Alpha Books, 1998), 176.

36 Diagnostic Classification Steering Committee. ed. Michael J. Thorpy. *The International Classification of Sleep Disorders: Diagnostic and Coding Manual* (Rochester, MN: American Sleep Disorders Association, 1990).

37 U.S. Dept. of Health and Human Services. *Sleep Disorders Publication*

No. ADM87-1541 (Washington, DC: U.S. Government Printing Office, 1987).

38 William C. Dement, M.D., Ph.D. and Christopher Vaughan. *The Promise of Sleep* (New York: Delacorte Press, 1999), 310.

39 Martin Moore-Ede, M.D., Ph.D., and Suzanne LeVert. *Complete Idiot's Guide to Getting a Good Night's Sleep* (New York: Alpha Books, 1998), 118.

40 Russel J. Reiter, Ph.D., and Jo Robinson. *Melatonin, Your Body's Natural Wonder Drug* (New York: Bantam, 1995), 124.

41 Ibid., 125.

42 H. Vafi, M.D., and Pamela Vafi. *How to Get a Great Night's Sleep* (Holbrook, MA: Bob Adams, 1994).

43 Dian Dincin Buchman, Ph.D. *The Complete Guide to Sleep* (New Canaan, CT: Keats Publishing, 1997), 43.

44 National Institutes of Health and National Heart, Lung, and Blood Institute. "Insomnia." *NIH Publication* No. 95-380. (Washington, DC: U.S. Department of Health and Human Services, 1995).

Chapter 3: Improve Your Diet

1 T. Chou. "Wake Up and Smell the Coffee: Caffeine, Coffee, and the Medical Consequences." *Western Journal of Medicine* 157:5 (1992), 544-553.

2 Elson M. Haas, M.D. *Staying Healthy With Nutrition* (Berkeley, CA: Celestial Arts, 1992), 941.

3 Kenneth Rifkin, N.D., R.Ac. Personal communication.

4 Elliot D. Abravanel, M.D., and Elizabeth King. *Dr. Abravanel's Anti-Craving Weight Loss Diet* (New York: Bantam, 1990), 53-57.

5 H.J. Rinkel et al. *Food Allergy* (Springfield, IL: Charles C. Thomas, 1950).

6 Stephen Langer, M.D., with James F. Scheer. *Solved: The Riddle of Weight Loss* (Rochester, VT: Healing Arts Press, 1989), 39.

7 Ralph Golan, M.D. *Optimal Wellness* (New

York: Ballantine, 1995), 193.

8 J.E. Pizzorno and M.T. Murray. *A Textbook of Natural Medicine* (Seattle, WA: John Bastyr University, 1989).

9 National Sleep Foundation. "1999 Omnibus Sleep in America Poll." Available from: National Sleep Foundation, 1522 K Street NW, Suite 500, Washington, DC 20005; fax: 202-347-3472; website: www.sleepfoundation.org.

10 B.M. Stone. "Sleep and Low Doses of Alcohol." *Electroencephalography and Clinical Neurophysiology* 48:6 (1980), 706-709.

11 H.P. Landolt et al. "Late-Afternoon Ethanol Intake Affects Nocturnal Sleep and the Sleep EEG in Middle-Aged Men." *Journal of Clinical Psychopharmacology* 16:6 (1996), 428-436.

12 Elson M. Haas, M.D. *Staying Healthy With Nutrition* (Berkeley, CA: Celestial Arts, 1992), 952.

13 Dian Dincin Buchman, Ph.D. *The Complete Guide to Sleep* (New Canaan, CT: Keats Publishing, 1997), 45.

14 National Sleep Foundation. "1999 Omnibus Sleep in America Poll." Available from: National Sleep Foundation, 1522 K Street NW, Suite 500, Washington, DC 20005; fax: 202-347-3472; website: www.sleepfoundation.org.

15 Stanley Coren. *Sleep Thieves* (New York: Free Press, 1996), 135.

16 R. Sandyk. "L-Tryptophan in the Treatment if Restless Legs Syndrome." *American Journal of Psychiatry* 143:3 (1986), 554-555.

17 G.S. Kelly. "Folates: Supplemental Forms and Therapeutic Applications." *Alternative Medicine Review* 3:3 (1998), 208-220.

18 S. Ayres and R. Mihan. "Restless Legs Syndrome : Response to Vitamin E." *Journal of Applied Nutrition* 25 (1973), 8-15.

19 H.S. Pall et al. "Restless Legs Syndrome." *Neurology* 37:8 (1987),

1436. S.T. O'Keefe, K. Gavin, and J.N. Lavan. "Iron Status and Restless Legs Syndrome in the Elderly." *Age and Aging* 23:3 (1994), 200-203.

20 Arthur Winter, M.D., F.I.C.S., and Ruth Winter, M.S. *Smart Food* (New York: St. Martin's Griffin, 1999), 77.

21 Stephen Langer, M.D., with James F. Scheer. *Solved: The Riddle of Weight Loss* (Rochester, VT: Healing Arts Press, 1989), 51.

22 Ralph Golan, M.D. *Optimal Wellness* (New York: Ballantine Books, 1995).

23 Stephen Langer, M.D., with James F. Scheer. *Solved: The Riddle of Weight Loss* (Rochester, VT: Healing Arts Press, 1989), 52.

24 Ralph Golan, M.D. *Optimal Wellness* (New York: Ballantine Books, 1995).

25 Peter Hauri, Ph.D., and Shirley Linde, Ph.D. "Three Things Every Insomniac Should Do." *No More Sleepless Nights* (New York: John Wiley & Sons, 1990), 52.

26 Ann Louise Gittleman, M.S., C.N.S. "Perimenopause—When Signs of 'The Change' Come Too Early." *Alternative Medicine* 26 (October/November 1998), 84-92.

27 Richard N. Podell, M.D., F.A.C.P., and William Proctor. *The G-Index Diet* (New York: Warner, 1993).

28 Ann Louise Gittleman, M.S. *Supernutrition for Women* (New York: Bantam, 1991), 68.

29 A. Kahn et al. "Insomnia and Cow's Milk Allergy in Infants." *Pediatrics* 76:6 (1985), 880-884.

30 James Braly, M.D. *Dr. Braly's Food Allergy and Nutrition Revolution* (New Canaan, CT: Keats Publishing, 1992), 60.

31 Roger Fritz, Ph.D. "What Would You Do For a Good Night's Sleep?" *Sleep Disorders: America's Hidden Nightmare* (Naperville, IL: National Sleep Alert, 1993), 122-123.

32 James F. Balch, M.D. and Phyllis A. Balch, C.N.C. *Prescription for Nutritional Healing* (Garden City Park, NY: Avery

Publishing Group, 1997), 351.

33 David S. Ludwig, M.D., Ph.D., et al. "Dietary Fiber, Weight Gain, and Cardiovascular Disease Risk Factors in Young Adults." *Journal of the American Medical Association* 282:16 (1999), 1539-1546.

34 R.L. Walford et al. "The Calorically Restricted Low-Fat Nutrient-Dense Diet in Biosphere 2 Significantly Lowers Blood Glucose, Total Leukocyte Count, Cholesterol, and Blood Pressure in Humans." *Proceedings of the National Academy of Sciences* 89:23 (1992), 11533-11537.

35 Linda Lizotte, R.D., C.D.N. "Healthy Eating Basics." Available from: Designs for Health, 211 Pondway Lane, Trumbull, CT 06611; tel: 203-371-4383; fax: 530-618-6730.

36 R.L. Walford and M. Crew. "How Dietary Restriction Retards Aging: An Integrative Hypothesis." *Growth, Development, and Aging* 53:4 (1989), 139-140.

37 J.R. DiPalma and W.S. Thayer. "Use of Niacin as a Drug." *Annual Review of Nutrition* 11 (1991), 169-187.

38 P.J. Bingley et al. "Nicotinamide and Insulin Secretion in Normal Subjects." *Diabetiologia* 36 (1993), 675-677.

39 M.R. Werbach, M.D. *Nutritional Influences on Illness* (Tarzana, CA: Third Line Press, 1993).

40 J. Martineau et al. "Vitamin B6, Magnesium, and Combined B6-Magnesium: Therapeutic Effects in Childhood Autism." *Biological Psychiatry* 20 (1985), 467-468.

41 M. Cohen and A. Bendich. "Safety of Pyridoxine: A Review of Human and Animal Studies." *Toxicology Letters* 34 (1986), 129-139.

42 L.M. Tierney, Jr., M.D., et al. *Current Medical Diagnosis & Treatment* (Norwalk, CT: Appleton & Lange, 1993).

43 S. Ayres and R. Mihan. "Leg Cramps and 'Restless Leg' Syndrome Responsive to Vitamin E (Tocopheral)." *California Medicine* 111:2 (1969), 87-91.

44 J. Penland. "Effects of Trace Element Nutrition on Sleep Patterns in Adult Women." *FASEB Journal* 2 (1988), A434.

45 J. Thom et al. "The Influence of Refined Carbohydrate on Urinary Calcium Excretion." *British Journal of Urology* 50 (1978), 459-464.

46 R.P. Heaney and C.M. Weaver. "Calcium Absorption From Kale." *American Journal of Clinical Nutrition* 51 (1990), 656-657.

47 B.P. Bourgoin et al. "Lead Content in 70 Brands of Dietary Calcium Supplements." *American Journal of Public Health* 83 (1993), 1155-1160.

48 J.A. Harvey et al. "Superior Calcium Absorption From Calcium Citrate Than Calcium Carbonate Using External Forearm Counting." *Journal of the American College of Nutrition* 9 (1990), 583-587.

49 C. Zhou et al. "Clinical Observation of Treatment of Hypertension with Calcium." *American Journal of Hypertension* 7 (1994), 363-367.

50 B.M. Altura. "Basic Biochemistry and Physiology of Magnesium: A Brief Review." *Magnesium and Trace Elements* 10 (1991), 167-171.

51 T. Bohmer et al. "Bioavailability of Oral Magnesium Supplementation in Female Students Evaluated From Elimination of Magnesium in 24-Hour Urine." *Magnesium and Trace Elements* 9 (1990), 272-278. L. Gullestad et al. "Oral Versus Intravenous Magnesium Supplementation in Patients With Magnesium Deficiency." *Magnesium and Trace Elements* 10 (1991), 11-16.

52 J.S. Lindberg et al. "Magnesium Bioavailability From Magnesium Citrate and Magnesium Oxide." *Journal of the American College of Nutrition* 9 (1990), 48-55.

53 Betty Kamen, Ph.D. *The Chromium Connection* (Novato, CA: Nutrition Encounter, 1992), 118.

54 W.W. Campbell and R.A. Anderson. "Effects of Aerobic Exercise and Training on the Trace Minerals Chromium, Copper, and Zinc." *Sports Medicine* 4 (1987), 9-18.

55 Jeffrey S. Bland, Ph.D. "Take Your Vitamins." *Delicious!* 8:7 (October 1992), 61.

56 E.B. Finley and F.L. Cerklewski. "Influence of Ascorbic Acid Supplementation on Copper Status in Young Adult Men." *American Journal of Clinical Nutrition* 47 (1988), 96-101.

57 Michael A. Schmidt, D.C., C.N.S., and Jeffrey Bland, Ph.D. "Thyroid Gland as Sentinel: Interface Between Internal and External Environment." *Alternative Therapies* 3:1 (January 1997), 78-81

58 S.T. O'Keefe, K. Gaavin, and J.N. Lavan. "Iron Status and Restless Legs Syndrome in the Elderly." *Age and Aging* 23 (1994), 200-203.

59 V. Gordeuk et al. "Iron Overload: Causes and Consequences." *Annual Review of Nutrition* 7 (1987), 485-508. P. Biemond et al. "Intra-Articular Ferritin-Bound Iron in Rheumatoid Arthritis." *Arthritis and Rheumatism* 29 (1986), 1187-1193. J.T. Salonen et al. "High Stored Iron Levels are Associated With Excess Risk of Myocardial Infarction in Eastern Finnish Men." *Circulation* 86 (1992), 803-811.

60 Eric R. Braverman, M.D. *P.A.T.H. Wellness Manual* (Princeton, NJ: Princeton Associates for Total Health, 1995), 124.

61 James Perl, Ph.D. *Sleep Right in Five Nights* (New York: William Morrow/Quill, 1993), 236.

62 T.C. Birdsall. "5-Hydroxytryptophan: A Clinically Effective Serotonin Precursor." *Alternative Medicine Review* 3:4 (1998), 271-280.

63 R. Ursin. "The Effects of 5-Hydroxytryptophan and L-Tryptophan on Wakefulness and Sleep Patterns in the Cat." *Brain Research* 106:1 (1976), 105-115.

Chapter 4: Detoxify Your Body

1 The Burton Goldberg Group. *Alternative Medicine: The Definitive Guide* (Tiburon, CA: Future Medicine Publishing, 1993), 3.

2 Ibid., 4.

3 Joseph Pizzorno, N.D. *Total Wellness* (Rocklin, CA: Prima Publishing, 1996), 105.

4 William Lee Cowden, M.D., "Is Your Shower Toxic? Some Pollution Solutions." *Alternative Medicine* 29 (April/May 1999), 69.

5 W. Melillo. "How Safe is Mercury in Dentistry?" *Washington Post Weekly Journal of Medicine, Science and Society* (September 1991), 4. World Health Organization. *Environmental Health Criteria for Inorganic Mercury* (Geneva, Switzerland: World Health Organization, 1991), 118.

6 William J. Rea, M.D. *Chemical Sensitivity*, Vol. 3 (Boca Raton, FL: C.R.C. Lewis, 1996), 1555-1579.

7 D.N. Taylor et al. "Effects of Trichloroethylene in the Exploratory and Locomotor Activity in Rats Exposed During Development." *Science Total Environment* 47 (1985), 415-420. H.N. Arito, T. Suruta, K. Nakagaki, and S. Tanaka. "Partial Insomnia, Hyperactivity and Hyperdipsia Induced by Repeated Administration of Toluene in Rats: Their Relation to Brain Monoamine Metabolism." *Toxicology* 37:1-2 (1985), 99-110.

8 S. Ziff. "Consolidated Symptom Analysis of 1,569 Patients." *Bio-Probe Newsletter* 9:2 (March 1993), 7-8.

9 Jack Tips, N.D., Ph.D. *Your Liver...Your Lifeline* (Ogden, UT: Apple-A-Day Press, 1995), 13-15.

10 William G. Crook, M.D. *The Yeast Connection and the Woman* (Jackson, TN: Professional Books, 1995), 25. Simon Martin. *Candida: The Natural Way* (Boston, MA: Element Books, 1998), 7.

11 Burton Goldberg Group. *Alternative*

Medicine: The Definitive Guide (Tiburon, CA: Future Medicine Publishing, 1993), 587.

12 Hal Huggins, D.D.S. "Dental Toxins: Your Teeth May Be Making You Sick." Alternative Medicine 23 (April/May 1998), 48-54.

13 R.L. Siblerud, J. Motl, and E. Kienholz. "Psychometric Evidence That Mercury From Silver Dental Fillings May Be an Etiological Factor in Depression, Excessive Anger, and Anxiety." Psychological Reports 74:1 (1994), 67-80.

14 L.A. Toth and J.M. Krueger. "Effects of Microbial Challenge on Sleep in Rabbits." FASEB Journal 3:9 (1989), 2062-2066.

15 Jeffrey Bland, Ph.D., "Drugs and Liver Overload." Delicious! (May 1995), 48.

16 Stephen Langer, M.D., with James F. Scheer. Solved: The Riddle of Weight Loss (Rochester, VT: Healing Arts Press, 1989), 24.

17 Burton Goldberg Group. Alternative Medicine: The Definitive Guide (Tiburon, CA: Future Medicine Publishing, 1993), 588.

18 Simon Martin. Candida: The Natural Way (Boston, MA: Element Books, 1998), 10-11. This information is adapted from a Candida questionnaire developed by William Crook, M.D., and included in his book, The Yeast Connection Handbook (Jackson, TN: Professional Books, 1996), 15-19.

19 Stephen Langer, M.D., with James F. Scheer. Solved: The Riddle of Weight Loss (Rochester, VT: Healing Arts Press, 1989), 24.

20 Jack Tips, N.D., Ph.D. Conquer Candida and Restore Your Immune System (Austin, TX: Apple-A-Day Press, 1995), 68-69.

21 Ann Louise Gittleman, M.S. Guess What Came To Dinner: Parasites and Your Health (Garden City Park, NY: Avery Publishing Group, 1993), 80-86. Hermann Bueno, M.D. Uninvited Guests

(New Canaan, CT: Keats: 1996), 33.

22 Ann Louise Gittleman, M.S. Guess What Came To Dinner: Parasites and Your Health (Garden City Park, NY: Avery Publishing Group, 1993), 94-95. Gary Null, Ph.D. The Woman's Encyclopedia of Natural Healing (New York: Seven Stories, 1996), 285. Pavel I. Yutsis, M.D. "Intestinal Parasites at Large." Explore! 7:1 (1996), 27-31.

23 Ann Louise Gittleman, M.S. Guess What Came To Dinner: Parasites and Your Health (Garden City Park, NY: Avery Publishing Group, 1993), 97.

24 Ibid., 96.

25 L.K.T. Lam et al. "Isolation and Identification of Kahweol Palmitate and Cafestol Palmitate as Active Constituents of Green Coffee Beans That Enhance Glutathione-S-Transferase Activity in the Mouse." Cancer Research 42 (1982), 1193-1198.

26 Howard Straus. "Coffee Corner." Gerson Healing Newsletter 11:5 (1996), 9-11.

27 Eugene Zampieron, N.D., and Ellen Kamhi, Ph.D., R.N. The Natural Medicine Chest (New York: M. Evans, 1999), 52-54.

28 Giovanni Maciocia, C.Ac. The Practice of Chinese Medicine (London: Churchill Livingstone, 1994), 285.

Chapter 5: Resetting the Body Clock

1 Roberto Refinetti, Ph.D. Circadian Physiology (Boca Raton, FL: CRC Press, 2000), 140.

2 Richard M. Coleman. Wide Awake at 3:00 a.m. (New York: W.H. Freeman, 1986), 6.

3 T. H. Monk, M.L. Moline, and R.C. Graeber. "Inducing Jet Lag in the Laboratory: Patterns of Adjustment to an Acute Shift in Routine." Aviation Space and Environmental Medicine 59 (1998), 703-710. See also: A.R. Wever. "Phase Shifts of Human Circadian Rhythms Due to Shifts of Artificial

Zeitgebers." *Chronobiologia* 7 (1980), 303-327.

4 Angela Lorio. "Shift Workers Must Defy Their Circadian Rhythm." *Medical Tribune* (November 27, 1997), 7.

5 Richard M. Coleman. *Wide Awake at 3:00 a.m.* (New York: W.H. Freeman, 1986), 59.

6 Ibid.

7 M. Melbin. *Night as Frontier: Colonizing the World After Dark* (New York: Free Press, 1987), 27.

8 Richard M. Coleman. *Wide Awake at 3:00 a.m.* (New York: W.H. Freeman, 1986), 59.

9 P.D. Peneve et al. "Chronic Circadian Desynchronization Decreases the Survival of Animals with Cardiomyopathic Heart Disease." *American Journal of Physiology* 275 (1998), H2334-H2337.

10 R.J. Reiter. "Static and Extremely Low Frequency Electromagnetic Field Exposure: Reported Effects on the Circadian Production of Melatonin." *Journal of Cellular Biochemistry* 51:4 (April 1993), 394-403.

11 R.C. Espiritu, D.F. Kripke, and O.J. Kaplan. "Low Illumination Experienced by San Diego Adultus: Association with Atypical Depressive Symptoms." *Biological Psychiatry* 35 (1994), 403-407.

12 M. Koller et al. "Personal Light Dosimetry in Permanent Night and Day Workers." *Chronobiology International* 10 (1993), 143-155.

13 Russel J. Reiter, Ph.D., and Jo Robinson. *Melatonin: Your Body's Natural Wonder Drug* (New York: Bantam Books, 1995), 162.

14 Ibid.

15 M.L. Roa, B. Muller-Oerlinghausen, and H.P. Volz. "Blood Serotonin, Serum Melatonin and Light Therapy in Healthy Subjects and in Patients with Nonseasonal Depression." *Acta Psychiatrica Scandinavica* 86 (1992), 127-132.

16 M. Koller et al. "Different Patterns of Light Exposure in Relation to Melatonin and Cortisol Rhythms and Sleep of Night Workers." *Journal of Pineal Research* 16:3 (April 1994), 127-135.

17 James Perl, Ph.D. *Sleep Right in Five Nights* (New York: William Morrow, 1993), 231.

18 W.F. Byerley et al. "Biological Effect of Bright Light." *Progress in Neuro-Psychopharmacology and Biological Psychiatry* 13:5 (1989), 683-686.

19 D. J. Kennaway et al. "Phase Delay of the Rhythm of 6-Sulphatoxy Melatonin Excretion by Artificial Light." *Journal of Pineal Research* 4:3 (1987), 315-320. See also: A.J. Lewy, T.A. Wehr, and F.K. Goodwin. "Light Suppresses Melatonin Secretion in Humans." *Science* (December 1980), 210.

20 Russel J. Reiter, Ph.D., and Jo Robinson. *Melatonin, Your Body's Natural Wonder Drug* (New York: Bantam Books, 1995), 165.

21 D.G.M. Murphy et al. "Seasonal Affective Disorder: Response to Light as Measured by Electroencephalogram, Melatonin Suppression, and Cerebral Blood Flow." *British Journal of Psychiatry* 163 (1993), 327-331.

22 M.L. Laakso et al. "One-Hour Exposure to Moderate Illuminance (500 Lux) Shifts the Human Melatonin Rhythm." *Journal of Pineal Research* 15:1 (August 1993), 21-26.

23 G. Copinschi, O. Van Reeth, and E. Van Cauter. "Biologic Rhythms: Effect of Aging on the Desynchronization of Endogenous Rhythmicity and Environmental Conditions." *Presse Medicale* 28:17 (May 1-8, 1999), 942-946.

24 I. Haimov et al. "Sleep Disorders and Melatonin Rhythms in Elderly People." *British Medical Journal* 309 (1994), 167.

25 Dorothy Castor, P.A.C., et al. "Effect of Sunlight on Sleep Patterns of the Elderly." *Journal of the American Academy of Physician Assistants* 4:4 (June 1991), 321-326.

26 P. Semm, T. Schneider, L. Vollrath. "Effects of an Earth-Strength Magnetic Field on Electrical Activity of Pineal Cells." *Nature* 288 (1980), 607-608.

27 T. Schneider et al. "Melatonon is Crucial for the Migratory Orientation of Pied Flycatchers (Ficedula Hypoleuca Pallas)." *Journal of Experimental Biology* 194:1 (September 1994), 255-262.

28 S. Reuss, P. Semm, and L. Vollrath. "Different Types of Magnetically Sensitive Cells in the Rat Pineal Gland." *Neuroscience Letters* 40:1 (September 19, 1983), 23-26.

29 R. Dubbels et al. "Melatonin Determination with a Newly Developed ELISA System: Inter-Individual Differences in the Response of the Human Pineal Gland to Magnetic Fields." In: G.J. Maestroni, A. Conti, and R.J. Reiter, ed. *Advances in Pineal Research* Vol. 7 (London: John Libbey, 1994), 27-33.

30 M. Kato. "Biological Influences of Electromagnetic Fields." *Hokkaido Igaku Zasshi* 70:4 (July 1995), 551-560.

31 M. Karasek et al. "Chronic Exposure to 2.9 mT, 40 Hz Magnetic Field Reduces Melatonin Concentrations in Humans." *Journal of Pineal Research* 25:4 (December 1998), 240-244.

32 D.H. Pfluger and C.E. Minder. "Effects of Exposure to 16.7 Hz Magnetic Fields on Urinary 6-Hydroxymelatonin Sulfate Excretion of Swiss Railway Workers." *Journal of Pineal Research* 21:2 (September 1996), 91-100.

33 Russel J. Reiter, Ph.D., and Jo Robinson. *Melatonin, Your Body's Natural Wonder Drug* (New York: Bantam Books, 1995), 173.

34 E.J. Sanchez-Barcelo et al. "Melatonin Suppression of Mammary Growth in Heifers." *Biology of Reproduction* 44:5 (May 1991), 875-879.

35 R. Luboshitzky. "Endocrine Activity During Sleep." *Journal of Pediatric*

Endocrinology and Metabolism 13:1 (January 2000), 13-20.

36 I. Modai et al. "Blood Levels of Melatonin, Serotonin, Cortisol, and Prolactin in Relation to the Circadian Rhythm of Platelet Serotonin Uptake." *Psychiatry Research* 43:2 (August 1992), 161-166.

37 O. Van Reeth et al. "Nocturnal Exercise Phase Delays Circadian Rhythms of Melatonin and Thyrotropin Secretion in Normal Men." *American Journal of Physiology* 266:6 Part 1 (June 1994), E964-E974.

38 P.J. Murphy, B.L. Myers, and P. Badia. "Nonsteroidal Anti-Inflammatory Drugs Alter Body Temperature and Suppress Melatonin in Humans." *Physiology and Behavior* 59:1 (January 1996), 133-139.

39 P.J. Murphy et al. "Nonsteriodal Anti-Inflammatory Drugs Affect Normal Sleep Patterns in Humans." *Physiology and Behavior* 55:6 (June 1994), 1063-1066.

40 K. Surrall et al. "Effect of Ibuprofen and Indomethacin on Human Plasma Melatonin." *Journal of Pharmacy and Pharmacology* 39:10 (October 1987), 840-843.

41 P.J. Murphy et al. "Nonsteriodal Anti-Inflammatory Drugs Affect Normal Sleep Patterns in Humans." *Physiology and Behavior* 55:6 (June 1994), 1063-1066.

42 A. C. Meyer, J. J. Nieuwenhuis, and B.J. Meyer. "Dihydropyridine Calcium Antagonist Depress the Amplitude of the Plasma Melatonin Cycle in Baboons." *Life Sciences* 39 (1986), 1563-1569.

43 M. Kabuto, I. Namura, and Y. Saitoh. "Nocturnal Enhancement of Plasma Melatonin Could Be Suppressed by Benzodiazepines in Humans." *Endocrinologia Japonica* 133:3 (1986), 405-414.

44 P. Monteleone et al. "Preliminary Observations on the Suppression of

Nocturnal Plasma Melatonin Levels by Short-Term Administration of Diazepam in Humans." *Journal of Pineal Research* 6:3 (1989), 253-258.

45 I. McIntyre, G.D. Burrows, and T.R. Norman. "Suppression of Plasma Melatonin by a Single Dose of the Benzodiazepine Alprozolam in Humans." *Biological Psychiatry* 24 (1988), 105-108. P. P. Hubain et al. "Alprazolam and Amitriptyline in the Treatment of Major Depressive Disorder: A Double-Blind Clinical and Sleep EEG Study." *Journal of Affective Disorders* 18:1 (January 1995), 67-73.

46 M. Kabuto, I. Namura, and Y. Saitoh. "Nocturnal Enhancement of Plasma Melatonin Could Be Suppressed by Benzodiazepines in Humans." *Endocrinologia Japonica* 133:3 (1986), 405-414.

47 Kenneth P. Wright, Jr., et al. "Caffeine and Light Effects on Nighttime Melatonin and Temperature Levels in Sleep-Deprived Humans." *Brain Research* 747 (1997), 78-84. See also: A.M. Babey, R.M. Palmour, and S.N. Young. "Caffeine and Propranolol Block the Increase in Rat Pineal Melatonin Produced by Stimulation of Adrenergic Receptors." *Neuroscience Letters* 176:1 (July 18, 1994), 93-96.

48 S. Rojdmark et al. "Inhibition of Melatonin Secretion by Ethanol in Man." *Metabolism* 42:8 (August 1993), 1047-1051. See also: C.L. Chik and A.K. Ho. "Ethanol Reduces Norepinephrine-Stimulated Melatonin Synthesis in Rat Pinealocytes." *Journal of Neurochemistry* 4:4 (October 1992), 12870-1286.

49 K. Honma, M. Kohsada, and S. Honma. "Effects of Vitamin B12 on Plasma Melatonin Rhythm in Humans: Increased Light Sensitivity and Phase-Advances the Circadian Clock." *Experientia* 48 (1992), 716-720. See also: Hiroshi Tioh et al. "Effects of Vitamin B12 and Bright Light on Circadian Rhythms." *The Japanese*

Journal of Psychiatry and Neurology 48:2 (1994), 502-505.

50 J. Daniel Kanofsky, M.D., M.P.H. "Magnesium Deficiency in Chronic Schizophrenia." *International Journal of Neuroscience* 61 (1991), 87-90.

51 Russel J. Reiter, Ph.D., and Jo Robinson *Melatonin: Your Body's Natural Wonder Drug* (New York: Bantam Books, 1995), 197.

52 James Perl, Ph.D. *Sleep Right in Five Nights* (New York: William Morrow, 1993), 232.

53 M.A. Carskadon, ed. *Encyclopedia of Sleep and Dreaming* (New York: Macmillan, 1993), 703.

54 Hiroshi Itoh et al. "Effects of Vitamin B12 and Circadian Rhythms." *The Japanese Journal of Psychiatry and Neurology* 48:2 (1994), 502-505. See also: Satoko Hashimoto et al. "Vitamin B12 Enhances the Phase-Response of Circadian Melatonin Rhythms to a Single Bright Light Exposure in Humans." *Neuroscience Letters* 220 (1996), 129-132.

55 Ron Lawrence, M.D., Ph.D., and Paul J. Rosch, M.D., F.A.C.P. *Magnet Therapy: The Pain Cure Alternative* (Rocklin, CA: Prima Publishing, 1998), 117.

56 R. Sandyk. "Resolution of Sleep Paralysis by Weak Electromagnetic Fields in a Patient with Multiple Sclerosis." *International Journal of Neuroscience* 90:3-4 (August 1997), 145-147.

57 Kathryn Reid et al. "Day-Time Melatonin Administration: Effects on Core Temperature and Sleep Onset Latency." *Journal of Sleep Research* 5 (1996), 150-154.

58 Lars Palm et al. "Long-Term Melatonin Treatment in Blind Children and Young Adults with Circadian Sleep-Wake Disturbances." *Developmental Medicine and Child Neurology* 39 (1997), 319-325.

59 J.S. Carman, R.M. Post, and F.K. Goodwin. "Negative Effects of Melatonin on Depression." *American*

Journal of Psychiatry 133:10 (1976), 1181-1186. See also: M.D. Steinhilber, M. Brungs, and C. Carlberg. "The Nuclear Receptor for Melatonon Represses 5-Lipoxygenase Gene Expression In Human B-Lymphocytes." Journal of Biological Chemistry 270:13 (1995), 7037-7040. I. Hansson, R. Holmdahl, and R. Mattson. "The Pineal Hormone Melatonin Exaggerates Development of Collagen-Induced Arthritis in Mice." Journal of Neuroimmunology 39 (1992), 23-30.

60 B. Voordouw et al. "Melatonin and Melatonin-Progestin Combinations Alter Pituitary-Ovarian Function in Women and Can Inhibit Ovulation." Journal of Clinical Endocrinology and Metabolism 74:1 (1992), 108-117.

61 G. J. Maestroni and A. Conti. "Anti-Stress Role of the Melatonin-Immuno-Opioid Network: Evidence for a Physiological Mechanism Involving T-Cell-derived, Immunoreactive B-Endorphin and Metenkephalin Binding the Thymic Opioid Receptors." International Journal of Neuroscience 61 (1991), 289-298.

62 Y.H. Watanabe et al. Nutrition Reports International 25 (1982), 733-741.

63 N. Zisapel. "The Use of Melatonin for the Treatment of Insomnia." Biological Signals 8:1-2 (January-April 1999), 84-89.

64 K. Petrie et al. "Effect of Melatonin on Jet Lag After Long Haul Flights." British Medicine Journal 298 (1989), 705-707.

65 Ray Sahelian, M.D. "Melatonin Isn't Just For Sleep Anymore." Let's Live (October 1995).

66 A. Lewy et al. "Melatonin, Light and Chronobiological Disorders." Photoperiodism, Melatonin and the Pineal (1985), 231-252.

67 Roger Field. "Melatonin May Relieve Sleep-Cycle Disorders." Medical Tribune (April 8, 1993), 2.

68 D. Kunz and F. Bes. "Melatonin as a Therapy in REM Sleep Behavior Disorder Patients: An Open-Labeled Pilot Study on the Possible Influence on REM-Sleep Regulation." Movement Disorders 14:3 (May 1999), 507-511.

69 D. Kunz and F. Bes. "Melatonin Effects in a Patient with Severe REM Sleep Behavior Disorder: Case Report and Theoretical Considerations." Neuropsychobiology 36:4 (1997), 211-214.

70 L.M. Rosen et al. "Prevalence of Seasonal Affective Disorder at Four Latitudes." Psychiatry Research 31 (1989), 131-144.

71 A. Wirz-Justic et al. "Natural Light Treatment of Seasonal Affective Disorder." Journal of Affective Disorders 37:2-3 (April 12, 1996), 109-120.

72 Y. Meesters et al. "Light Therapy for Seasonal Affective Disorder: The Effects of Timing." British Journal of Psychiatry 166 (1995), 607-612.

73 Alfred J. Lewy, M.D., Ph.D. "Treating Chronobiologic Sleep and Mood Disorders with Bright Light." Psychiatric Annals 17:10 (October 1987), 664-669.

Chapter 6: Resolve Emotional Issues

1 M. Scofield. Work Site Health Promotion (Philadelphia: Hanley & Belfus, 1990), 459.

2 Timothy D. Schellhardt. "Company Memo to Stressed-Out Employees: 'Deal With It'." The Wall Street Journal (October 2, 1996).

3 J.L. Marx. "The Immune System 'Belongs to the Body'." Science 277 (1985), 1190-1192.

4 Hans Selye, M.D. Stress Without Distress (New York: New American Library, 1975). J.D. Beasley and J. Swift. Kellogg Report: The Impact of Nutrition, Environment, and Lifestyle on the Health of Americans (Annandale-on-Hudson, NY: Institute of Health Policy and Practice, The Bard College Center, 1989).

5 L. Schindler, E. Hohenberger-Sieber, and

P. Pauli. "Correlates of Disordered Sleep: A Replication Study." *Zeitschrift fur Klinische Psychologie, Psychopathologie und Psychotherapie* 36:2 (1988), 118-129.

6 W.F. Waters et al. "Attention, Stress, and Negative Emotion in Persistent Sleep-Onset and Sleep-Maintenance Insomnia." *Sleep* 16:2 (1993), 128-136.

7 A.N. Vgontzas et al. "Chronic Insomnia and Activity of the Stress System: A Preliminary Study." *Journal of Psychosomatic Research* 45:1 (1998), 21-31.

8 Associated Press. "For Chronic Pain, Try to Relax." (October 19, 1995).

9 William Boericke, N.D. *Pocket Manual of Homeopathic Materia Medica* 9th ed. (New York: Boericke & Runyon, 1927), 179.

10 Brian Tracy. *The Psychology of Achievement* (Niles, IL: Nightingale-Conant Corporation, 1987), 4.

11 R. A. Chalmers et al., eds. *Scientific Research on Maharishi's Transcendental Meditation and TM-Sidih Program: Collected Papers*, Vol. 2-4 (Vlodrop, Netherlands: Maharishi Vedic University Press, 1989).

12 R.K. Wallace et al. "Physiological Effects of Transcendental Meditation." *Science* 167 (1970), 1751-1754. M.C. Dillbeck et al. "Physiological Differences between TM and Rest." *American Physiologist* 42 (1987), 879-881.

13 R. W. Cranson et al. "Transcendental Meditation and Improved Performance on Intelligence-Related Measures: A Longitudinal Study." *Personality and Individual Differences* 12 (1991), 1105-1116.

14 D.H. Shapiro and R.N. Walsh. *Meditation: Classic and Contemporary Perspectives* (New York: Aldine, 1984).

15 N. Miller. "Learning of Visceral and Glandular Responses." *Science* 163:866 (January 1969), 434-445.

16 Jean Callahan. "Relax." *Self* (June 1995), 130.

17 Lara Pizzorno, M.A. L.M.P. "The Healing Power of the Mind." *Delicious!* (May 1995), 20.

18 Peter Hauri, Ph.D., and Shirley Linde, Ph.D. *No More Sleepless Nights* (New York: John Wiley & Sons, 1990, 1991), 98.

19 N. Miller. "Learning of Visceral and Glandular Responses." *Science* 163:866 (January 1969), 434-445, 627.

20 Shad Helmsetter, Ph.D. *What to Say When You Talk To Yourself* (Scottsdale, AZ: Grindle Press/Audio, 1986).

21 Lawrence Paros, Ph.D., and Daniel L. Kirsch, Ph.D., D.A.A.P.M. "Cranial Electrotherapy Stimulation (CES): A Very Safe and Effective Non-Pharmacological Treatment for Anxiety." *MedScope Monthly* 3:1, 1-16, 24-27.

22 Eric Braverman, M.D. *PATH Wellness Manual* (Princeton, NJ: PATH, 1995), 171.

23 Daniel L. Kirsh, Ph.D., D.A.A.P.M., and Fred Lerner, Ph.D., D.A.A.P.M. "Electromedicine, the Other Side of Physiology." In: Richard S. Weiner, ed. *Pain Management: A Practical Guide for Clinicians* (Boca Raton, FL: CRC Press, 1998), Chapter 23, 2-3.

24 Terry Willard. "Insomnia: Wake Up to Ten Simple Solutions." *Herbs for Health* (January/February 1997), 37-39.

25 German Ministry of Health. *Valerian: Commission E Monographs for Phytomedicines* (Bonn, Germany: German Ministry of Health, 1985).

26 ESCOP, European Scientific Cooperative for Phytotherapy. *Valerian Root* (Meppel, The Netherlands: European Scientific Cooperative for Phytotherapy, 1990).

27 Simon Y. Mills, M.A. *The Dictionary of Modern Herbalism* (Rochester, VT: Healing Arts Press, 1988), 211.

28 P. Huard and M. Wong. *Chinese Medicine* (New York: World University Library/McGraw Hill, 1968).

29 Terry Williard. "Insomnia: Wake Up to Ten Simple Solutions" *Herbs for Health*

(January/February 1997), 38.

30 Linda White, M.D. "No More Tossing and Turning." *Vegetarian Times* (November 1996), 38.

31 Terry Willard. "Insomnia: Wake Up to Ten Simple Solutions." *Herbs for Health* (January/February 1997), 39.

32 Christopher Hobbs. "Valerian: A Literature Review." *HerbalGram* 21 (1989), 19-34.

33 German Ministry of Health. Passion Flower Leaves: Commission E Monographs for Phytomedicines (Bonn, Germany: German Ministry of Health, 1985).

34 S. Foster. *Passion Flower: Botanical Series* 314 (Austin, TX: American Botanical Council, 1993).

35 E. Lehmann et al. "Efficacy of a Special Kava Extract (*Piper methysticum*) in Patients with Anxiety, Tension, and Excitedness of Non-Mental Origin." *Phytomedicine* 3 (1996), 113-119.

36 H.P. Volz and M. Kieser. "Kava-Kava Extract WS 14490 Versus Placebo in Anxiety Disorders: A Randomized Placebo-Controlled 25-Week Outpatient Trial." *Pharmacopsychiatria* 30 (1997), 1-5.

37 Simon Y. Mills, M.A. *The Dictionary of Modern Herbalism* (Rochester, VT: Healing Arts Press, 1988), 58-59.

38 ESCOP, European Scientific Cooperative for Phytotherapy. *Valerian Root* (Meppel, The Netherlands: ESCOP, European Scientific Cooperative for Phytotherapy, 1990). S. Foster. *Chamomile: Botanical Series* 307 (Austin, TX: American Botanical Council, 1991).

39 O. Suzuki et al. "Inhibition of Monoamine Oxidase by Hypericin." *Planta Medica* 50 (1984), 272-274. H. Muldner and M. Zoller. "Antidepressive Effect of a Hypericum Extract Standardized to an Active Hypericine Complex: Biochemical and Clinical Studies." *Arzneimittelforschung* 34:8 (1984), 918-920.

40 Peter De Smet et al. "St. John's Wort as an Antidepressant." *British Medical Journal* 7052:313 (August 3, 1996), 241-242. Klaus Linde et al. "St. John's Wort for Depression—An Overview and Meta-Analysis of Randomized Clinical Trials." *British Medical Journal* 7052:313 (August 3, 1996), 253-258.

41 Lesley Tierra, L.Ac., Dip.Ac. *Healing With Chinese Herbs* (Freedom, CA: The Crossing Press, 1997).

42 Terry Willard. "Insomnia: Wake Up to Ten Simple Solutions." *Herbs for Health* (January/February 1997), 37.

43 Ibid., 39.

44 Andrew Lockie, M.D., and Nicola Geddes, M.D. *The Women's Guide to Homeopathy* (New York: St. Martin's, 1994), 238.

45 Peter Holmes, M.H., L.Ac. "Lavender Oil: A Study in Contradictions." *International Journal of Aromatherapy* 4:2 (Summer 1992), 20.

46 Patricia Kaminski and Richard Katz. *Flower Essence Repertory* (Nevada City, CA: Flower Essence Society, 1994), 203.

Chapter 7: Protection From a Toxic Environment

1 Lita Lee, Ph.D. *Radiation Protection Manual* (Redwood City, CA: Grassroots Network, 1990), 39.

2 Robert O. Becker, M.D. *Cross Currents: The Perils of Electropollution, The Promise of Electromedicine* (New York: Jeremy P. Tarcher, 1990), 276.

3 N. Wertheimer and E. Leeper. "Electrical Wiring Configurations and Childhood Cancer." *American Journal of Epidemiology* 109 (1979), 273-284.

4 J. Wolpay. *Biological Effects of Power Line Fields* (New York: New York State Power Lines Project, Scientific Advisory Panel, 1987).

5 Lita Lee, Ph.D. *Radiation Protection Manual* (Redwood City, CA: Grassroots Network, 1990), 34.

6 Robert O. Becker, M.D., and Gary Selden. *The Body Electric: Electromagnetism and the Foundation of Life* (New York: William Morrow and Sons, 1985).

7 Robert O. Becker, M.D. *Cross Currents: The Perils of Electropollution, The Promise of Electromedicine* (New York: Jeremy P. Tarcher, 1990), 160-166

8 John W. Gofman, M.D., Ph.D. *Radiation and Human Health* (New York: Pantheon Books, 1981, 1983).

9 Robert O. Becker, M.D., and Gary Selden. *The Body Electric: Electromagnetism and the Foundation of Life* (New York: William Morrow and Sons, 1985).

10 R. Edwards. "Leak Links Power Lines to Cancer." *New Scientist* 4 (October 7, 1995), 4.

11 C. Ezzell. "Power-Line Static. Debates Rage Over the Possible Hazards of Electromagnetic Fields." *Science News* 140 (September 1991), 202-203.

12 B.W. Wilson, C. Wright, and L.E. Anderson. "Evidence for an Effect of ELF Electromagnetic Fields on Human Pineal Gland Function." *Journal of Pineal Research* 9 (1990), 259-269.

13 D. Wartenberg. "EMFs: Cutting Through the Controversy." *Public Health Reports* 111:3 (May/June 1996), 204-217.

14 Robert O. Becker, M.D. *Cross Currents: The Perils of Electropollution, The Promise of Electromedicine* (New York: Jeremy P. Tarcher, 1990), 270.

15 Burton Goldberg Group. *Alternative Medicine: The Definitive Guide* (Tiburon, CA: Future Medicine Publishing, 1993), 332.

16 Russel J. Reiter, Ph.D., and Jo Robinson. *Melatonin: Your Body's Natural Wonder Drug* (New York: Bantam Books, 1995), 178.

17 B. Holmberg. "Magnetic Fields and Cancer: Animal and Cellular Evidence—An Overview." *Environmental Health Perspectives* 2:Suppl (1995), 63-67. See also: C. Decker. "ELF-Zapped Genes Speed DNA Transcription." *Science News* (April 14, 1990), 229.

18 M. Mevissen, A. Lerchl, and W. Loscher. "Study on Pineal Function and DMBA-Induced Breast Cancer Formation in Rats During Exposure to a 100-mG, 50-Hz Magnetic Field." *Journal of Toxicology and Environmental Health* 48 (1996), 169-185.

19 Robert O. Becker, M.D. *Cross Currents: The Perils of Electropollution, The Promise of Electromedicine* (New York: Jeremy P. Tarcher, 1990), 71.

20 Jane Thurnell-Read. *Geopathic Stress: How Earth Energies Affect Our Lives* (Rockport, MA: Element Books, 1996), 38.

21 U.S. Department of Health, Education, and Welfare. *Geomagnetism, Cancer, Weather, and Cosmic Radiation* (Salt Lake City, UT: U.S. Department of Health, Education, and Welfare, 1979).

22 Robert O. Becker, M.D. *Cross Currents: The Perils of Electropollution, The Promise of Electromedicine* (New York: Jeremy P. Tarcher, 1990), 220.

23 Master Lam Kam Chuen. *Feng Shui Handbook* (New York: Henry Holt, 1996), 42.

24 Sarah Rossbach. *Interior Design with Feng Shui* (New York: Penguin Books, 1987), 21.

25 Glenda Cassutt. "Energize Your Home for Good Health." *Natural Health* (May/June 1995), 95.

26 Richard Webster. *101 Feng-Shui Tips for the Home* (St. Paul, MN: Llewellyn, 1998). Kirsten M. Lagatree. *Feng Shui: Arranging Your Home to Change Your Life* (New York: Villard, 1996). Li Pak Tin and Helen Yeap. *Feng Shui: Secrets That Change Your Life* (York Beach, ME: Samuel Weiser, 1997).

27 Karen Kingston. *Creating Sacred Space with Feng Shui* (New York: Broadway Books, 1997).

28 Norman Ford. *The Sleep Rx: 75 Proven Ways to Get a Good Night's Sleep* (Englewood Cliffs, NJ: Prentice Hall, 1994), 209.

29 Don Eady. "Sleep Easy." *Alive* (January 1996), 32.

30 Tina Spangler. "Is Your Bedroom Making

You Sick?" *Natural Health* (May/June 1996), 82-85.

Chapter 8: Balancing Your Hormones

1 J.F. Owens and K.A. Matthews. "Sleep Disturbance in Healthy Middle-Aged Women." *Maturitas* 30:1 (1998), 41-50.

2 John R. Lee, M.D., with Virginia Hopkins. *What Your Doctor May Not Tell You About Menopause* (New York: Warner Books, 1996), 34.

3 John R. Lee, M.D., with Virginia Hopkins. *What Your Doctor May Not Tell You About Menopause* (New York: Warner Books, 1996), 131. John R. Lee, M.D., Jesse Hanley, M.D., and Virginia Hopkins. *What Your Doctor May Not Tell You About Premenopause* (New York: Warner Books, 1999), 184.

4 Giampiero Porzio et al. "HRT as First-Step Treatment of Insomnia in Postmenopausal Women." *European Menopause Journal* 4:4 (1997), 145-148.

5 P. Polo-Kentola et al. "When Does Estrogen Replacement Therapy Improve Sleep Quality?" *American Journal of Obstetrics and Gynecology* 178:5 (1998), 1002-1009.

6 K.P. Wright, Jr., and P. Badia. "Effects of Menstrual Cycle Phase and Oral Contraceptives on Alertness, Cognitive Performance, and Circadian Rhythms During Sleep Deprivation." *Behavioural Brain Research* 103:2 (1999), 185-194.

7 Theresa L. Crenshaw, M.D. *The Alchemy of Love and Lust* (New York: G.P. Putnam's Sons, 1996), 205.

8 Eugene Shippen, M.D., and William Fryer. *The Testosterone Syndrome* (New York: M. Evans, 1998), 91.

9 H.P. Roffwarg et al. "Plasma Testosterone and Sleep: Relationship to Sleep Stage Variables." *Psychosomatic Medicine* 44:1 (1982), 73-84.

10 R.C. Schiavi, D. White, and J. Mandeli. "Pituitary-Gonadal Function During Sleep in Healthy Aging Men." *Psychoneuroendocrinology* 17:6 (1992), 599-609.

11 Theo Colborn, Dianne Dumanoski, and John Peterson Myers. *Our Stolen Future* (New York: Dutton/Penguin Group, 1996).

12 Betty Kamen, Ph.D. "Thyroid and Stress Connections." *Hormone Replacement Therapy: Yes or No?* (Novato, CA: Nutrition Encounter, 1993), 196.

13 A.W. Meikle et al. "Effects of a Fat-Containing Meal on Sex Hormones in Men." *Metabolism* 39:9 (1990), 943-946.

14 C.D Hunt et al. "Effects of Dietary Zinc Depletion on Seminal Volume and Zinc Loss: Serum Testosterone Concentrations and Sperm Morphology in Young Men." *American Journal of Clinical Nutrition* 56:1 (1992), 148-157.

15 Joseph Pizzorno, N.D. *Total Wellness* (Rocklin, CA: Prima, 1996), 244.

16 Eugene Shippen, M.D., and William Fryer. *The Testosterone Syndrome* (New York: M. Evans, 1998), 49.

17 S.J. Brown. "Environmental Doctors Take Up Pollution Prevention Cause." *Family Practice* News (January 1, 1995), 6.

18 J. Yeh and A.J. Friedman. "Nicotine and Cotinine Inhibit Rat Testis Androgen Biosynthesis *in vitro*." *Journal of Steroid Biochemistry* 33:4A (1989), 627-630.

19 Joseph Pizzorno, N.D. *Total Wellness* (Rocklin, CA: Prima, 1996), 242.

20 Ibid., 236-237.

21 Albert Einstein Medical Center, Philadelphia, Pennsylvania. *Premier Years* (February 1996), 1-3.

22 Charles Morin, Ph.D. *Relief from Insomnia: Getting the Sleep of Your Dreams* (New York: Doubleday, 1996), 188-189.

23 Ibid., 190.

24 James Perl, Ph.D. *Sleep Right in Five Nights* (New York: William Morrow, 1993), 100-103.

25 Russel J. Reiter, Ph.D., and Jo Robinson. *Melatonin—Your Body's Natural Wonder Drug* (New York: Bantam, 1995), 8.

26 L. Haimov and P. Lavie. "Sleep Disorders and Melatonin Rhythms in Elderly People." *British Medical Journal* 309 (1994), 167.

27 John R. Lee, M.D., with Virginia Hopkins. *What Your Doctor May Not Tell You About Menopause* (New York: Warner Books, 1996), 300.

28 Michael Murray, N.D., and Joseph Pizzorno, N.D. *Encyclopedia of Natural Medicine* 2nd Ed. (Rocklin, CA: Prima, 1998), 636.

29 E.H. Brown and L.P. Walker, Pharm.D., M.Ac., D.H.M. "Diet, Exercise and Hormone Balance." *Menopause and Estrogen* (Berkeley, CA: Frog Ltd., 1996), 111-119.

30 John R. Lee, M.D., with Virginia Hopkins. *What Your Doctor May Not Tell You About Menopause* (New York: Warner Books, 1996), 317.

31 Ann Louise Gittleman, M.S., C.N.S. "Perimenopause—When Signs of 'The Change' Come Too Early." *Alternative Medicine* (October/November 1998), 84-92.

32 John R. Lee, M.D., with Virginia Hopkins. *What Your Doctor May Not Tell You About Menopause* (New York: Warner Books, 1996), 279-317.

33 John R. Lee, M.D. *Natural Progesterone: The Multiple Roles of a Remarkable Hormone* (Sebastopol, CA: BLL Publishing, 1993), 41.

34 John R. Lee, M.D., with Virginia Hopkins. *What Your Doctor May Not Tell You About Menopause* (New York: Warner Books, 1996), 263-278.

35 Jill Stansbury. "Fortifying Fertility With Vitamins and Herbs." *Nutrition Science News* 2:12 (December 1997), 606-612.

36 Linda Ojeda, Ph.D. *Menopause Without Medicine* (Alameda, CA: Hunter House, 1995), 101.

37 Harriet Beinfield, L.Ac. "Menopause East and West." *Body, Mind, Spirit* (June/July 1995), 24-26.

38 Eugene Shippen, M.D., and William Fryer. *The Testosterone Syndrome* (New York: M. Evans, 1998), 190-193.

39 "Staying Sexually Fit During Male Menopause." *Alternative Medicine Digest* 10 (1995), 10-13. Sandra Cabot, M.D. *Smart Medicine for Menopause* (Garden City Park, NY: Avery, 1995).

40 Julian Whitaker, M.D. "A Hormone Replacement Program for Men." *Health and Healing* 8:2 (February 1998), 1-4. Available from: Philips Publishing, Inc., 7811 Montrose Road, Potomac, MD 20854; tel: 800-539-8219; 12 issues/$69 in the U.S.

41 M.S. Fahim et al. "Effect of *Panax ginseng* on Testosterone Level and Prostate in Male Rats." *Archives of Andrology* 8:4 (1982), 261-263.

42 James A. Duke, Ph.D. *The Green Pharmacy* (Emmaus, PA: Rodale, 1997), 192.

43 A. Steiger. "Thyroid Gland and Sleep." *Acta Medica Austriaca* 26:4 (1999), 132-133.

44 Gary S. Ross, M.D. "Men's Health Issues in Clinical Practice: Andropause." *Biomedical Therapy* XV:3 (June 1997), 94-95.

Chapter 9: Correcting Structural Imbalances

1 S.J. Griffin and J. Trinder. "Physical Fitness, Exercise and Human Sleep." *Psychophysiology* 15:5 (1978), 447-450.

2 Benedict Carey. "The Sleep Solution." *Health* (July/August 1996), 74.

3 Karla Kubitz, M.D. "The Effects of Acute and Chronic Exercise on Sleep: A Meta-Analystic Review." *Sports Medicine* 21:4 (1996), 277-291.

4 Helen S. Driver et al. "Submaximal Exercise Effects on Sleep Patterns in Young Women Before and After an Aerobic Training Programme." *Physiologica Scandivavica* 133:Suppl 574 (1988), 3-13.

5 Ilkka Vuori et al. "Epidemiology of Exercise Effects on Sleep." *Acta Physiologica Scandinavica* 133:Suppl. 574 (1988), 3-7.

6. This is an adaptation of a program designed by Visual Health Information, P.O. Box 44646, Tacoma, WA 98444; tel: 253-536-4922; fax: 253-536-4944.

7 The President's Council on Physical Fitness and Sports, 200 Independence Avenue SW, Room 738-H, Washington, DC 20201; tel: 202-690-9000; fax: 202-690-5211; website: www.surgeon-general.gov/ophs/pcpfs.htm.

8 The President's Council on Physical Fitness and Sports, 200 Independence Avenue, SW, Room 738-H, Washington, DC 20201; tel: 202-690-9000 voice mail; fax: 202-690-5211; website: www.surgeongeneral.gov/ophs/pcpfs.htm. The Cooper Institute for Aerobic Research, 12330 Preston Road, Dallas, TX 75230; tel: 800-635-7050; fax: 972-341-3224; website: www.cooperinst.org.

9 R. Pate et al. "Physical Activity and Public Health: A Recommendation From the Centers for Disease Control and Prevention and the American College of Sports Medicine." *Journal of the American Medical Association* 65 (1995), 312-318.

10 Beryl Bender Birch. *Power Yoga* (New York: Simon & Schuster, 1995), 44-45.

11 For another description of NET treatments, see: K. Peterson. "Two Cases of Spinal Manipulation Performed While the Patient Contemplated an Associated Stress Event: The Effect of the Manipulation/ Contemplation on Serum Levels in Hypercholesterolemic Subjects." *Chiropractic Technique* 7:2 (May 1995).

12 The Bodywork KnowledgeBase is an abstracted collection of the world literature on massage compiled by Richard van Why, available from the American Massage Therapy Association.

13 John Yates, Ph.D. *A Physician's Guide to Therapeutic Massage* (Canada: Massage Therapist's Association of British Columbia, 1990).

14 The Bodywork KnowledgeBase is an abstracted collection of the world literature on massage compiled by Richard van Why, available from the American Massage Therapy Association.

15 William Collinge, M.P.H., Ph.D. *The American Holistic Health Association Complete Guide to Alternative Medicine* (New York: Warner Books, 1996), 270.

16 Philip Goldberg and Daniel Kaufman. *Everybody's Guide to Natural Sleep* (Los Angeles: Jeremy Tarcher, 1990), 192-193.

Index

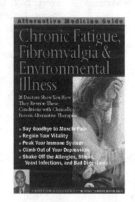
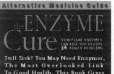
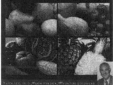
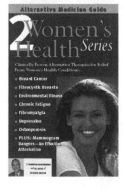
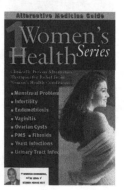
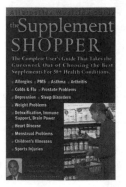

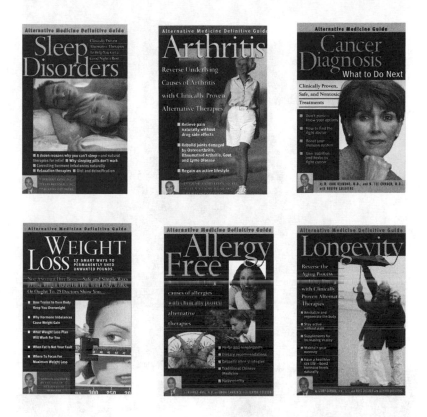

These titles are part of our *Alternative Medicine Guide* paperback series—healing-edge advice that may mean the difference between sickness and robust health. We distill the advice of hundreds of leading alternative physicians from all disciplines and put it into a consumer-helpful format—medical knowledge without the jargon. Essential reading before—or instead of—your next doctor's visit. Because you need to know your medical alternatives.

To order, call 800-841-BOOK or visit www.alternativemedicine.com. You can also find our books at your local health food store or bookstore.

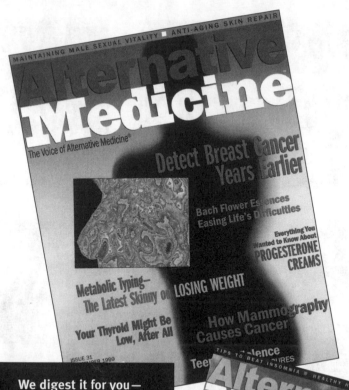

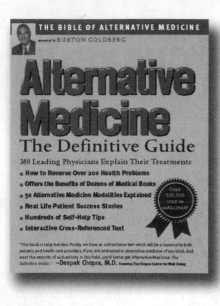